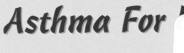

Asthma For Dummies®

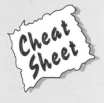

Cheat Sheet

D0515408

Major Myths about Asthma and/or Allergies

The following ideas are myths and misinformation that you may often hear about asthma and allergies. This listing isn't a true or false test — all these statements are incorrect! Refer to the chapters in parentheses for the real story about these topics.

- ✔ Moving to Arizona will cure my asthma and allergies (Chapter 10).
- ✔ A cat or dog with short hair is safer for my asthma than a long-haired pet (Chapter 10).
- ✔ Asthma is contagious (Chapter 1).
- ✔ I can't exercise because I have asthma (Chapter 9).
- ✔ I just have a recurring chest cold. I don't need to check for asthma (Chapters 2 and 7).
- ✔ My children don't need to be evaluated or treated for asthma because they'll outgrow it anyway (Chapter 18).
- ✔ My friends and family say that my asthma is all in my head (Chapter 1).
- ✔ The only medication I'll ever need for my asthma is a quick-relief, over-the-counter (OTC) rescue inhaler such as albuterol, Proventil, or Ventolin (Chapter 14).
- ✔ I get stomach cramps and diarrhea every time I drink milk, so I must be allergic to it (Chapter 8).
- ✔ *Allergic rhinitis* (hay fever) is just a minor annoyance and won't cause any serious problems (Chapter 13).
- ✔ I can take as many OTC medications as I want, because if I don't need a prescription for them, these products probably don't cause any side effects. Besides, my doctor didn't prescribe them, so it's none of his or her business if I'm taking them (Chapters 12 and 14).
- ✔ I should stop taking all my allergy and asthma medication while I'm pregnant (Chapter 19).
- ✔ I'll try to drop by my doctor's office for allergy shots when it's convenient for me. I don't need to stick to a regular schedule for immunotherapy (Chapter 11).
- ✔ I don't need to check with my doctor. I can just give my child half an adult dose of my asthma or allergy medication (Chapter 18).
- ✔ Nothing's going to happen during the flight, so why bother packing my asthma and allergy medications in my carry-on bag (Chapter 21)?
- ✔ I'll figure out how to use an epinephrine kit (for example, EpiPen) when I need it (Chapter 1).
- ✔ I can't do much to improve my asthma, so I'll have to settle for less and just live with my condition (Chapter 22).

For Dummies: Bestselling Book Series for Beginners

Asthma For Dummies®

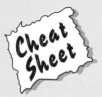

Problems That Asthma Patients Often Have

Asthma and allergic rhinitis can affect you in several ways:

- **Airways of lungs:** Asthma (Chapter 2), food hypersensitivities (Chapter 8), and *anaphylaxis* (a widespread, potentially life-threatening reaction that affects many organs simultaneously; Chapter 1)
- **Eyes:** Allergic conjunctivitis (Chapter 7)
- **Ears:** *Otitis media,* which is an inflammation of the middle ear, often leading to an ear infection — a frequent complication of allergic rhinitis (Chapter 13)
- **Gastrointestinal tract:** Food hypersensitivities (Chapter 8) and anaphylaxis (Chapter 1)
- **Nose:** Allergic rhinitis, which is the medical term for hay fever (Chapter 7)
- **Sinus:** Sinusitis — inflammation of the sinuses, a frequent complication of allergic rhinitis (Chapter 13)
- **Throat:** Allergic rhinitis and/or *pharyngitis* (a complication of postnasal drip associated with allergic rhinitis; Chapter 7), and food hypersensitivities (Chapter 8)

Dr. Berger's Top Ten List of Common Asthma Triggers

1. Animal dander — especially from cats and dogs (Chapters 5 and 10)
2. Dust mites (Chapter 10)
3. Mold spores and pollens from certain grasses, weeds, and trees (Chapter 10)
4. Exercise (Chapter 9)
5. Tobacco smoke (Chapter 5)
6. Air pollution and weather changes (Chapters 5 and 7)
7. Occupational irritants and allergens (Chapter 5)
8. Other ailments, including rhinitis (Chapter 7), sinusitis (Chapter 13), gastroesophageal reflux disease (GERD), and viral infections (Chapter 5)
9. Household products (Chapter 5)
10. Aspirin and other nonsteroidal anti-inflammatory drugs (NSAIDs) (Chapter 5)

For Dummies: Bestselling Book Series for Beginners

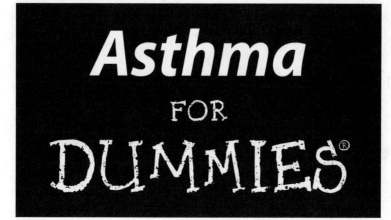

Asthma
FOR
DUMMIES®

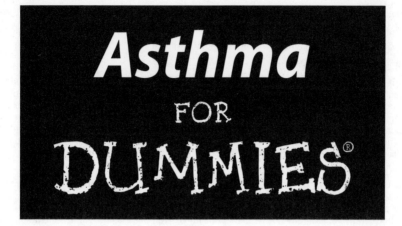

Asthma FOR DUMMIES®

by William E. Berger, MD, MBA

Foreword by Jackie Joyner-Kersee

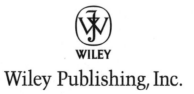

WILEY

Wiley Publishing, Inc.

Asthma For Dummies®

Published by
Wiley Publishing, Inc.
111 River St.
Hoboken, NJ 07030-5774
www.wiley.com

Copyright © 2004 by Wiley Publishing, Inc., Indianapolis, Indiana

Published simultaneously in Canada

For general information on our other products and services or to obtain technical support, please contact our Customer Care Department within the U.S. at 800-762-2974, outside the U.S. at 317-572-3993, or fax 317-572-4002.

Wiley also publishes its books in a variety of electronic formats. Some content that appears in print may not be available in electronic books.

Library of Congress Control Number: 2004103499

ISBN: 0-7645-4233-8

Manufactured in the United States of America

10 9 8 7 6 5 4 3

1B/RV/QW/QU/IN

WILEY

About the Author

William E. Berger, MD, MBA, is one of the nation's foremost experts on allergies and asthma. As a board-certified physician in two separate specialties (pediatrics and allergy and immunology), Dr. Berger has had extensive clinical experience in diagnosing and treating patients with allergies and asthma for more than 25 years. He holds dual appointments at the University of California, Irvine, as clinical professor in the College of Medicine, Department of Pediatrics, Division of Allergy and Immunology, and as adjunct professor of Health Care Management in the Graduate School of Management. In addition, he has also served as principal investigator in numerous clinical research projects.

Dr. Berger is a former member of the Joint Task Force on Practice Parameters that writes the national treatment guidelines for asthma and allergies. He has served as president of the American College of Allergy, Asthma, and Immunology and both the Orange County and California Societies of Allergy, Asthma, and Immunology. In recognition of his continued achievement in the specialty of treating allergic diseases, Dr. Berger was awarded the title Distinguished Fellow of the American College of Allergy, Asthma, and Immunology.

A former medical correspondent for the Orange County Newschannel, the Medical News Network, and ABC's *Mike and Maty Show,* Dr. Berger is also the author of many academic papers and lay press articles in the field of allergy, asthma, and immunology. He is a recognized international speaker in the field of allergy and asthma and is frequently invited to lecture at medical conferences and symposia held throughout the world. In addition, Dr. Berger has been the subject of medical reports on allergies and asthma that have appeared on CBS *Evening News,* ABC *World News Tonight,* Lifetime Medical Television, NBC *Dateline,* and Cable News Network (CNN). He has also been featured in medical articles published in *Time, The Wall Street Journal, USA Today,* the *Los Angeles Times,* and *The Orange County Register.*

Dr. Berger founded the Allergy and Asthma Associates of Southern California Medical Group in 1981 in Mission Viejo, California, where he currently practices both adult and pediatric allergy medicine. In 1995, Dr. Berger established the Southern California Research Center, focusing on respiratory and allergy clinical research studies.

Dedication

This book is dedicated to my wife Charlette, my son Michael, and my daughter Johanna, for their loving encouragement and their inspiring confidence that I would actually get the writing done on time.

Author's Acknowledgments

I especially want to thank acquisitions editor Natasha Graf, whose vision and foresight actually made this book possible. My project editor, Allyson Grove, kept me on track throughout the writing process and ensured that this book follows in the great line of the *For Dummies* tradition. I also greatly appreciate the artistry of Kathryn Born, our medical illustrator, whose drawings enhance the text, and the contributions of Chad Sievers, the copyeditor of this book.

I am also very grateful to the numerous other people who have made this book possible, most of all my indefatigable senior research editor, Carl Byron, who probably won't miss my midnight telephone calls to review the manuscript. Thanks also to Skye Herzog, agent extraordinaire, part-time psychologist, nurturer, and motivational expert. I am extremely grateful to Francene Lifson, executive director of the Southern California Chapter of the Asthma and Allergy Foundation of America, whose assistance was invaluable during the initial stages of this project.

A very special thanks to my friend, Olympic gold medalist Jackie Joyner-Kersee, the world's greatest female athlete, for writing the foreword to this book and for her unceasing efforts in raising awareness of the importance of early diagnosis and effective treatment of asthma. Jackie has inspired asthmatics throughout the world by proving that having asthma shouldn't prevent you from achieving your goals — no matter what they are.

I also want to express my deep-felt appreciation to Phil Lieberman, MD, who acted as technical editor for this book and who provided invaluable insights from his many years of experience in the field of allergy and immunology. Richard Nicklas, MD, and Bob Lanier, MD, also deserve my special thanks for taking time out from their busy schedules to review the manuscript and for providing excellent comments and suggestions.

Also, thanks to the following individuals who have been great friends, outstanding educators, and constant sources of inspiration due to their supreme dedication to providing excellent patient care: Brian Levine, MD; Eric Schenkel, MD; Joel Cristol, MD; Stanley Galant, MD; Sherwin Gillman, MD; Charles Siegel, MD; Bruce Prenner, MD; Joseph Bellanti, MD; Ira Finegold, MD; Don Mitchell, MD; John Zucker, MD; Tom Plaut, MD; and Mark Wohlgemuth, MD.

Thanks to my fellow members of the Joint Task Force on Practice Parameters in Allergy, Asthma, and Immunology, including Stanley Fineman, MD; Richard Nicklas, MD; I. Leonard Bernstein, MD; Joann Blessing-Moore, MD; Mark S.

Dykewicz, MD; Rufus Lee, MD; James Li, MD, PhD; Jay Portnoy, MD; Diane Schuller, MD; and Sheldon Spector, MD, all of whose extraordinary commitment and hard work in developing and maintaining the highest quality parameters for the care of our patients inspired me to write this book.

I greatly appreciate the information provided by allergy historians Sheldon Cohen, MD, and Guy Settipane, MD, whose research helped in developing Chapter 22.

As always, I place special value on the support and understanding of my clinical and research staff, my associates in practice, Mark Sugar, MD, Janis Davidson, RN, CPNP, and especially Ellen Schonfeld, RN, CPNP, who provided invaluable assistance in reviewing the manuscript and researching the illustrations for this book.

I am especially grateful to Georgia Beams and Jennifer Feaser, RN, who helped me start Allergy and Asthma Associates of Southern California in Mission Viejo more than 25 years ago (we were all 12 years old at the time!) and who have always provided me with their generous support and advice in whatever professional goals and endeavors I have pursued (including this book).

Nancy Sander, patient advocate and spokesperson and founder and president of Allergy and Asthma Network•Mothers of Asthmatics, also deserves my gratitude for her friendship, insights, and especially for her dedication to raising awareness about asthma and allergies.

Most of all, I would like to thank all of my patients for allowing me the privilege of caring for them and their children. Over the years, I've learned a great deal from them and am a better person and physician for the experience. As Ralph Waldo Emerson once wrote: "To know that even one life has breathed easier because you have lived: That is to have succeeded!"

Publisher's Acknowledgments

We're proud of this book; please send us your comments through our Dummies online registration form located at www.dummies.com/register/.

Some of the people who helped bring this book to market include the following:

Acquisitions, Editorial, and Media Development

Project Editor: Allyson Grove

(Previous Edition: Christine Meloy Beck)

Acquisitions Editor: Natasha Graf

Copy Editor: Chad R. Sievers

(Previous Edition: Billie A. Williams)

Assistant Editor: Holly Gastineau-Grimes

Technical Editor: Phillip Lieberman, MD

Editorial Manager: Michelle Hacker

Editorial Assistant: Elizabeth Rea

Cover Photos: © Spencer Rowell/Getty Images/Taxi

Cartoons: Rich Tennant, www.the5thwave.com

Production

Project Coordinator: Courtney MacIntyre

Layout and Graphics: Andrea Dahl, Stephanie D. Jumper, Michael Kruzil, Kristin McMullan, Jacque Schneider

Special Art: Kathryn Born

Proofreader: TECHBOOKS Production Services

Indexer: TECHBOOKS Production Services

Special Help
Georgette Beatty

Publishing and Editorial for Consumer Dummies

Diane Graves Steele, Vice President and Publisher, Consumer Dummies

Joyce Pepple, Acquisitions Director, Consumer Dummies

Kristin A. Cocks, Product Development Director, Consumer Dummies

Michael Spring, Vice President and Publisher, Travel

Brice Gosnell, Associate Publisher, Travel

Kelly Regan, Editorial Director, Travel

Publishing for Technology Dummies

Andy Cummings, Vice President and Publisher, Dummies Technology/General User

Composition Services

Gerry Fahey, Vice President of Production Services

Debbie Stailey, Director of Composition Services

Contents at a Glance

Table of Contents

· ·

Part II: Understanding Asthma Triggers 75

Chapter 5: Knowing Your Asthma Triggers 77

Foreword

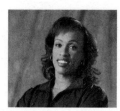

*W*hen I was first diagnosed with asthma back in college, I could have used a book like this. I really didn't know what asthma was all about or what I needed to do to manage it.

The truth is, I didn't take my asthma very seriously. I didn't want to think of myself — a serious athlete — as being sick. So I lived in denial. I took rescue medicine when my symptoms acted up, but mostly I tried to ignore it. I thought I could overcome it — that maybe it would go away on its own. Finally, after one particularly scary attack, it hit me: Instead of controlling my asthma, I was letting my asthma control me.

Now, I work with my doctor and manage my asthma daily. It's made a big difference. My symptoms are much less frequent, and I can do the things I want to do without being limited by my asthma.

The more I talk to people with this disease, the more I realize that my story is a very common one. If symptoms and attacks are interfering with your life or if you limit your activities in order to avoid asthma symptoms, keep in mind that things don't have to be this way.

That's why this book is so useful. It tells you everything you need to know about how to keep your asthma under control, so you don't have to go through what I went through.

Read it carefully and work with your doctor. Find out what you can do to help prevent symptoms from happening in the first place, and stick with it. Set your sights high, and never settle for less than your personal best.

It's not always easy, but you can do it. Take it from me: With the proper training and attitude, asthma doesn't have to slow you down.

Jackie Joyner-Kersee

— Jackie Joyner-Kersee

Introduction

"I feel like I'm breathing through a straw." "Oh, my aching sinuses." "I can't stop coughing." "My child keeps wheezing." If you've ever uttered words like these, you're not alone. Statements similar to these are some of the most frequent medical complaints that people in the United States and around the world report, and their complaints often describe asthma symptoms.

Asthma affects 17 million people in the United States and is the most common chronic childhood disease. Asthma also leads to more than 2 million emergency room visits and more than 9 million doctors' appointments per year. In fact, costs associated with asthma, including treatment, medications, and lost productivity, exceed $11 billion each year. The incidence of asthma is rising dramatically in the United States and across the globe, particularly in highly developed parts of the world, including Western Europe, Australia, and New Zealand. In fact, many experts now consider asthma a global epidemic.

But enough about facts and figures. I want to talk about you: How are you feeling? Do you, or someone you know, think that having asthma means that feeling unwell is normal and that your condition can never improve? Unfortunately, many people answer yes to this question. However, as I explain throughout this book, the plain, simple, and accurate medical truth is this: Although no cure exists for asthma, when you receive effective, appropriate care from your doctor, combined with your motivated participation as a patient, you can lead a normal, active, and fulfilling life.

About This Book

I wrote this book to give you sound, up-to-date, practical advice, based on my 25-plus years of experience with numerous patients, about dealing with your asthma effectively and appropriately. For that reason, I structure this book so that you can jump to sections that most directly apply to your medical condition. You don't need to read this book from cover to cover, although I won't object if you do. (Be careful, though, because when you start reading, you may have a really hard time putting it down!)

This book can also serve as a reference and source for information about the many facets of diagnosing, treating, and managing asthma. Although you may pick up this book for one aspect of asthma, you may realize later that other topics also apply to you or a loved one.

Don't worry about remembering where related subjects are in this book. I provide ample cross-references in every chapter that remind you where to look for the information you may need in other chapters or within other sections of the chapter that you're reading.

I intend the information in this book to empower you as a person with asthma, thus helping you to

✔ Set goals for your treatment

✔ Ensure that you receive the most appropriate and effective medical care for your respiratory condition

✔ Do your part as a patient by adhering to the treatment plan that you and your physician develop

Foolish Assumptions

I don't think I'm being too foolish, but I assume that you want substantive, scientifically accurate, relevant information about asthma, presented in everyday language, without a lot of medical mumbo-jumbo. In this book, you find straightforward explanations when I present important scientific aspects of asthma and when I use key medical terms. (You also get a chance to work on your Latin and Greek.)

If you've chosen to read my book, I know you're no dummy, so I'm willing to go out on a limb and make some further assumptions about you, dear reader:

✔ You or someone you care about suffers from asthma.

✔ You want to educate yourself about asthma as part of improving your medical condition (in consultation with your doctor, of course).

✔ You want to feel better.

✔ You really like doctors named Bill.

How This Book Is Organized

I structure this book in six parts to help you find the information you need as easily as possible.

Part 1: Asthma Basics

This part helps you determine what may affect you, explaining how asthma presents itself, the underlying immune system mechanisms involved in asthma, how you can — as well as why you should — get a proper diagnosis of your condition, and how to develop a long-term management plan.

Part 11: Understanding Asthma Triggers

In this part, you find an extensive discussion concerning the underlying inflammatory mechanism that characterizes asthma, what you need to know about how your doctor diagnoses your condition, and the important connections and coexistence between asthma and *allergic rhinitis* (hay fever). I also cover how to cope with food allergies and asthma, and deal with exercise-induced asthma (EIA).

Part 111: Treating Your Asthma

In Part III, I cover how to avoid allergens that cause allergic rhinitis, the many effects allergies can have on your body, how those effects occur, the types of complications frequently associated with allergic diseases, and what you and your doctor can do to effectively treat your allergic condition.

You also discover appropriate medications that you can take to control and prevent your symptoms. Likewise, I explain why *immunotherapy* (allergy shots) may successfully manage your allergic rhinitis long-term and treat your asthma.

Part 1V: Controlling Asthma with Medications

In this part, I detail the ways that medications are successfully used to manage asthma. Chapter 14 provides an overview of asthma treatment. I devote Chapters 15 and 16 to the controller (long-term) and rescue (short-relief) drugs that your doctor may prescribe for you. Chapter 17 presents my insights on upcoming drugs and therapies that may offer even more effective ways of treating asthma.

Part V: Special Asthma Conditions

In Part V, I discuss taking care of a child with asthma, continuing your asthma treatment during pregnancy, and managing asthma in the elderly.

Part VI: The Part of Tens

All *For Dummies* books contain one of these parts. The chapters in this part offer information that simply fits better in this more informal format, such as:

- ✔ What you need to take with you — and practical information and steps to remember — when traveling with asthma
- ✔ Examples of significant people, from ancient times to today, who have excelled in spite of their asthma

Appendix

The appendix at the back of the book is a compendium of valuable asthma and allergy resources, information on numerous important asthma and allergy organizations, and suppliers and manufacturers of environmental-control products that can greatly assist you in managing your condition. I also include listings of other important books and information sources about asthma and allergies, and, of course, a survey of quality asthma Web sites.

Icons Used in This Book

Throughout the margins of the book, you may notice the following icons. They're intended to catch your attention and alert you to the type of information I present in particular paragraphs. Here's what they mean:

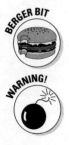

The Berger Bit icon represents me expressing my opinion.

A Warning icon advises you about potential problems, such as symptoms you shouldn't ignore or treatments that you may not want to undergo.

Myths and misconceptions abound about asthma. The Myth Buster icon indicates that I expose and correct mistaken beliefs that many people hold about asthma.

The Remember icon indicates things you shouldn't forget, because you may find the information useful in the future. (Now, where did I put my car keys?)

The See Your Doctor icon alerts you to matters that you should discuss with your physician.

To give you as complete a picture as possible, I occasionally get into more complex details of medical science. The Technical Stuff icon lets you know that's what I'm doing so that you can delve into the topic further — or skip it. You don't have to read these paragraphs to understand the subject at hand. (However, reading the information with these icons may give you a better handle on managing your medical condition, as well as provide some great material for impressing your friends at your next party.)

You can find plenty of helpful information and advice in paragraphs marked with the Tip icon.

Where to Go from Here

Although you can read this book from cover to cover if you want, I suggest turning to the table of contents (okay, check out Rich Tennant's cartoons first) and finding the sections that apply to your immediate concern. Then begin reading your way to better management of your asthma.

Part I
Asthma Basics

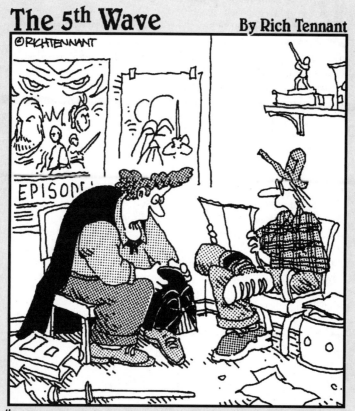

The 5th Wave   By Rich Tennant

"For years my family confused my asthma for a bad cold, bronchitis, or an obsessive need to do Darth Vader impersonations."

In this part . . .

You're experiencing respiratory symptoms that indicate you may have asthma, but you're not sure what your problem is. How do you figure out whether your ailment is asthma? Or if you're diagnosed with this medical condition, what does that mean in terms of your overall health? This part helps you determine what may be affecting you by explaining the signs and symptoms of asthma, the underlying mechanisms involved in this ailment, and how you can — as well as why you should — get a proper diagnosis of your condition.

In this part, you also find out what the vital elements of a successful asthma management plan are and how doctors use severity levels to manage your ailment. I also describe in detail the types of lung-function measurements that are crucial for assessing your asthma's severity, and how you can check your lung functions yourself at home with peak-flow monitoring. Additionally, this part discusses using a symptom record, monitoring your medication use, and evaluating your inhaler technique.

Chapter 1

Knowing What's Ailing You

*A*ccording to many experts, asthma is now a global epidemic, and its prevalence and severity continue to grow in many parts of the world, primarily in highly developed countries, including the United States, Western Europe, Australia, and New Zealand. More than 17 million people in the United States have some form of asthma. That equals three times the number of asthma cases diagnosed in 1960, despite major medical breakthroughs during the last 40 years in diagnosing and treating airway obstruction — the basis of this disease.

One of the most important factors in this rising incidence of asthma may be an increase of indoor air pollution (see Chapter 2 for more information). In addition, according to a growing number of researchers, asthma's pervasiveness in countries with the most advanced public health systems could also be due to a combination of factors popularly referred to as the *hygiene hypothesis*. This hypothesis proposes that although modern day hygiene in much of the developed world has greatly reduced the incidence of childhood diseases and dramatically improved the well-being of the overall population, people may still benefit — especially as children — from some exposure to key types of bacteria and infections. In other words, a little dirt early in life may be good. The idea is that the human immune system is thereby primed to develop responses mainly against bacterial, viral, and parasitic infections rather than against otherwise innocuous allergens and other substances that trigger most patients' asthma symptoms.

Asthma through the ages

Through the ages, asthma has affected people from all walks of life, in all parts of the world. The Roman emperor Caesar Augustus was only one of many historical figures (see Chapter 22) who suffered from this serious respiratory disease. As far back as 2,500 B.C., Chinese doctors documented cases of asthma, as did chroniclers in many subsequent civilizations, including those of ancient Greece. In fact, *asthma* is the ancient Greek word for a classic symptom of this disease: panting or breathlessness.

Proponents of the hygiene hypothesis point to lower rates of asthma as well as allergies that afflict many asthma patients — mainly *allergic rhinitis* (hay fever) and *atopic dermatitis* (allergic eczema) — in less developed and rural parts of the planet. In those areas, living environments aren't often as hygienic as in the so-called first world, and infectious childhood diseases are more common. Because the hygiene hypothesis is finding increased support among health professionals in North America, Europe, Australia, and New Zealand, and is also a hot topic with most of my patients, I discuss it further in Chapter 6.

Although the mortality rates of other serious illnesses are declining, deaths due to asthma continue to rise. More than 5,000 Americans — many between the ages of 5 and 34 — die each year because of asthma. Most of these deaths, however, are clearly preventable. With proper diagnosis, effective and timely treatment, and an asthma management plan that empowers a person with asthma (and the patient's family) to control symptoms of the disease, most asthma patients can lead fulfilling and productive lives, free from the worry of life-threatening asthma attacks.

Understanding the Relationship between Asthma and Allergies

The vast majority of asthma patients also suffer from certain types of allergic conditions. In fact, a relationship exists between asthma and these allergic ailments, and it's vital for asthmatics, their families, and healthcare providers to understand the connections between, for example, the characteristic coughing and wheezing of asthma, and the sneezing and nasal congestion of a typical hay fever attack.

Asthma denotes a specific disease process of the lungs, while *allergy* is a descriptive term for a wide variety of hypersensitivity disorders (meaning that you're excessively sensitive to one or more substances to which most people don't normally react). Asthma and allergy share a strong bond, often coexisting as partners in disease. Effectively managing your asthma also requires understanding how an allergic condition may be affecting you. But always remember that asthma is the disease and allergies are one of the main causes.

Symptoms of seemingly disparate ailments such as most cases of asthma, allergic rhinitis, and atopic dermatitis, as well as some food allergies (see Chapter 8), basically result from your immune system's similar, hyperreactive response to otherwise harmless substances that doctors refer to as *allergens*. Think of asthma and allergy as two distinct avenues with major intersections, like Broadway and 42nd Street or Hollywood and Vine. In order to be an aware and involved patient, you often have to travel down both pathways.

The word *allergy* is the ancient Greek term for an abnormal response or over-reaction. Contrary to popular belief, weak or deficient immune systems don't cause asthma or allergy ailments. Rather, your body's defenses work over-time, making your immune system too sensitive to substances that pose no real threat. That's why physicians often use the term hypersensitivity to refer to an allergy.

These are the main points to keep in mind when dealing with asthma and related allergies that cause it:

✔ **These ailments aren't infectious or contagious. You don't catch asthma or an allergy.** However, as I explain in "Sensitizing your immune system," later in this chapter, you may inherit a genetic predisposition to develop hypersensitivities that can eventually appear as asthma and/or allergies.

✔ **Asthma and allergies aren't like trends or shoe sizes. You don't really outgrow them.** Extensive studies over the past 15 years show that although your ailment can certainly vary in character and severity over your lifetime, asthma and allergies are ongoing physical conditions that are most likely always present in some form.

✔ **Allergic rhinitis often coexists with asthma and can affect your nose, ears, sinuses, eyes, and throat (see Chapter 7).**

✔ **Triggers of asthma and allergic rhinitis include allergens, such as pollens, animal dander, dust mites, mold spores, and, for some asthma patients, certain foods and drugs.** (See "Sensitizing your immune system," later in this chapter, for more detailed classifications of these items.)

✔ **Asthmatic reactions can also result from nonallergic triggers that act as irritants, including tobacco smoke, household cleaners, aerosol products, solvents, chemicals, fumes, gases, paints, smoke, and indoor and outdoor air pollution.**

✔ **Other forms of nonallergic triggers that primarily affect people with asthma are known as *precipitating factors*.** These factors include

- Other medical conditions, such as rhinitis, sinusitis, gastroesophageal reflux disease (GERD), and viral infections (colds, flu)

- Physical stimuli, such as exercise or variations in both air temperature and humidity levels

- Sensitivities to food additives such as sulfites, drugs such as beta-blockers (Inderal, Lopressor, Corgard, Timoptic), and aspirin and related over-the-counter nonsteroidal anti-inflammatory drugs (NSAIDs), such as ibuprofen (Advil, Motrin), ketoprofen (Actron, Orudis), naproxen (Aleve), and newer prescription NSAIDs known as COX-2 inhibitors, including celecoxib (Celebrex) and rofecoxib (Vioxx)

✔ **When allergies affect the lungs, the resulting coughing, wheezing, and shortness of breath often manifest as symptoms of asthma.** However, allergies can also affect other organs of the body at the same time. Therefore, although allergic reactions can trigger symptoms of asthma, they can also simultaneously trigger symptoms of other allergic disorders, such as allergic rhinitis (mainly affecting your nose) and allergic conjunctivitis (your eyes).

✔ **All that wheezes, coughs, sneezes, drips, runs, congests, waters, itches, erupts, or swells isn't always due to an allergic reaction.** That's why, as I explain in the section "Managing Asthma Effectively," later in this chapter, the first step to receiving effective treatment is to have your ailment properly diagnosed (see Chapter 2 for a full discussion).

✔ **Although the majority of people with asthma also have allergies (allergic rhinitis in most cases), some manifestations of asthma seem to develop without an allergic component.** In cases of adult-onset asthma, which often develops in people older than 40 and is less common than child-onset asthma, *atopy* (a genetic tendency toward developing allergic hypersensitivity; see the next section) doesn't appear to play an important role. Instead, precipitating factors such as sinusitis, GERD, nasal polyps, and sensitivities to aspirin and related NSAIDs are more likely to trigger this condition (see Chapter 5).

Triggering Asthma and Allergic Reactions

Your immune system acts as your second line of defense against foreign substances. (The main barrier against foreign substances is your largest organ — your skin. Tuck that away in your brain for your next Trivial Pursuit tournament!) Usually your immune system protects you against infectious bacteria, viruses, parasites, and other harmful agents by producing antibodies that recognize the invaders and fend them off without too much fuss.

In fact, most of the time, as long as your immune system works well, you may not even know that this constant, ongoing process takes place to ensure your survival and good health. However, with an allergic condition, your immune system overproduces antibodies against typically harmless or inoffensive substances such as pollens.

Sensitizing your immune system

A complex sensitization process, in which your immune system responds to allergens, causes allergic reactions that often affect asthma patients. Allergens that your immune system may respond to include the following:

- Dander from many animals, including cats, dogs, rabbits, birds, and horses, as well as gerbils and other pet rodents (see Chapters 5 and 10)
- Dust mites (see Chapter 10)
- Foods, including milk, eggs, peanuts, tree nuts, fish, shellfish, soy, and wheat (see Chapter 8)
- Mold spores (see Chapter 10)
- Pollens from certain grasses, weeds, and trees (see Chapter 10)

Approximately 10 percent of asthma patients also have sensitivities to aspirin, aspirin-containing compounds (such as Alka-Seltzer, Anacin, and Excedrin), and other NSAIDs.

Developing an allergic reaction

If you're predisposed to developing asthma and/or allergies, here's how a typical sensitization process and allergic reaction can develop, using ragweed pollen, one of the most common triggers of allergic rhinitis, as an example (you can find more details about this process in Chapter 6):

1. **Ragweed pollen enters your body, usually as a result of inhaling it through your nose.**

2. **Your immune system detects the presence of these foreign substances in your body and reacts by producing *IgE antibodies*, a special class of antibodies.**

3. **IgE antibodies attach themselves to the surfaces of mast cells that line tissues throughout your body, especially in your nose, eyes, lungs, and skin.**

4. **Your body designs IgE antibodies to counter specific substances.**

   Your immune system is a magnificent memory machine: Unlike you or me, it hardly ever forgets a face. After sensitization occurs, you'll likely experience allergies to that substance for most of your life. With ragweed, for example, your immune system produces specific IgE antibodies with receptor sites that allow ragweed allergens to cross-link two of the IgE ragweed-specific antibodies. The IgE antibodies work like a lock on the mast cell surface, and the allergen is the key. When the ragweed allergen connects with two IgE antibodies on the mast cell surface, the union of all three (allergen, antibody, and mast cell) results in the cell releasing its chemical contents.

5. **Unlocking the mast cell initiates the secretion of histamine, leukotrienes, and other potent chemical mediators of inflammation as a defensive response to the allergen.**

   In turn, the actions of these chemicals trigger the swelling and inflammation that result in familiar allergy symptoms.

All in the atopic family

Your genetically determined allergic predisposition (*atopy*) may present itself through different allergic conditions and target organs. This predisposition and a family history of allergies are the strongest predictors that you may develop asthma and/or other allergic conditions such as allergic rhinitis (hay fever), atopic dermatitis (allergic eczema), and food or drug hypersensitivities.

For example, your Uncle Ed may have allergic rhinitis, your sister Sally may suffer from recurrent sinus and ear infections, and cousin Al may have a childhood history of atopic dermatitis.

Some of your especially unlucky relatives may even be "blessed" with a combination of all these allergic conditions, plus asthma, over the course of their lifetime. (If you want to be the most popular member of your family, buy them a copy of this book.)

A typical atopic family history could consist of a person having atopic dermatitis as an infant, developing common atopic complications such as otitis media (ear infections — see Chapter 13) as a toddler, experiencing noticeable symptoms of allergic rhinitis in later childhood, and then developing asthma as a teenager.

Doctors frequently use antihistamines to relieve allergy symptoms because histamine plays such an important role in the inflammatory process. In addition, as I explain in Chapters 12 and 15, in the last two decades, government-funded and pharmaceutical researchers have developed more specialized drugs to counter and/or inhibit some of the more fundamental allergic processes. In particular, inhaled corticosteroids, mast cell stabilizers, leukotriene modifiers, and anti-IgE antibodies (see Chapter 15) provide new therapeutic approaches to preventing and controlling symptoms of asthma and other allergic reactions.

Previewing Asthma and Related Conditions

Consider this part of the chapter a preview of coming reactions. In the following sections, I summarize the significant features of the most common types of asthma, as well as hay fever and allergic eczema, and provide important details about distinguishing them from nonallergic conditions that are similar. I also include references to the chapters where I discuss these ailments in more detail.

Asthma: Breathing and wheezing

The most fundamental definition of asthma is a chronic, inflammatory airway disease of the lungs that causes breathing problems. However, in practice, asthma has many faces and is often difficult to recognize and properly diagnose. As a result, even though currently available prescription medications offer effective ways of relieving, preventing, and controlling the symptoms and underlying *inflammation* (redness, swelling, and congestion that characterize asthma), the disease continues to cause serious problems for many people worldwide.

Inflammation of the airways (bronchial tubes) is the most important underlying factor in asthma. In the vast majority of cases, if you have asthma, your symptoms may come and go, but the underlying inflammation usually persists.

Asthma's characteristic symptoms are

- Chest tightness
- Productive coughs (coughs that produce mucus)
- Shortness of breath
- Wheezing

Important symptoms of asthma in infancy and early childhood include wheezing, persistent coughing, and recurring or lingering chest colds. (Because of its symptoms, asthma in children is often misdiagnosed as recurring bronchitis, recurring chest colds, or lingering coughs.)

In an overwhelming number of cases, asthma is a manifestation of *atopy* (the genetic tendency toward developing hypersensitivity to allergens). In fact, many people with asthma also have allergic rhinitis. The hyperreactive response of the sensitized immune system to asthmatic triggers (typically inhalant allergens, such as dander and dust mites, as well as other substances, including irritants, that also trigger allergic rhinitis symptoms) causes the underlying airway inflammation (see Chapter 5 for a detailed explanation of this process).

Allergic rhinitis: Running away with your nose

Frequently referred to as hay fever, allergic rhinitis is the most common allergic disease in the United States. As many as 45 million Americans or more suffer from some form of this allergy, which often coexists with asthma. Trademark symptoms of allergic rhinitis include

- ✔ Runny nose with clear, watery discharge
- ✔ Sneezing
- ✔ Stuffy nose
- ✔ Postnasal drip
- ✔ Itchy nose, ears, palate, and throat

In addition, itchy and watery eyes, symptoms of allergic conjunctivitis, are often associated with allergic rhinitis. Infections of the middle ear (otitis media) and of the sinuses (sinusitis) are frequent complications of allergic rhinitis.

Part III includes several chapters on the many forms of allergic and nonallergic rhinitis, as well as the ways doctors diagnose and treat these ailments, important tips on avoiding triggers of various types of rhinitis, details on medications, and information on the complications of allergic rhinitis symptoms.

It's in your airways, not in your head

For centuries, many people believed that psychological factors such as anxiety, emotional disorders, or stress caused asthma. However, although these problems can *aggravate* asthma or allergies, they don't *cause* asthma or allergies. Unfortunately, I still hear about the friends and family of asthmatics who claim that asthma is all in the patient's head. Some of these people insist that if the person would just calm down, his or her condition would go away. Actually, instead of stress causing asthma, it can be the other way around: Breathing problems can cause stress. Stressing out because you can't breathe is a perfectly normal and understandable response.

Therefore, a proper diagnosis of asthma and/or allergies and early, aggressive treatment for these conditions are crucial. In most cases, you should be able to control your asthma and allergy condition so that it doesn't control you, thus enabling you to lead a full and active life. Forget the negative stereotypes of asthmatics and people with allergies as nerdy, weak, anxious types, forever coughing and blowing their noses. Asthma and allergies can affect anyone: from the captain of the school chess team to the captain of the football team, as well as everybody in between.

Atopic dermatitis: Scratching your itch

Also described as atopic eczema or allergic eczema, *atopic dermatitis* is an allergic condition that targets your skin. The simplest way to define this non-contagious skin condition is the itch that rashes (or the "itch that scratches").

"The itch that rashes" is a result of the itch-scratch cycle, the hallmark of atopic dermatitis. Scratching your dry skin causes it to rash, leading to more irritation and inflammation, further damaging your skin and making it even itchier — resulting in more scratching and increasingly irritated skin. Eventually, fissures and cracks can develop on your skin, allowing irritants, bacteria, and viruses to enter, often leading to complicating infections.

Atopic dermatitis frequently occurs with allergic rhinitis and can also precede other allergic symptoms. As such, atopic dermatitis can provide an early clue that you're at risk of developing other allergies and asthma.

Food hypersensitivities: Serving up allergens

Most adverse food reactions aren't the result of true *food hypersensitivities* (the more precise term for food allergies). In fact, various forms of food intolerance, food poisoning, and other nonallergic mechanisms cause the majority of reactions that most people blame on food allergies.

The most frequent triggers of actual food hypersensitivities are proteins in the following foods:

- ✔ Cow's milk, including products that contain casein and whey
- ✔ Eggs, especially egg whites
- ✔ Fish, both freshwater and saltwater
- ✔ Peanuts and other legumes, including soybeans, peas, lentils, beans, and foods containing these ingredients
- ✔ Shellfish, including shrimp, lobster, crab, clams, and oysters
- ✔ Tree nuts, including almonds, Brazil nuts, cashews, hazelnuts, and walnuts
- ✔ Wheat and other grains and cereals, such as corn, rice, barley, and oats

In cases in which mouth and lip swelling, wheezing, or hives occur immediately after consuming a particular food (peanuts, for example), you may easily deduce that an allergic process caused your reaction. However, in many other instances, distinguishing between food intolerance and true food hypersensitivity can require more extensive diagnostic procedures. If you're hungry for more information on adverse food reactions, see Chapter 8.

Drug hypersensitivities: Taking the wrong medicine

Certain drugs are prone to produce allergic reactions in susceptible individuals. The most frequent type of adverse allergic reactions to medications occurs with penicillin and its related compounds. Aspirin and related NSAIDs — including newer prescription NSAIDs, known as COX-2 inhibitors, such as celecoxib (Celebrex) and rofecoxib (Vioxx) — and other drugs can also trigger adverse reactions. However, as with adverse food reactions, most adverse drug reactions result from nonallergic mechanisms.

Although drug hypersensitivity reactions most frequently target the skin, adverse allergic reactions to drugs can affect any part of your body, including mucous membranes, lymph nodes, kidneys, liver, lungs, and joints. These reactions can include skin rashes, hives and *angioedema* (deep swellings), respiratory symptoms such as coughing or wheezing, fever (sometimes resulting in drug fever, occasionally with shaking chills and a skin rash), and low blood pressure and/or anemia, resulting from an adverse reaction that destroys your red blood cells.

In less frequent but more serious cases, an adverse drug reaction can result in *anaphylaxis,* a severe, potentially life-threatening response that affects many organs simultaneously (see the next section). In fact, penicillin injections cause most drug-related anaphylactic deaths in the United States. (Fortunately, the use of penicillin shots has significantly decreased in recent years.)

Anaphylaxis: Severe systemic symptoms

Anaphylaxis, an ultimate but thankfully rare form of allergic reaction that seldom affects asthma patients, is a severe, potentially life-threatening response that affects many organs simultaneously. The characteristic signs of anaphylaxis include

- ✔ Difficulty breathing
- ✔ Dizziness or fainting
- ✔ Dramatic itching over the entire body
- ✔ Flushing (sudden reddening of skin)
- ✔ Itchy rash or hives
- ✔ Nausea, vomiting, abdominal pain, and/or diarrhea
- ✔ Severe drop in blood pressure
- ✔ Swelling of the throat and/or tongue (limbs may also swell)

Significant causes of anaphylaxis in the United States include

- ✔ Foods — particularly peanuts and shellfish
- ✔ Venom from stinging insects of the *Hymenoptera* order (honeybees, yellow jackets, wasps, hornets, and fire ants)
- ✔ Drugs such as penicillin and related compounds
- ✔ Exercise, including food-dependent exercise-induced anaphylaxis (see Chapter 9 for more information)
- ✔ Latex, by direct contact with the skin or by inhalation (most often by breathing in corn starch powder used in some latex gloves — see Chapter 5)

In addition, pseudoallergic reactions caused by drugs such as aspirin or related OTC NSAIDs like ibuprofen (Advil, Motrin), ketoprofen (Actron, Orudis), naproxen (Aleve), and newer prescription NSAIDs, known as COX-2 inhibitors, including celecoxib (Celebrex) and rofecoxib (Vioxx), can (in some cases) lead to severe, potentially life-threatening reactions referred to as *anaphylactoid reactions.* These reactions are immediate, systemic reactions that closely resemble anaphylaxis but aren't caused by IgE-mediated allergic responses.

Dyeing your allergies

Inhaled corticosteroids, which are often used as asthma and allergic rhinitis treatments — including budesonide (Pulmicort, Rhinocort Aqua), fluticasone (Flovent, Flonase), and other inhaled corticosteroid products that I list in Chapter 15 — are extremely effective in suppressing the inflammatory process that is the hallmark of asthma. Keep in mind, however, that most asthma and allergy drugs treat the end result of a long, complex chain of immune system reactions but don't fundamentally prevent the underlying process causing your ailment. Therefore, if you stop taking your prescribed medications, the underlying disease process most likely restarts and your symptoms reappear.

I compare this process to dyeing your hair. You can change your hair color, but if you don't continue coloring it (like treating your asthma and allergies with your prescribed medicine), your new hair growth comes in with its original color, because you haven't really altered its underlying, genetically determined characteristics.

If you're at risk for anaphylaxis, be prepared to take emergency measures to prevent this type of extremely serious reaction. Consult with your doctor about prescribing an emergency kit (such as EpiPen) that contains an injectable dose of epinephrine.

Make sure that your doctor shows you how to use the kit. Finding out the proper technique for administering epinephrine in your physician's office is much more effective than trying it out for the first time while you're having a reaction.

Because anaphylaxis is such a serious issue and can result from various types of exposures, I address it throughout the book, wherever applicable.

Managing Asthma Effectively

In most parts of the world, asthma causes a wide range of problems for millions of people. Asthma can present as an occasional minor symptom, as a serious episode or attack, and even as a potentially life-threatening reaction (in the most severe and rare cases). However, thanks to recent medical breakthroughs, properly diagnosing what's ailing you and developing an appropriate and effective treatment plan for controlling your symptoms and managing your condition is now possible.

Effectively managing allergic conditions — particularly asthma and allergic rhinitis — frequently requires dealing with an assortment of symptoms, treatments, and preventive measures, because allergies and asthma and several related allergic conditions tend to be ailments with many faces. Think of a typical Chinese restaurant menu: You may need to order dishes from different columns in order to have a complete meal.

The basic components of effectively managing asthma and allergies include the following steps:

✔ **Getting a proper diagnosis.** Identifying the specific allergens, irritants, and/or precipitating factors that may trigger your ailment is a critical component of your diagnosis. Cough medicine isn't the treatment for your cough if you have asthma. First finding out why you're coughing (a cough may be the only obvious symptom of underlying asthma in certain patients) is vital so you can then take appropriate steps to effectively control and manage your condition.

✔ **Avoiding or reducing exposures to allergens, irritants, and precipitating factors that may trigger your asthma and/or allergies.** Effective avoidance and allergy-proofing measures (see Chapters 5 and 10) can significantly improve your quality of life and often reduce, or in certain cases eliminate, your need for medication.

✔ **Taking long-term preventive medications to control your underlying condition while appropriately using short-term medications when you experience flare-ups, episodes, or attacks.** (I provide extensive information on prescription and OTC asthma and allergy products in Chapters 12 and 14–16.)

✔ **Evaluating and monitoring your condition.** When you're initially evaluated, pulmonary testing should be done. At home, you can monitor your lung functions with a peak-flow meter (see Chapter 4 for details on managing asthma long-term).

✔ **Adhering to your treatment plan (see Chapter 2) and keeping yourself informed about all aspects of your condition.** Make sure you have an action plan to deal with any worsening of symptoms and read educational materials that your physician provides (especially this book!).

✔ **Keeping yourself in good general health to avoid developing more severe symptoms or potential complications of your ailment and to help you enjoy the highest quality of life possible.** Lead an active, healthy lifestyle, including eating right, getting plenty of exercise, and having regular checkups with your general physician.

Chapter 2

The Basics of Treating and Managing Your Asthma

Asthma isn't a recurring chest cold, a psychological disorder, a minor annoyance, or a condition that you usually outgrow. It's a multifaceted, chronic, inflammatory airway disease of the lungs that causes breathing problems and that requires proper diagnosis, early and aggressive treatment, and effective long-term management. Asthma is also unfortunately an ailment that many people — asthmatics themselves, family members, and even some doctors — may not recognize or may improperly diagnose, often as a chest cold or bronchitis.

Doctors don't yet clearly understand the origin of the airway inflammation that characterizes asthma. However, researchers have determined that this underlying inflammation often results in hyperresponsive ("twitchy"), constricted, and congested airways, which are increasingly liable to react to asthma triggers (see Chapter 5 for an extensive discussion of these triggers).

Understanding Who Gets Asthma and Why

The strongest predictor that an individual may develop asthma is a family history of allergies and asthma and/or *atopy,* an inherited tendency to develop hypersensitivities to allergic triggers. This tendency is almost always due to an overactive immune system that produces elevated levels of immunoglobulin E (IgE) antibodies to allergens. (See Chapter 6 for an extensive discussion of this process.)

The predisposition to asthma is inherited. This genetic inheritance can be a significant factor in developing the condition: Two-thirds of asthma patients have a family member who also has the disease.

Most cases of asthma are of an allergic nature (known as *allergic asthma*), and usually begin to manifest during childhood, affecting boys more often than girls. In fact, asthma is the most common chronic disease of childhood. Other allergic disorders, such as food allergies, atopic dermatitis (allergic eczema), or allergic rhinitis (hay fever), which are also indicators of atopy in young children, can precede this form of the ailment, often referred to as childhood-onset asthma.

Adult-onset asthma, which is less common than childhood-onset asthma, develops in adults older than 40, more often in women. Atopy doesn't appear to play a role in these cases. Rather, adult-onset asthma more often seems to be triggered by various nonallergic mechanisms, including sinusitis, upper respiratory infections, nasal polyps, gastroesophageal reflux disease (GERD), sensitivities to aspirin and related nonsteroidal anti-inflammatory drugs (NSAIDs), as well as occupational exposures to chemicals, such as those found in fumes, gases, resins, dust, and insecticides. However, many episodes seem to occur spontaneously without known triggers.

Keep these points in mind about asthma:

✔ Important symptoms of asthma in infancy and early childhood include persistent coughing, wheezing, and recurring or lingering chest colds.

✔ Inflammation of the airways is the single most important underlying factor in asthma. If you have asthma, your symptoms may come and go, but the underlying inflammation usually persists. Episodes of asthma symptoms can vary in length from minutes to hours and even from days to weeks, depending on your medical treatment (see Chapter 4), the severity of your symptoms (see Chapter 14), and the character of the triggering mechanism (see Chapter 5).

✔ Although no cure exists for asthma, in most cases you can manage and even reverse the effects of the disease. However, poorly managed or undertreated asthma may lead to loss of airway functions and, in some cases, irreversible lung damage as a result of airway remodeling. (I explain airway remodeling in the section "How airway obstruction develops," later in this chapter.)

✔ Early, aggressive treatment with appropriate medication is vital to effectively managing your asthma.

Why aren't these antibiotics curing my bronchitis?

Bronchitis is a general term for inflammation of the *bronchi*, or airways. (*Itis* is Greek for swelling or inflammation.) The most frequent causes of bronchial or airway inflammation are viral or bacterial infections, smoking, or asthma.

Because the coughing symptoms in different types of airway inflammation can appear similar and because bacterial infections of the airway are common, some patients who actually have asthma often are mistakenly treated with antibiotics. Although these drugs can clear bacterial infections of the airways, they don't relieve or control asthma symptoms.

If you experience lingering coughs, recurring colds, or similar symptoms that could indicate bronchitis, make sure that your doctor performs appropriate lung-function tests to check for reversible airflow obstruction, a hallmark of asthma. Performing such tests gives doctors the information they need to prescribe appropriate and effective treatment for your condition.

Identifying triggers, attacks, episodes, and symptoms

A wide variety of allergens, irritants, and other factors, such as colds, flu, exercise, and drug sensitivities, can trigger asthma symptoms — what you may refer to as *asthma attacks* or *asthma episodes*. (See Chapter 5 for more information about asthma triggers and how to avoid them.) Asthma symptoms can range from decreased tolerance to exercise to feeling completely out of breath and from persistent coughing to wheezing, chest tightness, or life-threatening respiratory distress. In many cases, a bothersome cough may be the only symptom of asthma that you even notice.

Experiencing asthma symptoms, whatever the intensity, means that your asthma isn't temporarily well controlled. Such symptoms may indicate that your asthma needs more effective management, as I explain in the section "Managing Your Asthma: Essential Steps," later in this chapter.

Realizing that asthma isn't in your head

Until recently, many healthcare providers and family members approached asthma as a nervous disorder, thought to be caused by anxiety and psychological stress. Doctors and researchers now know that this misconception has no basis in fact. Asthma occurs in your lungs' airways, not in your head. Although anxiety and stress can aggravate your asthma (as well as other illnesses), psychological factors don't cause your condition.

Uncovering the Many Facets of Asthma

Asthma can show up in various ways. The underlying mechanism causing many of the symptoms of asthma is due to a complex series of events involving many types of cells and tissue that reside in your lungs. I explain this process further in the section "Asthma and Your Airways," later in this chapter.

Because such a wide range of factors can precipitate asthma symptoms, and because certain triggers can cause stronger reactions in some asthma patients than in others, doctors often classify asthma according to the triggers that instigate your symptoms. Classifying asthma in this way can help you and your doctor understand the cause of your symptoms.

Allergies and asthma all over the world

According to numerous samples of populations in many countries, large numbers of people have allergic sensitivities that frequently increase their risk of developing symptoms associated with asthma. Here's a sampling of allergy and asthma surveys from the around the globe:

✔ Almost half the U.S. population has some sensitivity to allergens, and a third of homes in the United States contain conditions such as elevated humidity levels that frequently lead to significant sources of household allergens like molds and dust mites. (See Chapter 10 for practical and important tips on allergy-proofing your home.)

✔ Based on allergy skin testing (see Chapter 11), at least half of all children in Hong Kong and other Chinese cities demonstrate allergic sensitivities, especially to cockroach and dust mite allergens. Likewise, as many as one-quarter of schoolchildren in Costa Rica may have asthma.

✔ Studies in Germany found that at least one-third of Germans have sensitivities to pollens, dust mites, and other common inhalant allergens, while as many as a quarter of that country's population experiences symptoms of asthma and allergic rhinitis.

✔ Research in India shows that as many as one-fifth of Bombay residents have hyper-responsive airways, a significant indicator of asthma (see Chapter 5), and equivalent numbers also experience sensitivities to dust mites.

✔ Australia and New Zealand consistently report two of the highest incidences of childhood asthma in the world. In Australia, the prevalence of childhood asthma has been reported as high as more than 20 percent in certain childhood age groups, while in New Zealand, comparable studies reveal a prevalence of asthma of more than 16 percent in similar childhood age groups.

✔ If you're thinking of moving to the desert to escape your allergies, consider the significant numbers of allergists in the telephone directories of cities such as Phoenix or Tucson, and also consider this: Studies in Kuwait show that as many as a quarter of Kuwaitis experience some sensitivity to dust mites.

Although a certain precipitating factor may predominate in many asthma cases, multiple triggers affect the majority of people with asthma. For example, most asthmatics have exercise-induced asthma (EIA), sometimes known as exercise-induced bronchospasm (EIB) — which I explain in the "Exercise-induced asthma (EIA)" section — in addition to asthma that manifests from other triggers or precipitating factors. The next sections list the main asthma classifications that many doctors use.

Allergic asthma

Throughout the world, triggers of this common form of asthma include inhalant allergens, such as dust mites, animal dander, fungal spores, and pollens from trees, grasses, and weeds. If you suffer from allergic asthma, you may be sensitive to a combination of these allergens and probably suffer from allergic rhinitis (hay fever) and/or allergic conjunctivitis, which I explain in detail in Chapter 7.

Develop and implement — in consultation with your doctor — an effective allergy-proofing and avoidance-measure plan to limit your exposure to allergy triggers as part of your overall asthma management plan. (Chapter 5 explains how to avoid the many forms of asthma triggers and precipitating factors.)

Depending on your degree of sensitivity and levels of exposure to inhalant allergens, your doctor may also recommend allergy testing (which an allergist usually performs) to determine what triggers your allergic asthma and whether *immunotherapy* (allergy shots) may provide an appropriate and effective treatment for your condition.

Immunotherapy can, in certain cases, reduce your level of sensitivity to the allergens that affect you, thus decreasing your allergy and asthma symptoms. (To find out more about immunotherapy, turn to Chapter 11.)

Nonallergic asthma

Irritants, such as tobacco smoke, household cleaners, soaps, perfumes and scents, glue, aerosols, smoke from wood-burning appliances or fireplaces, fumes from unvented gas, oil, or kerosene stoves, and indoor and outdoor air pollutants can also trigger asthma.

Upper respiratory tract infections, such as the common cold and flu, as well as sinusitis, nasal polyps, GERD, and aspirin sensitivity (see "Aspirin-induced [and food-additive-induced] asthma," later in this chapter), may also aggravate airway inflammation and trigger asthma symptoms in some people.

Occupational asthma

Current estimates are that occupational asthma, which a wide range of allergens and irritants can trigger, affects as many as 15 percent of asthma patients in the United States. The precipitating factors in occupational asthma cases often include exposure to fumes, chemicals, gases, resins, metals, dust, insecticides, vapors, and other substances in the workplace that can induce or aggravate airway inflammation.

Exercise-induced asthma (EIA)

Symptoms of *exercise-induced asthma* (EIA) occur to varying degrees in a majority of asthmatics. Exercising that involves breathing cold, dry air — such as running outdoors in winter — may trigger EIA symptoms more often than activities that involve breathing warmer, humidified air, such as swimming in a heated pool.

Certain medications can help you prevent and control EIA symptoms (see Chapter 9) so that you can enjoy many types of exercise and sports activities, in spite of your condition. Chapter 15 provides information on these medical products, which you should take only according to your doctor's advice.

Aspirin-induced (and food-additive-induced) asthma

A significant number of people who have both asthma and nasal polyps may experience intensified asthma symptoms if they take aspirin and related medications, such as over-the-counter NSAIDs and newer prescription NSAIDs, known as COX-2 inhibitors, such as celecoxib (Celebrex) and rofecoxib (Vioxx). Some asthma sufferers may also experience intensified symptoms if they ingest *sulfites* (preservatives found in beer, wine, and many processed foods) or *tartrazine* (FDC yellow dye No. 5), which is used in many medications, foods, and vitamin products.

Asthma and Your Airways

Your airways are vital to your health. This network of bronchial tubes enables your lungs to absorb oxygen into the bloodstream and eliminate carbon dioxide — the process called *respiration,* or breathing. Most people take breathing for granted — you usually don't need to think about it, unless something interferes with this process by obstructing your airways.

The inflammatory response

In asthma, airway obstruction is most often the result of an underlying airway inflammation that leads to one or more of the following conditions (which I explain in the section "How airway obstruction develops," later in this chapter):

- ✔ Airway hyperresponsiveness
- ✔ Airway constriction
- ✔ Airway congestion

These airway conditions can become part of an overall, ongoing process known as the *inflammatory response.* This complex response can develop into a vicious cycle of worsening inflammation, hyperresponsiveness, constriction, and congestion, in which your airways become more and more sensitive and inflamed as a result of reacting to allergens, irritants, and other factors.

Burning your lungs

You need to realize that the ongoing, underlying airway inflammation is often so subtle that it can go unnoticed. Asthma symptoms are often just the tip of the iceberg. If you have asthma, the inflammation smolders away in your airways, whether or not you're actually experiencing symptoms.

Imagine if you had a rash or sunburn and only took pain relievers to deal with the discomfort, rather than staying out of the sun or treating the cause of the problem. The underlying airway inflammation in asthma is similar to having a sunburn in your bronchial tubes, as my good friend Nancy Sander, founder of the Allergy and Asthma Network/Mothers of Asthmatics (AANMA), likes to explain. If you suffer from asthma, the insides of your airways are often red and inflamed, and, as with a bad rash or sunburn, the top layer of airway tissue may peel.

What you can't see can hurt you

If your lungs were external organs — like gills — or if your body were transparent so that you could see what happens internally, more doctors would treat asthma earlier and more aggressively because you and your doctor could easily see how the underlying disease affects you.

As I explain in the section "Testing your lungs," later in the chapter, you need to make sure that your doctor performs appropriate pulmonary (lung) function tests if you have bouts of wheezing, recurring coughs, lingering colds, or other symptoms that could indicate an underlying respiratory ailment.

Breathing basics: How your lungs function

To better understand how asthma adversely affects your airways, consider what happens in normal breathing:

1. The air you inhale flows through your nose or mouth into your *trachea,* or windpipe.

2. Your trachea then divides into right and left main *bronchi* (or branches), splitting and funneling the air into each of your lungs.

3. The main bronchi continue branching, like tree branches, within your lungs, dividing into a network of airways called *bronchial tubes.* The outside of your bronchial tubes consists of layers of smooth, involuntary muscles that

relax and tighten your airways as you inhale and exhale. Doctors refer to the process of airway relaxation as *bronchodilation.* Likewise, doctors refer to the tightening, which helps your lungs push out air when you exhale, as *bronchoconstriction.*

4. Your network of airways ultimately leads to *alveoli,* tiny air sacs that look like small clusters of grapes. The alveoli contain blood vessels and provide the means for vital respiratory exchange: Oxygen from the air you inhale is absorbed into the bloodstream, while carbon dioxide gas from your blood exits as you exhale.

How airway obstruction develops

Here's an overview of how the mechanisms of asthma interact. Although I've itemized these processes to explain them, keep in mind that they are often ongoing events that can occur simultaneously in your lungs. As you read these descriptions, take a look at Figure 2-1, which compares a normal airway with an asthmatic airway.

✔ **Airway constriction:** When a trigger or precipitating factor irritates your airways, causing the release of chemical mediators such as histamine and leukotrienes (see Chapter 6) from the mast cells of the *epithelium* (the lining of the airway), the muscles around your bronchial tubes can tighten, leading to *airway constriction.* This process results in narrowing airways and breathing difficulty. Airway constriction can also occur in people who don't have asthma or allergies if they're exposed to substances that can harm their respiratory systems, such as poisonous gases or smoke from a burning building.

✔ **Airway hyperresponsiveness:** The underlying airway inflammation in asthma can cause *airway hyperresponsiveness* as the muscles around your bronchial tubes twitch or feel ticklish. This twitchy or ticklish feeling indicates that your muscles overreact and tighten, causing acute bronchoconstriction or bronchospasms even if you're exposed only to otherwise harmless substances, such as allergens and irritants, that rarely provoke reactions in people without asthma and allergies (see the section "Uncovering the Many Facets of Asthma," earlier in the chapter).

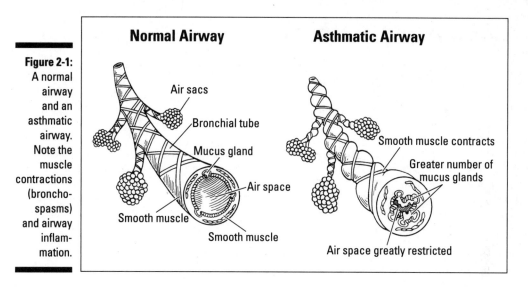

Figure 2-1: A normal airway and an asthmatic airway. Note the muscle contractions (broncho-spasms) and airway inflam-mation.

(Figure labels: Normal Airway — Asthmatic Airway; Air sacs; Bronchial tube; Mucus gland; Air space; Smooth muscle; Smooth muscle; Smooth muscle contracts; Greater number of mucus glands; Air space greatly restricted)

✔ **Airway congestion:** Mucus and fluids are released as part of the inflam-matory process and can accumulate in your airways, overwhelming the *cilia* (tiny hair-like projections from certain cells that sweep debris-laden mucus through your airways) and leading to *airway congestion*. This accumulation of mucus and fluids may make you feel the urge to cough up phlegm to relieve your chest congestion.

✔ **Airway edema:** The long-term release of inflammatory fluids in con-stricted, hyperresponsive, and congested airways can lead to *airway edema* (swelling of the airway), causing bronchial tubes to become more rigid and further interfering with airflow. In severe cases of airway con-gestion and edema, a chronic buildup of mucus secretion leads to the formation of mucus plugs in the airway, which limit airflow.

✔ **Airway remodeling:** If airway inflammation is left untreated or poorly managed for many years, the constant injury to your bronchial tubes due to ongoing airway constriction, airway hyperresponsiveness, and airway congestion can lead to *airway remodeling,* as scar tissue perma-nently replaces your normal airway tissue. As a result of airway remod-eling, airway obstruction can persist and may not respond to treatment, leading to the eventual loss of your airway function as well as potentially irreversible lung damage.

This vicious cycle of asthma can develop gradually, over hours or even days following exposure to triggers or precipitating factors. After this cycle is set in motion, you can suffer severe and long-lasting consequences.

Diagnosing Asthma

Effectively managing your asthma begins with your doctor correctly diagnosing your condition. In order to determine whether asthma causes your respiratory symptoms, your doctor should take your medical history, perform a physical exam, test your lung functions, and perform other tests, as I explain in the following sections.

The diagnostic processes that your doctor uses are crucial because, as my friend Nancy Sander notes, asthma isn't a neat little package of symptoms that you or your doctor can easily identify and eliminate. Asthma symptoms vary widely from patient to patient. In fact, your own symptoms may change over time. Make sure your doctor establishes these key points when diagnosing your asthma:

✔ You experience episodes of airway obstruction.

✔ Your airway obstruction is at least partially reversible (and can be improved through treatment).

✔ Your symptoms result from asthma, not from other conditions that I describe in "Considering other possible diagnoses," later in this chapter.

Taking your medical history

A careful, thorough medical history is vital in diagnosing the correct cause of your respiratory symptoms. For this reason, your doctor may ask several questions about your condition and your life. Keeping track of symptoms in a diary may help provide your doctor with details that can assist her with a proper diagnosis. Try to provide your doctor with as much information as possible about the following subjects:

✔ The type of symptoms you experience, which may include coughing, wheezing, shortness of breath, chest tightness, and productive coughs (coughs that bring up mucus).

✔ The pattern of your symptoms:

 • *Perennial* (year-round), seasonal, or perennial with seasonal worsening

 • Constant, episodic, or constant with episodic worsening

✔ The onset of your symptoms. At what rate do your symptoms develop — rapidly or slowly? And does that rate vary?

✔ The duration and frequency of your symptoms and whether the type and intensity of symptoms vary at different times of day and night. Especially note if your episodes awaken you from sleep or are more severe when you wake up in the morning.

✔ The impact that exercise or other physical exertion has on your symptoms.

✔ Your exposure to potential asthma triggers. In addition to the allergens, irritants, and precipitating factors that I list in the section "Uncovering the Many Facets of Asthma," earlier in this chapter, your doctor also needs to know about endocrine factors, such as adrenal or thyroid disease. Special considerations for women are pregnancy or changes in their menstrual cycles.

✔ The development of your disease, including any prior treatment and medications you've received or taken and their effectiveness. Your doctor particularly wants to know whether you presently take or have previously taken oral corticosteroids and, if so, the dosage and frequency of use.

✔ Your family history, especially whether parents, siblings, or close relatives suffer from asthma, allergic or nonallergic rhinitis, and other types of allergies, sinusitis, or nasal polyps.

✔ Your lifestyle, including

 • Your home's characteristics, such as its age and location, type of cooling and heating system, your basement's condition, whether you have a wood-burning stove, humidifier, carpet over concrete, mold and mildew, and the types of bedding, carpeting, and furniture coverings that you use.

 • Whether anyone smokes in your home or the other locations where you spend time, such as work or school.

 • Any history of substance abuse.

✔ The impact of the disease on you and your family, such as

 • Any life-threatening symptoms, emergency or urgent care treatments, or hospitalizations.

 • The number of days you (or your child with asthma) tend to miss from school or work, the disease's economic impact, and its effect on your recreational activities.

 • If your child has asthma, your doctor may ask you about the effects of the illness on your youngster's growth, development, behavior, and extent of participation in sports.

✔ Your knowledge, perception, and beliefs about asthma and long-term management of the disease, as well as your ability to cope with the illness.

✔ The level of support you receive from your family members and their abilities to recognize and assist you in case your symptoms suddenly worsen.

Examining your condition

A physical exam for suspected asthma usually focuses not only on your breathing passageways, but also on other characteristics and symptoms of atopic disease. The significant physical signs of asthma or allergy that your doctor looks for primarily include

- ✔ Chest deformity, such as an expanded or overinflated chest, as well as hunched shoulders
- ✔ Coughing, wheezing, shortness of breath, and other respiratory symptoms
- ✔ Increased nasal discharge, swelling, and the presence of nasal polyps
- ✔ Signs of sinus disease, such as thick or discolored nasal discharge
- ✔ Any allergic skin conditions, such as atopic dermatitis (eczema — in Chapter 1, I explain how this ailment and asthma can often be connected)

Testing your lungs

Many people are used to routinely taking their temperature or regularly having their doctor check their pulse and blood pressure, in addition to monitoring their blood sugar and cholesterol levels on a consistent basis. However, most people aren't yet in the habit of having routine pulmonary (lung) function tests, which may be why asthma is so frequently not diagnosed at an early stage but rather after a severe episode.

Objective pulmonary function tests are the most reliable means of assessing the extent to which your lung function is limited or affected. The following sections explain the most important tests that doctors use to diagnose asthma. (See Chapter 4 for a more detailed description of these tests.)

Spirometry

In order to determine whether you have airway obstruction and whether your condition is reversible (can improve with appropriate treatment), doctors often use a *spirometer* to measure the volume of air you exhale from your large and small airways before and 15 minutes after inhaling a short-acting inhaled beta$_2$-adrenergic bronchodilator. Figure 2-2 shows a patient using a spirometer.

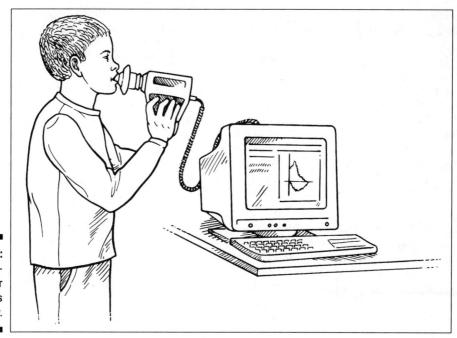

Figure 2-2:
A spirom-
eter
measures
airflow.

Spirometry provides many types of airflow measurements, including:

- ✓ **Forced vital capacity (FVC):** The maximum volume (in liters) of air that you can exhale after taking in as deep a breath as you can.

- ✓ **Forced expiratory volume (FEV1):** The volume (in liters) of air that you're able to exhale when you breathe out with maximal effort in the first second, as forcefully as possible. Physicians determine a reduction in FEV1 as the most common indicator of airway obstruction and in patients with symptoms of asthma. This test, the most important measurement in the diagnosis and management of asthma, generally measures obstruction of the large airways, although FEV1 can also reveal severe obstruction, if present, of the small airways. A baseline FEV1 (before using a bronchodilator) that is lower than normal but that increases by at least 12 percent 15 minutes after inhaling a short-acting bronchodilator (post-bronchodilator) allows your doctor to more conclusively establish the diagnosis of asthma.

- ✓ **Maximum midexpiratory flow rate (MMEF):** The middle part of your forced exhalation (in liters per second). This measurement is also referred to as the *forced expiratory flow rate between 25 and 75 percent* (FEF 25–75 percent) of FVC. A reduction in this measurement can indicate obstruction of the lungs' small airways.

BERGER BIT

The jaws of asthma

Picture one of those scary shark movies: People swim about peacefully on the ocean surface until suddenly, a fin breaks the waves (cue the ominous double basses and cellos) and a shark attacks a hapless swimmer. The shark doesn't just materialize out of nowhere; it's been lurking around underwater, probably for a long time. But the swimmers on the surface don't notice it until it's too late.

Your asthma episodes are similar to that shark attack (without the bite marks). If you rely only on short-acting inhaled beta$_2$-adrenergic bronchodilators — known as rescue medications —

to treat your asthma symptoms when they flare up, that's the equivalent of swimming in shark-infested waters, hoping that someone rescues you if the creature comes after you.

I constantly advise my patients (and you, throughout this book) to manage their asthma on a consistent, long-term preventive basis and to avoid a crisis-management approach. (The section "Managing Your Asthma: Essential Steps," later in this chapter, provides you with more details.) You can control your asthma; don't let your asthma control you!

Your doctor compares the values from the spirometry to the predicted normal reference values, based on your age, height, sex, and race, as established by the American Thoracic Society. The percent of the predicted normal value of your measured FEV1 is one of the major criteria your doctor uses to classify your level of asthma severity. (See Chapter 4 for information on the four levels of asthma severity.)

TIP

Doctors consider spirometry a valuable diagnostic tool for diagnosing childhood cases of asthma in children older than 4. However, for younger children, the test can be difficult, if not impossible, to perform. In those cases, your child's physician may decide that trying a peak-flow meter or other less complicated assessment process is more suitable. (See Chapter 18 for information on diagnosing asthma in infants and children.)

Peak-flow meters

Just as diabetics check their blood sugar levels with a monitoring device and people with hypertension take their own blood pressure, you can also keep an eye on your lung functions at home with a peak-flow meter. Peak-flow meters, which are available in a variety of shapes and sizes from different manufacturers (see the appendix), are convenient, portable, and easy-to-use devices for monitoring *peak expiratory flow rate* (PEFR), the maximum rate of air (in liters per minute) that you can force out of your large airways, as a measurement of lung function.

This measurement isn't as accurate as spirometry, but you can easily perform it at home. Measurements of PEFR are also a vital part of long-term management of your asthma, as I explain in more depth in Chapter 4.

Challenge tests

If spirometry indicates normal or near-normal lung functions but asthma continues to seem the most likely cause of your symptoms, your doctor may decide that a form of challenge test is necessary for a more conclusive diagnosis.

Challenge tests, also called bronchoprovocation, usually involve your doctor administering small doses of inhaled methacholine or histamine to you or making you exercise under his observation. The goal of such tests is to see whether these challenges cause obstructive changes in your airways, thus provoking mild asthma symptoms. Your doctor usually measures your lung functions before and after each test.

Considering other possible diagnoses

Although asthma causes most recurring episodes of coughing, wheezing, and shortness of breath, other disorders can cause these symptoms in some cases. With infants and children, underlying problems may include

✔ An upper respiratory disease, such as allergic rhinitis or sinusitis

✔ A swallowing mechanism problem or the effects of GERD

✔ Congenital heart disease, often leading to congestive heart failure

✔ An obstruction of large airways, possibly caused by

- A foreign object in the trachea or main bronchi, such as a small piece of popcorn that your child may have accidentally inhaled

- Problems of the *larynx* (the cartilaginous portion of the upper respiratory tract that contains the vocal cords) or with the vocal cords themselves

- Benign or malignant tumors or enlarged lymph nodes

✔ An obstruction of the small airways, as a result of

- Cystic fibrosis

- Abnormal development of the bronchi and lungs

- Viral infection of the *bronchioles* (small bronchi)

With adult cases, underlying problems may include

✔ Chronic bronchitis and/or emphysema, collectively referred to as *chronic obstructive pulmonary disease* (COPD)

✔ Pulmonary embolism (a blood clot, air bubble, bacteria mass, or other mass that can clog a blood vessel)

✔ Heart disease

✔ Problems of the vocal cords or the larynx (vocal cord dysfunction)

✔ Benign or malignant tumors in the airways

✔ A cough reaction due to drugs such as ACE inhibitors that you may be using to treat other conditions, such as hypertension

Classifying asthma severity

If your doctor diagnoses you with asthma based on your medical history, the physical exam, and appropriate tests, studies, and assessments, he also needs to define your condition's severity. Physicians classify asthma — whether allergic or nonallergic — according to four levels of severity.

Experts from different fields of medicine have developed these severity classifications, which provide the basis for "stepwise" management of asthma. I explain stepwise management and asthma severity levels in detail in Chapter 4.

Referring to a specialist for diagnosis

In order to diagnose your condition, you or your physician should consider consulting an asthma specialist, such as an allergist or *pulmonologist* (lung doctor), when

✔ Your diagnosis is difficult to establish.

✔ Your diagnosis requires specialized testing, such as allergy testing (see Chapter 11), bronchoprovocation (see the section "Testing your lungs," earlier in this chapter), or *bronchoscopy* (an exam of the interior of your bronchi using a slender, flexible fiber-optic bronchoscope).

✔ Your doctor advises you to consider allergy shots; see Chapter 11.

✔ Other conditions, such as sinusitis, nasal polyps, severe rhinitis, GERD, chronic bronchitis and/or emphysema (COPD), vocal cord problems, or *aspergillosis* (a fungal infection that can affect the lungs), complicate your condition or diagnosis.

✔ You don't seem to be doing as well as you'd like.

✔ You aren't able to regularly sleep through the night without being awakened by your asthma.

✔ You can't exercise as you'd like to because of asthma.

✔ You need to use an asthma inhaler for quick relief on a daily basis or in the middle of the night.

✔ You've experienced a previous emergency room visit or hospitalization for asthma (see Chapter 5) or anaphylaxis (see Chapter 1).

Managing Your Asthma: Essential Steps

If you're diagnosed with asthma, you and your doctor need to develop and implement appropriate long-term and emergency-management plans to effectively treat your condition. In my experience, motivated patients (with family members) who address their conditions through this type of thorough, individualized process almost always lead fulfilling and productive lives.

Going over the basics

Your asthma management plan requires your full participation in order to work most effectively. One of the most important ways for you to actively participate in your asthma treatment is to find out about not only the disease's complexities, but also medications, self-monitoring, allergies, triggers, and precipitating factors.

Your asthma management plan should address the following key areas:

✔ **Assessment and monitoring of your lung functions:** In addition to helping diagnose asthma, certain tests and assessments are vital in tracking how your condition develops and responds to prescribed treatment. See the section "Testing your lungs," earlier in the chapter, and Chapter 4 for more information.

✔ **Avoidance measures:** Ways of avoiding and controlling your exposure to asthma triggers and precipitating factors.

✔ **Medication:** Using appropriate medication to prevent symptoms if you're exposed to allergens, irritants, and other asthma triggers.

 • **Long-term pharmacotherapy:** This involves using medications to prevent symptoms by treating the underlying airway inflammation, congestion, constriction, and hyperresponsiveness.

 • **Short-term pharmacotherapy:** This involves using fast-acting rescue medications when your condition suddenly deteriorates.

✔ **Knowing when an attack is serious:** This is based on frequency of rescue inhaler use, decrease in peak-flow values, and increased night-time awakenings.

✔ **Determining what to do if you have a serious attack:** You should know how to adjust your medication in response to a worsening of symptoms and when to call for medical help if your condition continues to deteriorate.

✔ **An ongoing process of education for you and your family about asthma:** This process can involve information and resources that your doctor, clinic staff, and patient support groups provide or recommend, as well as relevant books, newsletters, videos, and other helpful materials that you and your family gather.

Determining your asthma therapy goals

Your asthma management plan should be results-oriented. I advise developing an overall goal, in consultation with your doctor, that aims for the highest attainable improvement of lung functions and enables you to maintain near-normal levels of exercise and other physical activities.

Other results that you should expect from asthma therapy include

✔ Preventing chronic and troublesome symptoms of asthma, such as coughing, shortness of breath, wheezing (especially upon awakening in the morning), and episodes that disturb your sleep at night

✔ Preventing recurring aggravation of symptoms

✔ Minimizing the need for emergency care and hospitalization

✔ Providing the most effective medication therapy that results in minimal or no adverse side effects

Based on the previous goals, if you feel that your doctor isn't providing adequate and effective treatment for your condition, consult an asthma specialist, such as an allergist or pulmonologist. Too often, people receive referrals only after their symptoms have gotten out of control. In my experience, after patients receive appropriate care for their asthma and understand that, in most cases, their asthma management goals are clearly achievable, they usually lead normal lives and don't tolerate going back to being frequently ill with asthma attacks.

In addition, you or your physician may also want to consider consulting an asthma specialist if

✔ You've suffered a life-threatening asthma attack.

✔ You're not meeting the goals of your asthma therapy.

✔ You require more education and guidance on possible treatment complications, the avoidance and control of triggers and precipitating factors, and your asthma management program.

✔ You have severe persistent asthma that requires constant daily use of preventive medications and frequent use of short-acting inhaled beta$_2$-adrenergic (beta$_2$-agonist) bronchodilators.

✔ Your condition requires continuous use of oral corticosteroids, high-dose inhaled corticosteroids, or more than two bursts of oral corticosteroids within one year.

✔ You have a child under age 3 who has moderate persistent or severe persistent asthma (see Chapter 4) and requires constant use of preventive medication and frequent use of short-acting inhaled beta$_2$-adrenergic bronchodilators.

✔ You care for a person with asthma who experiences significant psychological, emotional, or family problems that interfere with or prevent that person from following an appropriate asthma management plan. Such experiences can lead to worsening asthma symptoms, which pose a threat to the patient's health. In this event, have him or her undergo an evaluation by a mental health professional.

Handling emergencies

In addition to instructing you on how to monitor your symptoms to recognize early warning signs of a worsening condition, your doctor should also

✔ Give you a written action plan that you can follow in case your condition deteriorates. Children with asthma need a plan that they can use at school, daycare, or summer camp. Your written action plan must clearly instruct you on how to adjust your medications in response to particular signs, symptoms, and PEFR levels, as well as tell you when to call for medical help.

✔ Instruct you to seek medical help early if your episode is severe, if medication doesn't provide rapid, sustained improvement, or if your condition continues to deteriorate.

✔ Advise you to keep on hand appropriate medications, peak-flow meters, and inhalant devices, such as nebulizers, to treat severe episodes at home if you suffer from moderate-to-severe persistent asthma or have a history of severe asthma attacks.

✔ Warn you against trying to manage severe episodes with home remedies, such as drinking large amounts of water, breathing steam or moist air (from a hot shower), taking OTC medications such as antihistamines, cold and flu remedies, and pain relievers, or using OTC bronchodilators.

Although these types of inhalers can sometimes provide temporary relief of airway constriction, they certainly aren't the preferable approach when appropriate medical care is required for treating acute asthma emergencies. (See Chapter 15 for information on effective use of asthma controller medications.)

Managing asthma at school

If your child has asthma, inform teachers, administrators, and the school nurse. Take the following steps to ensure that your child's school days are as healthy, safe, and fulfilling as possible:

✔ Meet with school staff to inform them about any medications that your child may need to take while on campus, as well as any physical activity restrictions that your doctor may advise. (With proper management of their conditions, most children with asthma can participate in sports and physical education classes.)

✔ File treatment authorization forms with the school office and discuss what school personnel need to do in case of an asthma emergency. Provide phone numbers and other avenues for school personnel to reach you and your child's physician in the event of an emergency.

✔ Inform school personnel of allergens and irritants that can trigger your child's asthma symptoms and request that the school remove the sources of those triggers if possible.

For more information on managing childhood asthma, turn to Chapter 18.

Chapter 3

Dealing with Doctor Visits

• •

In This Chapter

▶ Preparing for your first asthma appointment

▶ Understanding the various tests your doctor may order

▶ Making a proper diagnosis and starting the appropriate treatment

▶ Understanding insurance issues and paying for treatment

▶ Knowing what to expect from your physician

• •

Seeing a doctor, whether an asthma specialist or your own family practitioner, is something to take seriously. You and your physician are partners in treating your medical condition. Developing and maintaining that partnership is one of the most important aspects of effectively managing and treating your asthma or any other serious ailment.

The effectiveness of your treatment depends not so much on the length of time you spend in your doctor's office, but rather on the quality of that time. As much as I enjoy seeing my patients and as much as they may delight in my winning personality, the real reason they're in my office is to get better. In my experience, patients who derive the greatest benefit from treatment are those who understand how to get the most out of their doctor visits. Some tips for getting the most out of your doctor visits include

✔ Preparing ahead of time.

✔ Communicating well with your doctor about your condition and your treatment.

✔ Understanding all aspects of your treatment plan, including the medications your doctor prescribes, and determining the most effective ways of avoiding asthma and allergy triggers. (Chapters 5 and 10 offer more information on avoiding asthma and allergy triggers.)

✔ Participating in developing treatment goals with your doctor.

✔ Adhering to your treatment plan. You're the most important factor in your own treatment process. Your good health and your quality of life clearly depend on your full and active participation in the treatment process.

Preparing for Your First Visit

When it comes to making a proper diagnosis of asthma, your primary care physician (PCP) may refer you to a specialist, such as an allergist and/or a pulmonologist. Your first visit will likely consist of the following items:

- ✔ Taking a thorough medical history (see the following sections), covering any and all ailments in your life, not just those that you think involve asthma.

- ✔ Performing a physical examination. Depending on your condition, on your past medical history, and especially on why your PCP referred you, your physical exam may focus only on the areas that your asthma or allergy symptoms affect, or your exam may also include a more comprehensive evaluation. (See the section "Looking for signs of asthma and allergies," later in this chapter, for more information on the signs and symptoms your doctor may be looking for, depending on your medical history.)

- ✔ Allergy skin testing (depending on your medical history and medical exam) for specific allergic sensitivities and/or other appropriate tests and lab procedures (such as pulmonary function tests for asthma, as I explain in "Assessing asthma with spirometry," later in this chapter).

- ✔ Prescribing and teaching you how to use appropriate medications and/or instructing you about effective environmental control steps that you can take to avoid or reduce exposure to your asthma or allergy triggers, thus reducing your symptoms.

Doing your homework

Identifying the underlying cause of your asthma provides the best approach to effectively treating your ailment. However, as I explain in Chapter 6, because of the complexity of asthma and allergic diseases, getting to the root of what's ailing you is usually more than a matter of just performing medical tests (such as blood tests or X-rays) and interpreting the results.

Although medical science has recently seen impressive breakthroughs in diagnosing and treating various diseases (especially with ongoing research in developing new medications), the first step an asthma or allergy specialist still takes to treat your condition is obtaining your complete medical history. The specialist uses your medical history as the foundation of your medical evaluation.

The doctor you're consulting for your asthma usually requests that you provide very specific medical information at your first visit. After taking your medical history, your specialist may also perform an appropriate medical exam. Subsequently, she may also order tests and procedures to confirm your diagnosis and to more precisely identify the specific triggers of your asthma and/or allergy symptoms, as well as to determine your sensitivity levels to those triggers. (Check out Part III to find out how allergies affect asthma.)

Preparing for an initial consultation with a specialist shouldn't stress you out the way school exams or job interviews may sometimes affect you. However, you need to spend some time before your appointment gathering and reviewing information that your specialist needs in order to make a specific diagnosis of your condition. Prepare to provide your doctor with, and to discuss in detail during your consultation, the following key information:

- ✔ Your symptoms, both those that seem to be caused by asthma and/or an allergic condition and any others, even if they seem unrelated, such as

    - • How many nights a month your asthma awakens you from sleep

    - • How many times, on average, you have to use a quick-relief inhaler to treat increased symptoms during a 24-hour period

    - • Your ability to exercise and exert yourself physically

    - • Any known triggers of your respiratory symptoms (see Chapter 5 for a full discussion of asthma triggers)

- ✔ Any other medical conditions for which you've been treated or are presently being treated

- ✔ Any medications you're taking, whether prescription or over-the-counter (OTC)

- ✔ Your medical history, as well as that of your family

- ✔ Details about other factors, such as your home, work, or school environment that may contribute to your medical condition

I provide detailed examples of the information your doctor will request, based on these general categories, in the "Telling your story" section, later in this chapter.

You may also have questions about your medical condition. Asking your physician about your concerns during your initial consultation is certainly appropriate. Remember, there's no such thing as a stupid question when you're asking about your medical history, diagnosis, or treatment.

You may think that an issue you raise is obvious, insignificant, or irrelevant, but bringing it up may further clarify the nature of your ailment for your doctor. The best way to find out is to go ahead and ask him or her. A good physician appreciates the fact that you've taken the time to formulate your own questions. I advise writing down your inquiries ahead of time and giving them to your doctor at the beginning of your appointment so that he or she can focus on the most important issues affecting your health during your office visit.

Patient, know thyself

Providing your doctor with the information that she requests about your medical history enables you to take part in the process of diagnosing and treating your medical problems. While assembling their medical histories and related details, many of my patients have discovered patterns and connections between symptoms, triggers, and environmental factors (for example, a sudden change in the weather, usually from hot to cold) that they hadn't realized before.

Gaining this type of self-knowledge not only helps your physician make a diagnosis, but it can also help you make more informed choices about your treatment options, as well as assist you in avoiding the triggers and precipitating factors of your asthma symptoms.

Filling out forms ahead of time

Many doctors (including myself) send patients a questionnaire to fill out prior to their initial consultation. The level of detail that these questionnaires require varies, depending on the symptoms you experience and the type of consultation you seek. Doctors don't send out these forms because they love paperwork, but rather because they want to ensure that your first appointment is productive.

In most cases, you can expect to spend between one and two hours at your first appointment. You may have a hectic life, but it's important to plan your schedule so that you can arrive at your physician's office on time. Remember to bring all requested forms, documents, and other materials, including your insurance and/or other payment information. (See "Paying for Your Care," later in this chapter.)

Telling your story

Whatever way it's gathered, you probably need to provide the following information at your first appointment with your asthma and allergy specialist:

- ✔ Your name, address, telephone number, and other contact information.
- ✔ Your age, gender, marital status, and information about family members living with you. (If you're making an appointment for your child, list your own and your spouse's age and those of any other children in your household.)
- ✔ The name of your referring physician (or other person who referred you).
- ✔ The major medical problems that affect you, and their duration.

✔ The symptoms you're experiencing and the specific areas or organs of your body that are affected. Providing details of when and in what circumstances these symptoms occur is often vital to establishing an accurate diagnosis.

✔ For women, let your physician know if you think or know you are pregnant or if you're planning to become pregnant.

✔ Aggravating factors that seem to make your condition worse. For example, if you notice that your respiratory symptoms — such as coughing, wheezing, or shortness of breath — are more severe when you visit people who have pets or when you're around smokers, make sure you tell your physician.

✔ The names of all the medications you're currently taking, including products that you use specifically for your condition, as well as other drugs, such as OTC preparations or herbal remedies that you take to relieve minor aches and pains. Because gathering this information all at once can be a challenge, I advise keeping a drug record that you can refer to when consulting with a new doctor, as I explain in "Recording your symptoms and medications," later in this chapter.

✔ If you've been treated or evaluated previously for the same condition, provide your new doctor with information on the results of these consultations and treatments. (Bringing the results from any tests you've had in the past may also save you the trouble — and cost — of repeating those procedures.)

✔ Providing accurate information on any other illnesses and related treatments you've had is also vital to evaluating your current condition.

✔ Your family history is very important in determining your diagnosis, so take time to list this information to the best of your ability (see "Taking your family history," later in this chapter). Likewise, if you fill out this form for a child, provide information on specific childhood factors, such as birth history, immunizations, and childhood illnesses (for example, bronchiolitis and/or croup).

✔ Your career, occupation, school (or daycare for children) you attend, and your hobbies or recreational activities are also important factors in figuring out what's ailing you.

✔ Your dietary history, including any special diets you follow, major food groups you avoid, and whether you've been diagnosed with any food allergies. (Check out Chapter 8 to discover why people with asthma should be aware of food allergies.)

✔ Doctors aren't census takers (or private detectives, for that matter), but your specialist needs to know about your home because many things in your domestic environment can trigger or aggravate asthma and/or allergy symptoms, particularly dust, animal dander, molds, and tobacco smoke. Therefore, provide your doctor with information on the following items:

- A list of the people living with you and any habits they may have, such as smoking or keeping pets that can affect your condition.

- A list of any plants you have in your home and where in the home they're located.

- Your home's condition, including its location, age, the principal construction materials, the building's air circulation system, the condition of the basement, and the type of carpets and furnishings you have. Your doctor may also ask about your yard, garden, and surrounding vegetation.

- Your bedroom's condition, including what the ventilation's like, whether it's a breeding ground for dust mites (and who knows what else!), and so on. Don't get the wrong idea, though. You most likely spend the majority of your life in your bedroom (even more time than on the golf course, in my case), so exposure to allergens (such as dust mites; see Chapter 10) in your bedroom can often play a significant role in the severity of your asthma or allergy symptoms.

Recording your symptoms and medications

Keeping a daily symptom diary (see Chapter 4) can provide valuable information that your physician can use when assessing your condition. A typical daily symptom diary is usually a table with columns and rows where you can record items, such as your daily symptoms, medications you take, your peak expiratory flow rate (PEFR, used to monitor asthma; see Chapter 2), and your observations about possible triggers or suspected exposures.

In addition to keeping a symptom diary, I also recommend establishing a medication record that lists all the drugs — prescription, OTC, and herbal remedies — that you take over your lifetime. Recording your medications is similar to recording checks in your check register.

Your medication record should include the brand and generic names of all drugs you've used and currently take, including OTC vitamins and supplements — some of which are as potent as conventional medical products that the Food and Drug Administration (FDA) regulates and which are available only by prescription. In addition, note the conditions you treat or have treated with particular drugs and the effectiveness and/or results of taking those products.

If you're unsure of the actual drugs that you use (perhaps the label is difficult to decipher), bring the medication with you in its original container. Also, ask your pharmacist, PCP, or other doctors for a list of medications they've prescribed for any of your medical conditions.

Focusing on foods

In addition to causing digestive problems such as nausea, vomiting, or diarrhea, hypersensitivities (allergies) to certain foods can trigger symptoms throughout your body. Food hypersensitivity symptoms can include stuffy nose, skin rashes and hives, headaches, respiratory problems (such as coughing, wheezing, and shortness of breath), and general fatigue.

If your doctor suspects that food hypersensitivity causes your symptoms, she may advise you to keep a detailed food diary to bring to your initial specialist consultation. Your food diary can help your specialist determine whether your problem is a food allergy or the result of another type of adverse food reaction, such as a food intolerance. (See Chapter 8 for information on keeping a food diary and details about how food allergies relate to asthma.)

Taking your family history

Because heredity often plays an important role in determining your likelihood of developing asthma or allergies, your physician usually asks about your family medical history. You don't need to become the next Alex Haley to research this information, but you should make sure that you know which relative (mother, brother, uncle, and so on) had a particular disease or condition. Letting your doctor know whether your parents, siblings, or close relatives have had asthma, and/or allergic conditions such as allergic rhinitis (hay fever), atopic dermatitis (eczema), and food or drug allergies, is especially important.

In addition, because other medical conditions that run in families can influence your treatment, your physician also needs to know whether any of your family members suffer from (or had) illnesses such as diabetes, high blood pressure, heart disease, cystic fibrosis, and cancer.

Knowing What Tests Your Doctor May Perform

After you and your physician review all the important information that I discuss in the previous section, she will need to examine you and possibly order some further testing. The following section explains what the next steps may be.

Looking for signs of asthma and allergies

After discussing your medical history, your physician will also probably examine you for physical signs of your asthma or allergies. The areas that your doctor usually checks vary based on your medical history, as well as the type of symptoms you have. Areas that your doctor may investigate include the following:

- Eyes, ears, nose, throat, and sinuses. Physicians often check for redness and watering of eyes, appearance of your eardrums, swelling of your nasal lining, amount and character of nasal discharge, presence of nasal polyps, size and color of tonsils, tender or swollen lymph nodes in your neck area, and possible tenderness over your sinus areas.

- Your chest and torso, to look for expanded or overinflated lungs and hunched shoulders, which can signal breathing difficulties.

- Your lungs (with a stethoscope), to check for wheezing, other abnormal breath sounds, and the character of your airflow.

- Your skin, to check for dry, red, itchy, and damaged skin (such as seen in *atopic dermatitis*—eczema), which can often indicate your predisposition to allergies and asthma (see Chapter 1).

- If your doctor suspects *allergic rhinitis* (hay fever) as part of your problem, she may also look for distinctive combinations of gestures and facial features, particularly in children and adolescents, as I detail in Chapter 7.

Testing for asthma and allergies

In order to confirm or more precisely identify the underlying cause of your symptoms, your doctor may advise certain tests and procedures. The types of diagnostic studies that your specialist performs depend on your medical history and the results of your physical examination. In the following sections, I provide an overview of the most frequently used tests and procedures.

Allergy skin testing

Allergists consider skin testing the gold standard for identifying sensitivities to certain types of allergens that can trigger symptoms of asthma. In some cases, allergy skin testing can also indicate your level of sensitivity to the particular allergen. Allergy skin tests are usually most useful for identifying sensitivities to pollen, dust mites, molds, animal dander, insect stings, food hypersensitivities, and, if necessary, for penicillin hypersensitivities.

Skin testing for allergies in the doctor's office generally involves placing a drop of a suspected allergen on your skin and then pricking, puncturing, or scratching your skin with a device to see whether the allergen produces a reaction. If you're allergic to the administered allergen, your skin usually reacts in a way that resembles a mosquito bite or small hive.

A positive reaction can help identify the cause of your allergic reactions and may also indicate your sensitivity level to that allergic trigger. (See Chapter 11 to find out more about allergy skin testing.)

Using RAST for allergy testing

Your allergist may recommend using *radioallergensorbent testing* (RAST) for diagnosing your allergic sensitivities and their connection to your asthma symptoms. Although RAST isn't as precise, practical, comprehensive, or cost-effective as allergy skin testing, your doctor may advise using this procedure under specific circumstances. See Chapter 11 for more information on RAST.

Assessing asthma with spirometry

If your symptoms include coughing, wheezing, and shortness of breath, your doctor should assess your lung functions with spirometry to evaluate whether asthma is the underlying cause of your condition.

A *spirometer* is a sophisticated machine that measures airflow from your large and small airways before and after you inhale a short-acting bronchodilator. For adults and children older than age 4 or 5, this procedure provides the most accurate way of determining whether airway obstruction exists and whether your condition is reversible (meaning that it improves after taking appropriate medication). Your doctor may also advise other lung-function tests if she suspects that other coexisting respiratory conditions may cause or affect your symptoms (see Chapter 5).

Other procedures for diagnosing asthma and allergies

Confirming an asthma or allergy diagnosis may also involve additional studies and tests, such as:

- ✔ **Bronchoprovocation.** In some cases, spirometry may indicate normal or near-normal lung functions, although asthma nonetheless seems the most likely cause of your symptoms. Therefore, your doctor may advise bronchoprovocation to more precisely diagnose your condition. These types of tests usually involve exercising for several minutes (on a stationary bicycle or treadmill in your doctor's office) or inhaling a small dose of methacholine or histamine (see Chapter 2), in order to determine whether mild asthma symptoms occur as a result of bronchial constriction. This test allows doctors to diagnose individuals whose asthma otherwise isn't apparent, but whose symptoms appear as a response to these challenges due to the hyperreactivity of their airways.

✔ **A chest and/or sinus X-ray or a CAT scan of the sinuses (see Chapter 13).** Your doctor may also order these types of imaging tests to determine whether other disorders, such as chronic bronchitis and emphysema — collectively referred to as *chronic obstructive pulmonary disease* (COPD), pneumonia, or sinusitis (sinus infection) may be part of your medical condition.

✔ **Rhinoscopy.** Your doctor may use a fiber-optic scope with a light for examining your nose, sinuses, and back of your throat. This technique is useful for investigating causes of nasal obstruction or blockage, post-nasal drainage, and the condition of the sinuses.

✔ **Nasal smear.** Although not considered a definitive diagnostic test, a nasal smear can help your doctor determine whether you suffer from allergic rhinitis. This procedure generally involves taking secretions from your nose, usually with a flexible, plastic device, which your doctor then examines under a microscope for levels of *eosinophils* (a type of white blood cell — see Chapter 6). Elevated counts of eosinophils can indicate an allergic condition.

✔ **Blood test.** Your physician may also look for an elevated count of eosinophils in your blood stream. This may indicate an allergic condition, and the test may help in distinguishing asthma from other respiratory conditions that can also present as coughing and shortness of breath.

✔ **Tympanometry.** Doctors often use this procedure, which measures your eardrum response to various pressure levels, to determine whether you have *otitis media* (inflammation of the middle ear, often associated with ear infections) — a frequent complication of both sinusitis and allergic rhinitis.

✔ **Thyroid function test.** Because *hypothyroidism* (an underactive thyroid) can cause chronic nasal congestion similar to a severe case of allergic rhinitis, your doctor may order this test to rule out an alternate diagnosis.

 ✔ **Elimination diet.** If skin testing for food allergies isn't conclusive, your doctor may advise an elimination diet (which you should only undertake under your physician's supervision), removing suspected highly allergenic foods from what you eat, in order to confirm what's triggering your adverse food reactions. (For more food for thought on food allergies and asthma, turn to Chapter 8.)

 ✔ **Oral food challenges.** These tests involve ingesting — under medical supervision — very small quantities of foods that contain suspected allergens. They should be performed only if your previous adverse food reactions haven't been life-threatening.

Following Up: Second and Subsequent Visits

Your second visit with an asthma or allergy specialist usually takes place one to two weeks after your initial consultation. This return visit is every bit as important as your first appointment, so make sure that you take with you any information, records, or documents your physician may require, based on your previous appointment.

When scheduling your follow-up visit, ask your doctor's office how much time the physician expects to spend with you, so you can plan your day accordingly.

Getting a diagnosis: What happens next?

At the conclusion of your initial consultation or at a separate second consultation, your doctor will go over the results of your tests, explain your diagnosis, and review your treatment plan.

Always ask for a specific diagnosis when you see a specialist.

Depending on your diagnosis and medical condition, your physician may take all or some of the following steps during your second visit (or third, in some cases):

- ✔ **Review the effectiveness of medications that he prescribed for you at your previous visit.** In some cases, your doctor may need to adjust your medications and dosages.

- ✔ **Provide you with a summary of the most important findings of your initial consultation.** You should also ask for recommendations concerning additional educational materials (such as this book!).

- ✔ **Provide you with a written treatment plan.** Make sure that you understand this plan and can adhere to it. If you have concerns or questions about your advised treatment, talk to your physician about them.

- ✔ **Give you handouts with written instructions on avoiding the allergens, irritants, and/or precipitating factors that may trigger your asthma or allergies.**

Considering allergy shots

If your medical history and skin testing provide clear evidence that you're allergic to certain allergens that trigger your asthma symptoms and can't be easily avoided, your doctor may advise you to consider *immunotherapy* (allergy shots). If your physician suggests immunotherapy, he should make sure that you understand the commitment that this treatment requires.

Immunotherapy isn't a quick fix, and it requires a significant investment of time on your part. For inhalant allergens, it may take up to one year of allergy shots before you and your doctor can determine whether you're clearly benefiting from the therapy. Your adherence to the program is the key for effective immunotherapy, meaning that you need to maintain the injection schedule that your allergist prescribes as much as possible (see Chapter 11 for an extensive discussion of this topic).

Paying for Your Care

Here's the fun part: dealing with your medical bills. Make sure that you read and understand your physician's financial policy before your first appointment so that you know and understand what your payment terms are.

The terms of financial policies usually depend on the level and type of health insurance you carry. If you're covered by Medicare or a contracted insurance plan, such as a health maintenance organization (HMO), you generally aren't billed, although you may need to make a small co-payment at the time of your visit (usually between $5 and $20).

However, you may need to pay out-of-pocket for your first office visit (at the time of your appointment) if any of the following applies to you:

✔ You don't carry health insurance.

✔ You have a private health insurance policy.

✔ You aren't covered by an insurance plan, such as an HMO, that contracts with your doctor's practice.

✔ You can't (or don't) provide your doctor's office with insurance information. (Make sure you have all requested healthcare documents and records with you when you see your physician.)

Dealing with insurance issues

With the movement toward managed care, seeing a specialist is frequently more difficult for patients. Having a first-rate health insurance policy, one that provides full access to the physicians you need to see, when you need to see them, is preferable. If you have the opportunity to choose among several medical coverage plans, paying a little bit more for a policy that allows direct access to specialists when you need them is well worth the extra investment. (Just like in most other purchases, you get what you pay for!)

I strongly advise my patients not to sell themselves short by buying insurance solely on the basis of price. A low-cost plan may work just fine when you're in good health and don't really require much specialty medical care. However, if you develop a serious medical problem, you may find that many of these low-cost plans cover expert treatment only after your ailment deteriorates into a potentially irreversible or life-threatening condition.

Gatekeeping and your treatment

Good primary care practitioners on the front lines of healthcare are essential to the well-being of much of the world's population, especially in the United States. In the United States, however, these doctors often work under difficult circumstances because of the limitations and deficiencies of the health insurance financing system.

In many cases, HMOs attempt to control their costs by providing bonuses and other incentives to PCPs (often known as *gatekeepers*) who limit referrals to specialists. *Capitation,* which involves giving these doctors restricted budgets for treating patients, has led to many complaints by both patients and PCPs alike.

According to the *New England Journal of Medicine,* at least one-quarter of PCPs worry that they're treating complicated conditions that specialists could handle better. Many PCPs, who receive a larger proportion of their income through capitation and who serve as gatekeepers for large numbers of patients, think their practice is too broad. These doctors are often required to treat people with more complex conditions than they treated in the past.

Getting the care you need and deserve

If your PCP tells you that no other treatment is available for your condition, he may actually mean there's nothing more that he can do for you in your managed care setting. If this situation happens to you and/or you're dissatisfied with the medical care you're receiving, consider taking the following steps:

- ✔ **Find out whether your HMO provides bonuses or other forms of incentives for limiting referrals.** Although you may feel uncomfortable asking your PCP about this topic, you have a right to know about the policies that directly affect the delivery and quality of your healthcare.

- ✔ **Become your own advocate.** Read up on the current issues regarding healthcare and understand your rights (as well as your responsibilities) as a patient. Especially if your child has asthma, an excellent place to start is by reading *A Parent's Guide to Asthma: How You Can Help Your Child Control Asthma at Home, School, and Play* (Plume/Penguin, 1994), by my friend Nancy Sander, the founder of the Allergy and Asthma Network/Mothers of Asthmatics. (I list more valuable information resources in the appendix.)

- ✔ **If a managed care plan that you're considering lists an impressive roster of specialists, make sure you can consult with these experts when you need them.** Some HMOs don't let you see a specialist until you're hospitalized, which is one hospitalization too many, in my opinion.

Working Well with Your Doctor

Expectations of treatment can vary from one individual to another, often depending on different people's priorities in life, so make sure you clearly communicate your own personal expectations to your doctor. Ask your doctor what you should expect to achieve from the treatment he prescribes for you, and participate in setting and developing your own individualized treatment goals.

The vast majority of people with asthma can lead normal lives. With effective, appropriate care from your doctor and your own motivated participation as a patient, your treatment plan can enable you to lead a full and active life. However, if following your plan properly doesn't allow you to participate fully in the activities and pursuits that matter to you, openly communicate your concerns to your physician and together adjust your plan to maximize the effectiveness of your treatment.

Chapter 4

Managing Asthma Long-Term

. . . .

In This Chapter

▶ Understanding what long-term asthma management involves

▶ Identifying the four levels of asthma severity

▶ Taking the stepwise approach to treatment

▶ Evaluating your lungs

▶ Figuring out self-management

▶ Enhancing your life and overall health

. . . .

*R*ather than letting your asthma control you, the key to controlling your asthma is to treat it on a consistent and preventive basis. Doing so means managing your asthma for the long term, rather than dealing with symptoms and episodes only temporarily. Developing and sticking to a long-term asthma management strategy is a priceless investment in your overall health and quality of life, especially if you have persistent asthma. The fundamental point is to address the root cause of your symptoms — the underlying airway inflammation that characterizes asthma.

BERGER BIT

In most cases, I find that after patients realize how much better they can feel by effectively managing their asthma on a long-term basis, they don't put up with going back to the ineffective, short-term, crisis-management ways of dealing with their disease.

Seeing What a Long-Term Management Plan Includes

A comprehensive long-term management plan for persistent asthma should include the following elements:

✔ Objective testing and monitoring of your lung functions to initially diagnose your condition and to continuously assess the effectiveness of your treatment (see Chapter 2 and the sections "Assessing Your Lungs" and "Taking Stock of Your Condition," later in this chapter, for more information).

✔ Avoiding and controlling exposures to asthma triggers and precipitating factors (see Chapter 5).

✔ Developing a safe and effective pharmacotherapy program that results in minimal or no adverse side effects. The program includes taking appropriate long-term preventive medications on a routine basis to control your asthma and using appropriate short-term, quick-relief rescue medications if your symptoms suddenly get worse (see Chapter 16).

✔ Initiating pharmacotherapy with a *stepwise* (step-up or step-down) approach. (See the "Using the Stepwise Approach" section, later in this chapter, for details.)

✔ Consulting with an asthma specialist, such as an allergist or *pulmonologist* (lung doctor), when advisable (see Chapter 2).

✔ Tailoring your asthma management plan to your specific circumstances and condition and continuing education for you and your family about asthma and your specific condition (see "Understanding Self-Management," later in this chapter).

"Outgrowing" your asthma: Fact or fiction

Asthma isn't something that you usually outgrow. Extensive studies over the past 15 years have shown that asthma is an ongoing physical condition that doesn't just disappear forever when you feel better. Your asthma can vary in its symptoms and severity during your lifetime. However, just like the color of your eyes or your individual fingerprint pattern, when you have asthma, it remains as another of your distinctive, although unseen, physical characteristics.

When you have asthma, the airways of your lungs get bigger as you grow, so mild airway obstruction may not affect you as much as you get older. Also, as you mature, your sensitivities may not be sufficient to cause clinical symptoms that you notice. However, people who feel that they "outgrew" their asthma as children or teenagers commonly experience symptoms of the disease later in life, particularly in response to certain triggers (see Chapter 5 for more on asthma triggers).

Focusing on the Four Levels of Asthma Severity

Experts from different fields of medicine have classified the severity of asthma — whether allergic or nonallergic — into four levels. These asthma severity levels provide the basis for the stepwise management of the disease.

Bear in mind, however, that these levels of severity aren't permanent or static. Asthma is a condition that can change throughout your life. The primary goal of the stepwise approach that I describe in this chapter is to get your asthma to the lowest classification possible. Therefore, effectively treating your condition is crucial: Otherwise, your asthma severity may move up the classification scale to the point where you could potentially suffer from severe, relentless symptoms that adversely affect your quality of life.

As described in the National Institutes of Health (NIH) Guidelines for the Diagnosis and Management of Asthma, the four levels of asthma severity are

- ✓ **Mild intermittent.** Symptoms occur no more than twice a week during the day and no more than twice a month at night. Lung-function testing (see Chapter 2) shows 80 percent or greater of the predicted normal value, compared to reference values based on your age, height, sex, and race, as established by the American Thoracic Society. In addition, your peak expiratory flow rate (PEFR; see Chapter 2) shouldn't vary by more than 20 percent during episodes and from the morning to the evening. Between episodes, you may be *asymptomatic* (not have noticeable symptoms), and your PEFR should be normal. If your asthma is at this level, a worsening of symptoms is usually brief, lasting a few hours to a few days, with variations of intensity.

- ✓ **Mild persistent.** Symptoms occur more than twice a week during the day, but less than once a day, and more than twice a month at night. Lung-function testing shows 80 percent or greater of the predicted normal value. Your PEFR may vary between 20 and 30 percent. If your asthma is at this level of severity, then worsening of symptoms can begin to affect your activities.

- ✓ **Moderate persistent.** Symptoms occur daily and more than once a week at night, requiring daily use of a short-acting bronchodilator. Lung-function testing shows a 60 to 80 percent range of the normal predicted value. Your PEFR can vary more than 30 percent. Symptoms can worsen at least twice a week, with episodes lasting for days and affecting your activities.

> ✔ **Severe persistent.** Symptoms occur continuously during the day and fre-
> quently at night, limiting physical activity. Lung-function testing is 60
> percent or less of the normal predicted value. Your PEFR may vary more
> than 30 percent, and frequent aggravations of your condition can
> develop.

When diagnosing your condition, your doctor should identify your asthma's
severity level. Check to see which of the severity levels your condition most
resembles, based on the definitions that I list in this section. Your own symptoms and lung functions may not always fit neatly into one of these particular
severity levels. Your doctor, therefore, should evaluate your individual condition and develop a treatment plan for you based on the specific characteristics of your asthma. Keep in mind, however, that based on symptom criteria
and the results of lung-function testing, the vast majority of asthma patients
have some form of persistent asthma — mild, moderate, or severe — requiring long-term control therapy.

If the symptoms you're experiencing seem to indicate that you have persistent
asthma, I strongly advise having your lung functions evaluated by *spirometry* if
you haven't already done so (see "Assessing Your Lungs," later in this chapter).
For a spirometry evaluation, you may need to ask your doctor for a referral to
an asthma specialist, such as an allergist or pulmonologist, because in many
cases, primary care physicians don't have easy access to office spirometers.

Using the Stepwise Approach

Asthma severity levels are steps in the staircase to controlling asthma, as
shown in Figure 4-1. The basic concept of stepwise management is to initially
prescribe long-term and quick-relief medications, based on the severity level
that's one step higher than the severity level you're experiencing (see Table
4-1). By using this approach, your doctor can usually help you gain rapid control over your symptoms. After your condition has been under control for a
month (in most cases), your physician can reduce the level of your medications by one level (*step down*).

Using the stepwise approach to asthma management means that you *step up*
your medication therapy to gain control, and then *step down* your medical
treatment to maintain control. Like waltzing, after you and your doctor
master the steps, you can move around life's dance floor with the ease and
grace of Fred Astaire or Ginger Rogers. Regular monitoring of your PEFR and
follow-up visits with your doctor, however, are vital to ensuring that you stay
in step, as I explain in the next section.

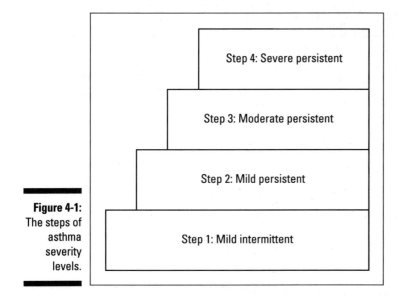

Figure 4-1:
The steps of asthma severity levels.

Step 4: Severe persistent

Step 3: Moderate persistent

Step 2: Mild persistent

Step 1: Mild intermittent

The information in Table 4-1 is based on the NIH Guidelines for the Diagnosis and Management of Asthma. Please remember that these are guidelines. Your doctor should always evaluate your own specific condition and prescribe individualized treatment accordingly.

Table 4-1	Stepwise Approach for Managing Asthma in Adults and Children Older Than 5	
Step	**Long-Term Control**	**Quick Relief**
Step 1: Mild intermittent	**No daily medication needed**	**Short-acting bronchodilator:** Inhaled beta$_2$-adrenergics as needed for symptoms. Intensity of treatment may vary depending on the severity of your symptoms. (If you're using a short-acting inhaled beta$_2$-adrenergics more than twice a week, you may need to initiate long-term control therapy. Consult your doctor in this case.)

(continued)

Table 4-1 *(continued)*

Step	Long-Term Control	Quick Relief
Step 2: Mild persistent	**One daily medication:** Anti-inflammatory medication, either inhaled corticosteroid (low dose) or mast cell stabilizers, such as cromolyn or nedocromil. Your doctor may also consider anti-leukotriene modifiers such as zafirlukast and montelukast. Your physician may also consider a methylxanthine product such as sustained-release theophylline as an alternative treatment, but not as preferred therapy.	**Short-acting bronchodilator:** Inhaled beta$_2$-adrenergics as needed for symptoms. Intensity of treatment may vary depend ing on the severity of your symptoms. (If you're using a short-acting inhaled beta$_2$-adrenergics more than twice a week, you may need additional long-term control therapy. Consult your doctor in this case.)
Step 3*: Moderate persistent	**Daily medication:** Anti-inflammatory medication, inhaled corticosteroid (medium dose), or inhaled corticosteroid (low to medium dose), adding a long-acting bronchodilator, especially for nighttime symptoms — either long-acting inhaled beta$_2$-adrenergics, sustained release theophylline, or long-acting beta$_2$-adrenergic tablets. **If needed:** Anti-inflammatory medication, inhaled corticosteroid (medium-high dose), and long-acting bronchodilator, especially for nighttime symptoms — either long-acting inhaled beta$_2$-adrenergics, sustained release theophylline, or long-acting beta$_2$-adrenergic tablets.	**Short-acting bronchodilator:** Inhaled beta$_2$-adrenergics as needed for symptoms. Intensity of treatment may vary depending on the severity of your symptoms. (If you're using a short-acting inhaled beta$_2$-adrenergic more than twice a week, you may need additional long-term control therapy. Consult your doctor in this case.)

Step	Long-Term Control	Quick Relief
Step 4*: Severe persistent	**Daily medication:** Anti-inflammatory medication, inhaled corticosteroid (high dose), and long-acting bronchodilator — either long-acting inhaled beta$_2$-adrenergics, sustained release theophylline, or long-acting beta$_2$-adrenergic tablets; and if required, long-term use of corticosteroid tablets or syrup.	**Short-acting bronchodilator:** Inhaled beta$_2$-adrenergics as needed for symptoms. Intensity of treatment may vary depending on the severity of your symptoms. (If you're using a short-acting inhaled beta$_2$-adrenergic more than twice a week, you may need additional long-term control therapy. Consult your doctor in this case.)

*If your asthma severity is at Step 3 or Step 4, consult an asthma specialist, such as an allergist or pulmonologist (lung doctor), to achieve better control of your condition.

Stepping down

If you're on long-term maintenance control at any level, your doctor should review your treatment every one to six months. A gradual stepwise reduction in treatment may be possible after your symptoms are under good control, meaning that you feel good, have maintained improved lung function, and experience no asthma symptoms.

The goal of the stepwise approach is to use early and aggressive treatment to gain rapid control over your asthma symptoms, thus allowing your doctor to reduce your medication to the lowest level required to maintain control of your condition.

Stepping up

If you find yourself frequently resorting to your quick-relief medications, your symptoms aren't under control, and your doctor should consider increasing your treatment by one step. In assessing whether to step up your therapy, your doctor will probably evaluate the following aspects of your current treatment step:

✔ Your inhaler technique. (See "Evaluating your inhaler technique," later in this chapter.)

✔ Your level of adherence in taking the medications that your doctor prescribes.

Taking your prescriptions as your doctor instructs is vital. If you're having trouble with a product (because of potential side effects) or you don't understand your doctor's instructions, tell your physician so that he can take appropriate measures.

✔ Your exposure level to asthma triggers, such as allergens and irritants and precipitating factors, such as viral infections and other medical conditions. Control your exposure to asthma triggers and precipitating factors as much as possible, no matter what step of treatment you're receiving. (See Chapter 5 for information on controlling asthma triggers.)

Make sure that your asthma management plan clearly explains at what point you should contact your physician if your symptoms worsen.

Treating severe episodes in stepwise management

Your doctor may consider prescribing a rescue course of oral corticosteroids at any step if you suddenly experience a severe asthma episode and your condition abruptly deteriorates. (Chapter 16 provides more information on oral corticosteroids.)

In some cases, severe episodes can occur even if your asthma is classified as intermittent. In many instances, patients with intermittent asthma may experience severe and potentially life-threatening episodes, often because of upper respiratory viral infections (such as the flu or colds), even though these patients may otherwise have long periods of normal or near-normal lung functions and few clinically perceptible asthma symptoms.

Assessing Your Lungs

Objective measurements of your lung functions are essential for monitoring your asthma's severity. Just as you check the oil level in your car on a regular basis (rather than waiting for the flashing red warning light), you and your doctor should also regularly check your airways to determine whether you're at the right step of asthma medication. In addition to recording your asthma symptoms in a daily symptom diary (see "Keeping symptom records," later in this chapter), you should also obtain objective measurements of lung functions with spirometry and peak-flow monitoring.

What your doctor should do: Spirometry

A *spirometer* is a sophisticated machine that your doctor or asthma specialist, such as an allergist or pulmonologist, uses for measuring airflow from your large and small airways before and 15 minutes after you've inhaled a short-acting bronchodilator. The spirometer helps your asthma specialist diagnose whether you have asthma and also allows your physician to follow your asthma's clinical course.

For adults and children older than age 4 or 5, spirometry currently provides the most accurate way of determining whether airway obstruction exists and whether it's reversible. For information on other types of lung-function tests your doctor may recommend and to find out more about diagnosing asthma in children under age 4, see Chapter 2.

What you can do: Peak-flow monitoring

Peak-flow meters (see Figure 4-2) allow you to keep an eye on your lung functions at home. The readings from this handy tool can be vital in diagnosing asthma and its severity and can also help your doctor prescribe medications and monitor your treatment's effectiveness. Peak-flow monitoring can also provide important early warning signs that an asthma episode is approaching.

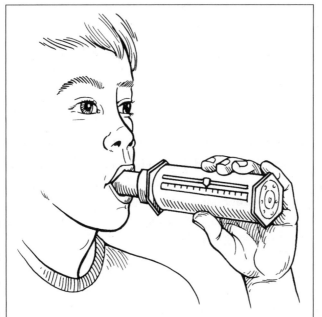

Figure 4-2:
A patient
using a
peak-flow
meter.

Children older than 4 or 5 who have asthma generally can also use this small, hand-held device to measure their own PEFR. If your kids constantly question your judgment (as mine do about almost everything), using a peak-flow meter can help youngsters understand when their condition may require them to limit their activities. If your child understands that the PEFR — not just you or your doctor — is advising him or her not to go to soccer practice on that particular day because of worsening asthma symptoms and a resulting PEFR reduction, you may have more success in helping to control your child's asthma.

Explaining and using peak-flow meters for children

I often advise parents to explain to their kids that when their peak-flow rate is down, it's like having an injury in their lungs. You can reinforce this analogy by telling your child that although the underlying airway inflammation isn't visible — unlike the injury to a sprained ankle, for example — the problem still needs proper treatment, just as a sprain needs to heal before resuming normal activities.

By the same token, when your child's PEFR is between 80 to 100 percent of his or her personal best, you can breathe easier about encouraging sports and other physical activities that are vital aspects of improving their overall health and fitness, including their lung functions. Make sure, however, that you and your child know how to manage potential symptoms of exercise-induced asthma (EIA), as I explain in Chapter 18.

Using a peak-flow meter at home

Consider these basic instructions and tips for using most types of peak-flow meters (several different makes and models are currently available). Remember, however, to follow the instructions that come with your specific device. Ask your doctor for specific advice on the most effective way you can use your peak-flow meter to assess your condition.

Generally, you use a peak-flow meter by following these steps:

1. **Move the sliding indicator at the base of the peak-flow meter to zero.**

2. **Stand up and take a deep breath to fully inflate your lungs.**

3. **Put the mouthpiece of the peak-flow meter into your mouth and close your lips tightly around it.**

4. **Blow as hard and as fast as possible, like you're blowing out the candles on your birthday cake.**

5. **Read the dial where the red indicator stopped. The number opposite the indicator is your peak-flow rate.**

6. **Reset the indicator to zero and repeat the process twice more.**

7. **Record the highest number that you reach.**

Finding your personal best peak-flow number

Your personal best peak-flow number is a measurement that reflects the highest number you can expect to achieve over a two- to three-week period after a course of aggressive treatment has produced good control of your asthma symptoms. Your best number is usually the result of step-up therapy.

To determine your personal best peak-flow number, take two peak-flow readings a day during an entire week when you're doing well and record the best result. Take one reading prior to taking medication in the morning and another reading between noon and 2 p.m. after taking an inhaled short-acting bronchodilator. Compare your personal best peak-flow number with the measurement that your physician predicts, which is based on national studies for children or adults of particular heights, sexes, and ages. This number can help you determine how your measurements compare with the norm. When your asthma is well controlled, your PEFR should consistently read between 80 and 100 percent of your personal best.

If your peak-flow measurements fall below 80 percent, early and aggressive intervention with medications and strict avoidance of potential asthma triggers may be necessary to prevent worsening symptoms. Ignoring a declining peak-flow reading can lead to serious symptoms and may result in the need for emergency treatment.

Reading green, yellow, and red peak-flow color zones

The peak-flow zone system involves green, yellow, and red areas, which are similar to a traffic signal. Using your peak-flow meter on a regular basis enables you and your doctor to treat symptoms before your condition deteriorates further.

You or your doctor may want to place small pieces of colored tape next to the actual numbers on your peak-flow meter, corresponding with the green, yellow, and red zones that your doctor provides as a graph on your written asthma peak-flow diary. (See "Keeping symptom records," later in the chapter, for more about asthma diaries.)

Table 4-2 explains how to read the peak-flow color zones.

Table 4-2	The Peak-Flow Color Zone System	
Zone	*Meaning*	*Points to Consider*
Green zone	Readings in this area are *safe.*	When your reading falls into the green zone, you've achieved 80 to 100 percent of your personal best peak flow. No asthma symptoms are present, and your treatment plan is controlling your asthma. If your readings consistently remain in the green zone, you and your doctor may consider reducing daily medications.
Yellow zone	Readings in this area indicate *caution.*	When your readings fall into the yellow zone, you're achieving only 50 to 80 percent of your personal best peak flow. An asthma attack may be present, and your symptoms may worsen. You may need to step up your medication temporarily.
Red zone	Readings in this area mean *medical alert.*	Readings in the red zone mean that you've fallen below 50 percent of your personal best peak flow. These readings often signal the start of a moderate to severe asthma attack.

If your readings are often in the yellow zone, even after taking the appropriate quick-relief medication that your asthma management plan specifies, contact your doctor. If your readings are in the red zone, use your quick-relief bronchodilator and anti-inflammatory medications immediately (based on your specific and individualized asthma management plan) and contact your doctor if your PEFR doesn't immediately return to and remain in the yellow or green zone.

Taking Stock of Your Condition

In addition to obtaining an objective measurement of your lung function with measuring devices, another important aspect of controlling your asthma is keeping track of a variety of other indicators. Your most valuable tracking device is usually a daily symptom diary. In fact, you should develop a rating system (in consultation with your doctor) for your diary that assesses your symptoms on a scale of 0 to 3, ranging from no symptoms to severe symptoms.

Keeping symptom records

Besides serving as a record of your PEFR readings, your daily symptom diary should monitor and record the following:

✔ Your signs and symptoms, as well as their severity

✔ Any coughing that you experience

✔ Any incidence of wheezing

✔ Nasal congestion

✔ Disturbances in your sleep, such as coughing and/or wheezing that awaken you

✔ Any symptoms that affect your ability to function normally or reduce normal activities

✔ Any time you miss school or work because of symptoms

✔ Frequency of use of your short-acting beta$_2$-adrenergic bronchodilator (rescue medication)

Tracking serious symptoms

Your daily symptom diary is also the place to monitor occurrences of symptoms that are severe enough to make you seek unscheduled office visits, after-hours treatments, emergency room visits, and hospitalizations. Therefore, you also want to note the date and kind of treatment that you seek.

Be sure to record the following types of serious symptoms:

✔ Breathlessness or panting while at rest

✔ The need to remain in an upright position in order to breathe

✔ Difficulty speaking

✔ Agitation or confusion

✔ An increased breathing rate of more than 30 breaths per minute

✔ Loud wheezing while inhaling and/or exhaling

✔ An elevated pulse rate of more than 120 heartbeats per minute

Furthermore, record exposures to triggers and/or precipitating factors that may have caused asthma flare-ups, including

- ✔ Irritants, such as chemicals or cigarette or fireplace smoke

- ✔ Allergens, such as plant pollen, household dust, molds, and animal fur

- ✔ Air pollution

- ✔ Exercise (Chapter 9 provides more information on exercise-induced asthma)

- ✔ Sudden changes in the weather, particularly cold temperatures and chilly winds

- ✔ Reactions to beta-blockers (such as Inderal or Timoptic), aspirin, and related products, including nonsteroidal anti-inflammatory drugs (NSAIDs) and food additives — particularly sulfites (see Chapter 5)

- ✔ Other medical conditions, such as upper respiratory viral infections (colds and flu), gastroesophageal reflux disease (GERD), and sinusitis (see Chapter 5)

Monitoring your medication use

Recording all the side effects that you experience when taking your prescribed medication is also important. Various asthma medications include many levels of side effects that a person can potentially experience. However, in most cases, patients who understand their asthma management plan and take their medications according to instructions have few, if any, adverse side effects. The tables in Chapter 15 provide extensive details on asthma medication products.

I need to emphasize how important it is to know and remember the names of your medications, especially if you're an older adult with multiple prescriptions. Patients telling me they're using a "white inhaler" or taking a "yellow pill" aren't providing the most helpful information in my quest to provide the best care possible and prevent potential adverse drug interactions with medications prescribed by another physician.

Evaluating your inhaler technique

Your doctor should show you the correct way to use your inhaler (see Chapter 15 for detailed instructions on using inhalers) and have you demonstrate your inhaler technique at each office visit. In the best of cases when using inhalers, only 10 to 20 percent of the topical inhaled drug gets into the areas of your lungs where it can really do some good. Because such small amounts of inhaler medications actually reach the airways of your lungs, understanding how to use your inhaler properly is vital to your treatment. Improper inhaler use is often the reason why some patients have difficulty controlling their asthma symptoms.

Understanding Self-Management

It takes two (at least) to treat asthma. You and your physician (as well as your other healthcare providers) are partners in controlling your asthma. Other members of your asthma partnership can include nurses, pharmacists, and other health professionals who treat you or assist you in understanding and finding out more about effectively managing your condition.

If you have asthma, your family also — in a sense — has the condition. Asthma isn't contagious; rather, your family also has the condition because you all may need to deal with the various issues associated with your medical condition's treatment. In fact, studies show that family support can be a major positive factor in the success of any asthma treatment plan. Particularly important to your asthma treatment is making sure that the people you live with (as well as co-workers, fellow students, or anyone you're around much of the time) help you reduce your exposure to asthma triggers and to precipitating factors. I explain in detail the most common triggers and precipitating factors to avoid in Chapter 5.

If your child has asthma, you should also be a partner with your child's doctor and other medical professionals in the management of your youngster's condition. (Chapter 18 provides details on managing asthma in children.)

Working with your doctor

Participate in developing treatment goals with your doctor. Make sure that you understand how your asthma management plan works and that you can openly communicate with your doctor about the effects and results of your treatment.

Making sure that your plan is tailored to your specific, individualized needs, as well as your family's, is also very important. Doing so can include taking into account any cultural beliefs and practices that can have an impact on your perception of asthma and of medication therapy. Openly discuss any such issues with your physician, so that together, you can develop an approach to asthma management that empowers you to take control of your condition. Ensuring that your plan is tailored to fit you and your family results in a more motivated patient, which almost always means a healthier individual.

Evaluating for the long term

Successfully managing your asthma also means constantly assessing your asthma management plan to determine whether it provides you with the means to achieve your asthma management goals.

Always keep in mind that asthma is a variable, complex, multifaceted condition. Just as many other aspects of your life can change and vary over time, your asthma may also manifest in different ways throughout your life. Remember: Your goal is lifetime management of your condition.

Becoming an expert about your asthma

The education process concerning asthma and its treatment should begin as soon as you're diagnosed. I believe that your doctor should make sure that you have a thorough understanding of all aspects of your condition. Ignorance is not bliss when it comes to managing your asthma effectively. Your process of education should include factors such as the following:

✔ Knowing the basic facts about asthma.

✔ Understanding the level of your asthma severity, how it affects you, and advisable treatment methods.

✔ Teaching you all the elements of asthma self-management, including basic facts about the disease and your specific condition, proper use of various inhalers and nebulizers, self-monitoring skills, and effective ways of avoiding triggers and allergy-proofing your home.

✔ Developing a written individualized daily and emergency self-management plan with your input (see Chapter 2).

✔ Determining the level of support you receive from family and friends in treating your asthma. It's also important for your doctor to help you identify an asthma partner from among your family members, relatives, or friends. This person should find out how asthma affects you and should understand your asthma management plan so that he or she can provide assistance (if necessary) if your condition suddenly worsens. I advise including your asthma partner in doctor visits when appropriate.

✔ Asking your doctor and/or other members of your asthma management team for guidance in setting priorities when implementing your asthma management plan. If you need to make environmental changes in your life, such as allergy-proofing your home (which may include relocating a pet, taking up the carpets, installing air filtration devices, and many other steps that I explain in Chapter 5), you may want advice on which steps you need to take soonest and which steps can wait.

Improving Your Quality of Life

Taking asthma medication doesn't mean that you can afford to ignore other aspects of your health. Effectively managing your asthma for the long term also requires being healthy overall. The better you take care of yourself, the more success you'll have in treating your asthma and living a full, normal life.

Consider these important, common-sense guidelines when developing an asthma management plan:

- **Eating right.** A healthy, well-balanced diet is especially important for people who have asthma. Include fresh fruits, meats, fish, grains, and vegetables in your diet.

- **Sleeping well.** If you experience asthma symptoms during the night that disturb your sleep, tell your doctor. These types of symptoms should be treated, and they may indicate that you're susceptible to precipitating factors, such as GERD, or asthma triggers such as dust mites in your bedroom (see Chapter 5).

- **Staying fit.** When patients are in good physical condition, their asthma is often easier to control. You don't have to sit on life's sidelines just because you have asthma. Your doctor can prescribe medications that you can take preventively to control symptoms of EIA, thus enabling you to enjoy many types of exercise and sports activities in spite of your asthma. (Chapter 9 provides information on appropriate products for controlling EIA.)

- **Reducing stress.** By effectively controlling your asthma, you'll feel less anxious about your condition, thus reducing the overall levels of stress in your life and further helping you manage your asthma.

Expecting the Best

With effective, appropriate care from your doctor and your own motivated participation as a patient, your asthma management plan can enable you to lead a full and active life. However, if properly following your asthma management plan still doesn't allow you to participate fully in the activities and pursuits that matter to you, openly communicate this to your physician so that she can adjust your plan and maximize the effectiveness of your treatment.

If, as sometimes happens, your doctor deals only with your asthma symptoms — instead of initiating the type of long-term approach that I discuss in this chapter — you may want to consider requesting a referral to an asthma specialist. Expect to effectively control your asthma, and your doctor should certainly help you achieve this goal.

Part II

Understanding Asthma Triggers

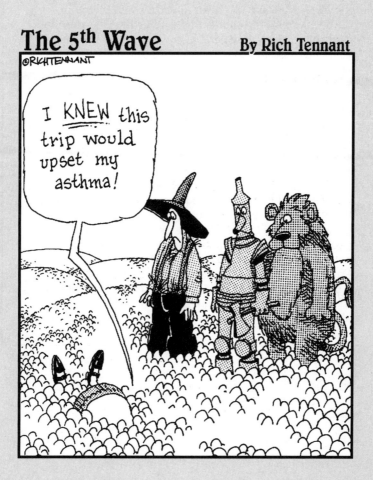

The 5th Wave   By Rich Tennant

In this part . . .

You don't need to be Cyrano de Bergerac or Jimmy Durante to know that your nose is a special organ of your body. If you have symptoms that indicate *allergic rhinitis* (hay fever), you need to understand that your allergy has a strong connection with asthma. Furthermore, it can often have more serious consequences than just annoying sneezing, a runny nose, a scratchy throat, and watery eyes.

Chapters 5, 6, and 7 offer detailed information on the various allergic and nonallergic triggers of respiratory symptoms, explain how to effectively avoid or at least reduce your exposure to them, and discuss how asthma and allergies are so closely linked.

For some asthmatics, respiratory symptoms can be triggered not just by exposure to airborne allergens and other types of inhalant triggers, but also by allergic reactions to certain foods. But are the adverse reactions that many people may experience at times to various dishes the result of food allergies? Mostly, no, as I explain in Chapter 8. In Chapter 9, I explain what triggers symptoms of exercise-induced asthma (EIA) and the ways you can prevent it, so that you can keep yourself in great physical shape while also keeping your respiratory symptoms at bay.

Chapter 5

Knowing Your Asthma Triggers

· ·

In This Chapter

▶ Identifying what's triggering your asthma symptoms

▶ Avoiding inhalant allergens

▶ Focusing on triggers in your home

▶ Recognizing triggers in your workplace

▶ Steering clear of food and drug triggers

▶ Dealing with other conditions that can aggravate your asthma

· ·

*W*ater covers two-thirds of the world's surface. If you have asthma, it may seem at times that the rest of the planet consists of nothing but asthma triggers. Throughout the world and in virtually every aspect of people's everyday lives, countless precipitating factors — allergens, irritants, or other medical conditions — can induce asthma symptoms.

Avoiding or limiting your exposure to these precipitating factors is vital for managing your condition. Avoiding asthma triggers can help you experience fewer respiratory symptoms and potentially allow you to reduce your need for medication, especially rescue drugs such as short-acting beta$_2$-adrenergic (beta$_2$-agonist) bronchodilators. (See Chapters 14, 15, and 16 for details on asthma medications.)

Although certain triggers frequently dominate each individual's asthma, controlling your condition often requires dealing with a host of precipitating factors — an especially common situation if you have allergic asthma, one of the most frequent types of asthma. Allergic asthma is usually associated with *allergic rhinitis* (hay fever) and/or allergic conjunctivitis (see Chapter 2 for details of allergic asthma).

If the prospect of dealing with a world full of asthma triggers seems daunting, don't despair. Throughout this chapter, I provide information and tips, based on extensive experience and the latest research findings, that can help you — in consultation with your doctor — implement practical and effective measures for avoiding or reducing exposure to your asthma triggers.

Recognizing What Triggers Your Asthma

One of the most important steps you need to take to effectively manage your asthma is to identify what triggers the symptoms of your condition. These triggers (see Figure 5-1) include

- ✔ Inhalant allergens, including animal danders, dust mite and cockroach allergens, some mold spores, and certain airborne pollens of grasses, weeds, and trees (see Chapter 10).

- ✔ Occupational irritants and allergens, found primarily in the workplace, that induce occupational asthma (see the section "Working Out Workplace Exposures," later in this chapter) or aggravate an already existing form of the disease.

- ✔ Other irritants that you inhale, such as tobacco smoke, household products, and indoor and outdoor air pollution.

- ✔ Nonallergic triggers, including exercise and physical stimuli such as variations in air temperature and humidity levels.

- ✔ Other medical conditions, including rhinitis, sinusitis, gastroesophageal reflux disease (GERD), and viral infections; sensitivities to aspirin, beta-blockers, and other drugs; and sensitivities to food additives — particularly sulfites.

- ✔ Emotional activities, such as crying, laughing, or even yelling. Although emotions aren't the direct triggers of asthma symptoms — and clearly asthma isn't an "emotional problem" — activities associated with emotions (happy or sad) can induce coughing or wheezing in people with pre-existing hyperreactive airways (see Chapter 2), as well as in individuals who don't have asthma but who may suffer from other respiratory disorders. For example, your friend with a bad cold may say, "Please don't make me laugh; if I do, I'll start coughing."

Evaluating triggers

In order to determine what triggers your asthma symptoms and your sensitivity levels to those triggers, your doctor should take a thorough medical history. Keeping an asthma diary (see Chapter 4) can assist in your doctor's assessment by providing details of your symptoms and your exposures to potential triggers. Prepare to give your doctor specific information about the respiratory symptoms that you experience.

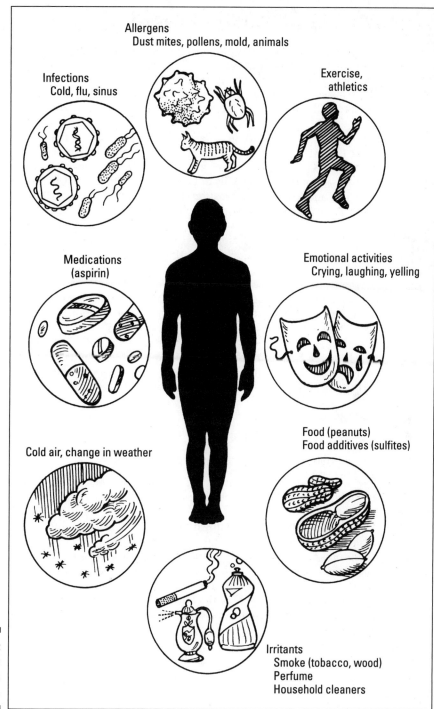

Allergens
Dust mites, pollens, mold, animals

Infections
Cold, flu, sinus

Exercise,
athletics

Medications
(aspirin)

Emotional activities
Crying, laughing, yelling

Food (peanuts)
Food additives (sulfites)

Cold air, change in weather

Irritants
Smoke (tobacco, wood)
Perfume
Household cleaners

Figure 5-1:
Common
asthma
triggers.

Testing for allergic triggers

Many asthma patients experience *perennial* (year-round) symptoms that worsen during particular seasons. Because such a wide range of triggers can contribute to perennial asthma episodes, provide your doctor with a record of the seasonal patterns of your symptoms. Your record contains valuable clues to help your doctor narrow down the factors that affect your condition.

For example, if your asthma consistently worsens during late summer and fall in the eastern parts of the United States, your physician may suspect ragweed or mold as a prime cause of the allergic reactions that aggravate your condition. However, doctors usually advise allergy testing (see Chapter 11 for a complete explanation of allergy testing) to investigate other possible causes and to confirm the diagnosis and determine appropriate treatment.

If you have persistent asthma (see Chapter 4) with year-round symptoms that occur primarily indoors, allergy testing can help your doctor identify several of the triggers, such as dust mites, that may be affecting you.

Nocturnal or *nighttime asthma,* which often shows up as a nighttime cough, wheezing, and/or shortness of breath, that disturbs your sleep and may require you to use your short-acting adrenergic bronchodilator (see Chapter 14) can often be severe. Allergens in your bedroom, postnasal drip from allergic rhinitis (see Chapter 7), or chronic sinus problems (such as sinusitis; see Chapter 13) often trigger this condition. Other mechanisms that can trigger nocturnal asthma include

- ✔ GERD
- ✔ Airway cooling and drying
- ✔ Increased bronchial airway hyperreactivity
- ✔ A delayed reaction (known as a *late-phase reaction;* see Chapter 6) to allergens that you've been exposed to previously during the day

The *circadian rhythm* (also known as *diurnal variation*), which is your body's internal clock, may also affect your asthma, making you more susceptible to symptoms in the early morning hours (around 3 to 5 a.m.). During the late evening and early morning hours, a decrease in plasma levels of *adrenal gland* (glands above your kidneys) *hormones,* such as *cortisol,* a hormone produced by the *cortex* (outer layer) of the adrenal gland, normally occurs. At the same time, a decrease in plasma epinephrine and an increase in plasma histamine also occur.

Controlling Inhalant Allergens

Inhalant allergen triggers, also known as *aeroallergens,* are probably the most familiar asthma precipitants because they're also associated with allergic rhinitis and similar conditions (see Chapter 7). If you have allergic asthma, reducing your exposure to inhalant allergens is the first and most important step to take — in consultation with your doctor — to manage your condition.

The following list details the most common inhalant allergens to look out for:

- ✔ **Animal allergens.** Pet dander, which also may contain traces of saliva, is a potent trigger of symptoms for many people with asthma. Although household dogs and cats are the most common sources of these allergens, all warm-blooded animals, such as horses, rabbits, small rodents, and birds, produce dander — regardless of hair length — that can cause allergic reactions and aggravate your asthma. Urine from these animals is also a source of allergens. Animal dander also serves as a food supply (along with dead human skin scales) for dust mites, as I explain in Chapter 10.

- ✔ **Dust mites.** Dust mites abound almost everywhere humans settle, and they thrive especially well in mattresses, carpets, upholstered furniture, bed covers, linens, clothes, and soft toys. Although eradicating these dusty denizens is virtually impossible, you can take practical and effective steps to minimize exposure to the allergens that dust mites produce.

  See Chapter 10 for more dirt on dust mites, and Chapter 11 for details on measures to control these creatures.

- ✔ **Cockroaches.** As if you need another reason to avoid cockroaches, exposure to allergens from cockroach droppings (yuck!) in house dust can trigger and aggravate your asthma symptoms. Studies show that inner-city children who unfortunately are exposed to high levels of cockroach allergens, especially in the bedroom, can develop increasingly severe asthma.

  Many asthmatic patients of inner-city clinics have tested positive for cockroach allergens (through allergy skin testing) but have improved after immunotherapy with cockroach allergen extract. (See Chapter 11 for more information on allergy skin testing and immunotherapy.)

  To control cockroach allergens in your home, include these key measures:

  - • Exterminate cockroach infestations. During the fumigation process, stay out of your home, and allow it to air out for several hours before re-entering. (This advice applies to anyone, regardless of whether or not you have asthma.)

  - • Clean your entire home thoroughly after extermination.

- Set roach traps.

- Seal any cracks or other conduits into your home to prevent rein-festation.

- Keep your kitchen clean by washing dishes and cookware promptly and by emptying garbage and recycling containers (including old newspapers) often, and avoid leaving food out.

✔ **Mold.** The airborne spores that molds (fungi) release in typically damp areas of many homes, particularly from basements, bathrooms, air condi-tioners, garbage containers, and under carpeting, can trigger allergy and asthma symptoms when you inhale them. Mold can also thrive in leaf piles, compost heaps, cut grass, fertilizer, hay, and barns. Airborne mold spores are more numerous than pollen grains and don't have a limited season. Depending on where you live, you may receive exposure to air-borne spores during many parts of the year, based on levels of humidity.

See Chapter 10 for more moldy matters, including tips on translating mold counts and what you can do to reduce mold exposures.

✔ **Pollen.** From spring through fall, many varieties of trees, grasses, and weeds release pollens that can trigger symptoms of allergic rhinitis and/or allergic conjunctivitis. These reactions can also affect your asthma, aggravating the underlying airway inflammation.

Many people primarily associate pollens with outdoor exposure. However, because most pollens are wind-borne, they can often make their way indoors and trigger allergy and asthma symptoms in your home.

See Chapter 11 for steps you can take to avoid excessive exposure to pollen, especially during periods of high pollination, and see Chapter 10 for more pollen particulars, including tips on pollen counts.

Clearing the Air at Home

Indoor environments at home, work, and school and in cars as well as other enclosed means of transportation can often provide far more significant sources of asthma triggers than the outdoors, because most enclosures con-centrate irritants and allergens. Therefore, you should seriously consider the effects of indoor air pollution because it can induce or aggravate allergies and asthma.

Household irritants

The most significant irritant triggers of asthma in many households are

- ✔ Tobacco smoke (see the next section)
- ✔ Fumes and scents from household cleaners, strongly scented soaps, perfumes, glues, and aerosols
- ✔ Smoke from wood-burning appliances or fireplaces
- ✔ Fumes from unvented gas, oil, or kerosene stoves

Other sources of indoor air pollution include pollens and mold spores that get inside, especially on windy days when windows and doors are open. These allergenic materials can also infiltrate your home via your clothing and hair. In fact, if you have allergic asthma, you may wake up congested and wheezing in the morning because allergenic materials find their way into your house so easily. (The pollen or mold spores in your hair probably wound up on your pillow, so you spent the night breathing those allergens into your lungs.)

No smoking, please

As far as truly irritating irritants go, tobacco smoke is the No.1 indoor air pollutant. Secondhand smoke has been associated with an increase in the following adverse effects: persistent wheezing associated with asthma, hospital admissions for respiratory infections, earlier onset of respiratory allergies, decreased lung function, and even increased incidence of *otitis media with effusion* (inflammation of the middle ear; see Chapter 13).

Tobacco smoke frequently precipitates asthma symptoms in children. In fact, numerous studies show that parental smoking, especially by the mother, is a major risk factor in the development of asthma in infants, who are exposed to the smoke during the first few months of life. Therefore, don't smoke and make sure that those people around you don't smoke, especially if you have children.

Filters and air-cleaning devices

The quality of the air you breathe indoors largely depends on the condition of your heating, ventilation, and air-conditioning (HVAC) system, as well as the air and particles that circulate throughout it.

If you're exposed to airborne allergens and irritants, such as animal dander, mold spores, pollen, and tobacco smoke, consider using air filters on your HVAC ducts to reduce the level of allergy and asthma triggers circulating through your home. Keep in mind, however, that these filters don't remove substances that have already settled in bedding, carpeting, and furniture — especially dust mite allergens. Dust mite allergens are generally larger than other airborne allergens and irritants, and they usually fall from the air within a few minutes after being stirred up in dust or air currents.

The two types of air filtration systems often recommended by doctors for reducing indoor levels of airborne allergens and irritants are

- ✔ **High Efficiency Particulate Arrester (HEPA):** These filters are designed to absorb and contain 99.97 percent of all particles larger than 0.3 microns (one-three hundredth the width of a human hair). If the unit truly operates at that level, only 3 out of 10,000 particles get into your indoor environment. Vacuum cleaners and air purifiers with HEPA and ULPA filters (see the next section for more information) can play a vital part in allergy-proofing your home.

- ✔ **Ultra Low Penetration Air (ULPA):** This system filters more thoroughly than the HEPA process and is designed to absorb and contain 99.99 percent of all particles larger than 0.12 microns.

If your home doesn't have a central HVAC system, you can purchase stand-alone HEPA and ULPA air cleaners for use in individual rooms. The appendix provides information on finding and purchasing these items.

Vacuum cleaning is also vital for reducing your exposure to allergens and irritants at home. However, many standard vacuum cleaners only absorb larger particles, and they allow many allergens to escape in the exhaust. This is often why you may experience asthma symptoms after housework: The vacuuming may actually have made matters worse for you by simply stirring up triggering substances that you then inhaled.

In order to avoid stirring up asthma triggers when you vacuum, ask your doctor whether she thinks investing in a vacuum cleaner that uses a HEPA or ULPA filtration process may work for you. You can find more information on HEPA- or ULPA-filtered vacuums in the appendix.

Working Out Workplace Exposures

Exposures to many types of chemicals and dust in workplace environments can induce different forms of occupational asthma. In many cases, people who have asthma but haven't yet developed obvious symptoms of the disease may experience asthma episodes for the first time as a result of exposure to occupational triggers. Allergic and nonallergic triggers can play a part in occupational asthma, which may account for as many as 15 percent of all new asthma cases each year in the United States.

Targeting workplace triggers

Doctors and other healthcare professionals typically associate occupational asthma with exposure to the following workplace triggers:

- **Industrial irritants:** These irritants can include chemicals, fumes, gases, aerosols, paints, smoke, and other substances you primarily find in the workplace. Tobacco smoke in the workplace can cause many asthma symptoms. Likewise, other irritants in the workplace can include perfumes, food odors, and even co-workers who use heavily scented perfumes and colognes.

- **Occupational allergens:** Many occupations involve exposure to or contact with substances made of plant materials, food products, and other items that contain allergenic extracts that can trigger allergic reactions, thus inducing occupational asthma in sensitized people. For example, "Baker's asthma" can occur in workers who receive constant respiratory exposure to the allergens contained in flour. (Eating the resulting baked food usually doesn't produce symptoms in these workers, however.) Latex is another common occupational allergen, as I explain in the sidebar "Latex and your lungs."

- **Physical stimuli:** These stimuli include conditions in your workplace, especially variations in temperature and humidity, such as heat and cold extremes or air that's especially dry or humid.

Diagnosing and treating workplace triggers

Your physician should distinguish between asthma that results from exposure to certain substances in the workplace, school, or other frequented locations (other than your home) and a pre-existing condition that is aggravated by occupational allergens and irritants. This determination is vital to developing appropriate and effective methods of avoiding or reducing your exposure to occupational substances that may affect your asthma.

Latex and your lungs

Latex is increasingly a part of the environment in most medical facilities, due to the need for more aggressive infection control. This rubber compound is found particularly in medical gloves and other medical equipment, such as latex ports in intravenous tubing for administration of fluids and medications.

Because many surgical gloves contain cornstarch powder that's coated with latex allergen, healthcare workers often inhale airborne allergen latex particles. These exposures can result in allergens from the rubber compounds sensitizing medical personnel. Thus, latex has become one of the most frequent causes of occupational allergy and asthma in the healthcare industry. In addition, patients being treated in medical facilities can also receive exposures and be sensitized to latex.

These exposures can lead to serious symptoms of allergic rhinitis, asthma, *urticaria* (hives), *angioedema* (deep swellings), and, in extreme cases, *anaphylaxis* (a potentially life-threatening reaction that affects many organs simultaneously).

The allergens in many natural rubber latex products (including condoms and diaphragms) typically cause Type I immediate hypersensitivity IgE-mediated reactions. (I explain this mechanism in Chapter 6.) For this reason, the FDA now requires labeling of all medical devices or packaging containing natural rubber latex. Parents should be aware that latex-sensitive children can be at risk for severe respiratory reactions from rubber balloons.

If you're at risk for allergic reactions to latex exposure, make sure that any physician who treats you knows this fact so that you can, ideally, receive medical/dental care in a latex-free environment — a setting in which no latex gloves are used and no latex accessories (such as catheters, adhesives, tourniquets, and anesthesia equipment) come into contact with you. Similarly, if your occupation involves contact with latex, find out what you can do to avoid or minimize your exposure to this allergen. In healthcare settings, powder-free latex gloves and non-latex gloves and other medical articles are increasingly becoming available. Using these alternative products can often substantially reduce the risk that you may suffer an allergic reaction to latex.

Additionally, wear a MedicAlert bracelet or pendant to alert medical personnel not to use latex articles in the event that you're unconscious or unable to communicate during a medical emergency. (The appendix provides information on obtaining these bracelets and pendants.) If you've experienced a serious allergic reaction to latex, also ask your doctor whether an emergency epinephrine kit, such as an EpiPen or Twinject, with an injectable dose of epinephrine, is advisable for you.

Diagnosing your occupational asthma is important for your long-term health and the effective management of your disease. The sooner you can effectively avoid or reduce your exposure to triggers at work, the better you can control your asthma.

In diagnosing a case of occupational asthma, your doctor may first need to assess the following factors:

> ✔ **The pattern of your symptoms.** Symptoms that improve when you're away from work strongly suggest that your problem is indeed work-related.
>
> ✔ **Your co-workers.** Do your co-workers suffer from similar symptoms?
>
> ✔ **The degree of exposure.** Did your first noticeable asthma episode at work occur after a particularly significant exposure, such as a spill of chemicals or other industrial substances?

Depending on your condition's severity, your doctor may prescribe medications that control your asthma symptoms at work. In most cases, however, for this treatment to be effective, your doctor will probably advise you to find ways of avoiding or at least reducing your exposure to workplace triggers.

Avoiding Drug and Food Triggers

Some people with asthma also suffer from sensitivities — sometimes potentially life-threatening — to certain foods and medications. In the following sections, I explain the most significant sensitivities that can adversely affect your asthma and what you can do to avoid them.

Aspirin sensitivities

Approximately 10 percent of asthma patients experience some level of sensitivity to aspirin, aspirin-containing compounds (such as Alka-Seltzer, Anacin, and Excedrin), and nonsteroidal anti-inflammatory drugs (NSAIDs). If your medical history includes nasal polyps and sinusitis in addition to asthma and aspirin sensitivity, use acetaminophen-based products such as Tylenol instead of aspirin or NSAIDs for the relief of common aches and pains.

A more serious form of aspirin sensitivity is the *aspirin triad*. This condition affects aspirin-intolerant patients who have asthma and chronic nasal polyps as well as a history of sinusitis. If you suffer from the aspirin triad, adverse reactions to aspirin, aspirin-containing compounds, NSAIDs, and newer prescription NSAIDs, known as COX-2 inhibitors, including celecoxib (Celebrex) and rofecoxib (Vioxx), can result in severe or potentially life-threatening asthma attacks.

I strongly advise anyone with this level of sensitivity to wear a MedicAlert bracelet or pendant. This device alerts medical personnel not to administer any medication to which you are sensitive if you're unconscious or unable to communicate during a medical emergency. See the appendix for more information on MedicAlert bracelets and pendants.

Beta-blockers

Doctors frequently prescribe oral beta-blocker medications, including Inderal, Lopressor, and Corgard, to treat conditions such as migraine headache, high blood pressure, angina, or hyperthyroidism, and beta-blocker eye drops for eye conditions, such as glaucoma. If you have one of these disorders and you also have asthma, know that taking beta-blockers can worsen your asthma symptoms by blocking the beta$_2$-adrenergic receptor sites in your airways that cause bronchodilation, thus making your asthma less responsive to beta$_2$-adrenergic (beta$_2$-agonist) bronchodilators.

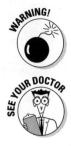

Occasionally, taking beta-blockers can trigger asthma episodes in susceptible individuals who haven't previously experienced any respiratory symptoms.

Because beta-blockers may trigger asthma symptoms, make sure that any doctor you consult for any of the conditions I mention in this section knows that you have asthma and/or has your complete medical history. If beta-blockers aren't advisable, your doctor may prescribe alternative forms of medication therapy, such as other families of anti-hypertensives or other types of anti-migraine drugs.

Sensitivities to sulfites and other additives

Sulfites are often used as antioxidants to preserve beverages, such as beer and wine, and foods like dried fruit, shrimp, and potatoes. These antioxidants are also often used in salad bars and in guacamole. Exposure to these food additives can trigger severe asthma symptoms — including potentially life-threatening *bronchospasm* (constriction of the airways) — in as many as 10 percent of people who have severe persistent asthma when these individuals inhale sulfite fumes from treated foods. Severe asthmatics who require long-term treatment with oral corticosteroids (see Chapter 15) are more likely to be sulfite-sensitive and may be especially at risk for severe adverse reactions to these additives.

If you're sensitive to sulfites, avoid consuming beer, wine, and processed foods. Also, carry rescue medication, such as an EpiPen, Twinject, and/or a short-acting inhaled bronchodilator, with you in the event that you unintentionally ingest food or liquids that contain sulfites. Eating more fresh foods, instead of processed foods, particularly fruits and vegetables, is a good idea anyway, regardless of whether or not you have asthma.

Tartrazine (FDC yellow dye No. 5), used in many medications, foods, and vitamin products, has been reported to possibly cause adverse reactions in asthmatics. If you're sensitive to this food additive, check the labels on liquid medications, such as cough syrups and other liquid cold and flu remedies, to see whether they contain tartrazine or sulfites. When in doubt, ask your pharmacist.

Food allergies

Some people with asthma develop hypersensitivities to certain foods. However, although certain foods have the potential to cause anaphylaxis, they don't appear to significantly increase the underlying airway inflammation that's characteristic of asthma in most patients.

 If your infant or young child has food allergies, your child may have a tendency to develop other allergy-related problems. In this case, your doctor should evaluate your child for possible signs of asthma and other atopic diseases, such as allergic rhinitis and atopic dermatitis.

 If you've experienced an episode of anaphylaxis, ask your doctor whether an emergency epinephrine kit, such as an EpiPen (or EpiPen Jr. for children under 66 pounds) or Twinject, is advisable for you. Wear a MedicAlert bracelet or necklace in case you're unable to speak during a reaction. The appendix provides more information on obtaining these items.

If you're hungering for details on food allergies, turn to Chapter 8.

Other Medical Conditions and Asthma

In addition to the triggers that I discuss previously in this chapter, certain activities, illnesses, and syndromes can also induce your asthma symptoms or make them worse. Managing these precipitating factors is as vital to effectively controlling your asthma as is avoiding allergens and irritants.

Rhinitis and sinusitis

Poorly managing allergic and nonallergic forms of rhinitis can lead to *sinusitis*. This infection of the sinuses can also aggravate your asthma symptoms, especially if it isn't responsive to repeated courses of antibiotic treatment. If so, sinus surgery may be necessary to treat sinusitis and reestablish control over asthma symptoms. Studies show that asthma patients who effectively manage their rhinitis and/or sinusitis can significantly improve their asthma symptoms.

Because your respiratory tract is essentially a continuum — or as I like to say, the united airway — treating your nose and sinuses can actually help treat the underlying inflammation that characterizes asthma. In fact, when dealing with serious respiratory diseases such as asthma, doctors increasingly consider it vital to treat the whole patient — not just the patient's lungs. For more information on dealing with sinusitis and other rhinitis complications, turn to Chapter 13.

Gastroesophageal reflux disease (GERD)

The digestive disorder *gastroesophageal reflux disease* (GERD) occurs when the valve that separates the esophagus from the stomach doesn't function properly. As a result, stomach acid and undigested food can wash up into the esophagus (and occasionally, through inhalation, into the respiratory tract) from the stomach in individuals who suffer from GERD. You can see a cross-section of the organs involved in GERD in Figure 5-2.

Patients who suffer from GERD often burp during and after meals, complain of an acid taste in their mouth, and feel a burning sensation in their throat or chest, symptoms that they typically describe as heartburn or indigestion.

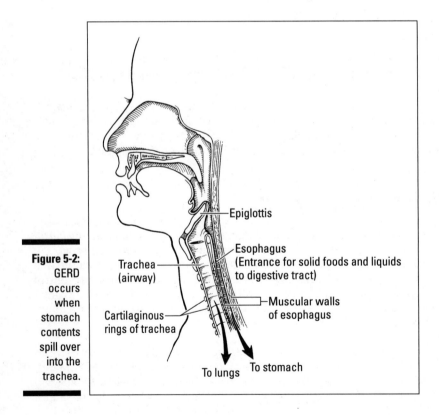

Figure 5-2:
GERD
occurs
when
stomach
contents
spill over
into the
trachea.

Epiglottis

Esophagus
(Entrance for solid foods and liquids
to digestive tract)

Trachea
(airway)

Muscular walls
of esophagus

Cartilaginous
rings of trachea

To lungs   To stomach

GERD is a trigger of asthma symptoms in a large number of asthmatics and is, in particular, a major trigger of adult-onset asthma (see Chapter 2) in patients whose asthma symptoms (coughing, wheezing, shortness of breath) aren't usually associated with allergic triggers. If you're asthmatic, the flow of acidic digestive contents into your respiratory airways can make your underlying airway inflammation worse. GERD, with or without inhalation of stomach contents, has also been associated with increased bronchospasm and chronic cough due to irritation of the esophagus. Conversely, when asthma is active, it can also aggravate GERD, and some of the drugs used to treat asthma, such as long-acting beta$_2$-adrenergic bronchodilators and oral theophylline (see Chapter 15 for details on long-term asthma medications), can also worsen GERD symptoms.

If you have frequent heartburn and poorly controlled asthma, particularly with episodes that occur at night and disturb your sleep, your doctor should investigate the possibility that GERD contributes to your asthma symptoms.

To help alleviate the effects of GERD, your doctor may advise the following:

- ✔ Avoid eating or drinking within three hours of going to bed.

- ✔ Avoid heavy meals and minimize dietary fat. Also, try to eat several small meals over the course of the day instead of fewer, larger meals.

- ✔ Eliminate or cut down on the consumption of chocolate, peppermint, alcoholic beverages, coffee, tea, and colas and carbonated beverages.

- ✔ Avoid or reduce smoking and the use of any tobacco products.

- ✔ Try elevating the head of your bed, by using 6- to 8-inch blocks, so that your stomach contents are less likely to rise to the point that you can inhale them while sleeping. Adding pillows under your head can also be of some benefit.

- ✔ To control the digestive problems that result from your GERD symptoms, use appropriate over-the-counter (OTC) products, including Zantac, Tagamet, Axid, Prilosec OTC, and Pepcid AC. Your physician may also prescribe other medications, such as Nexium, Protonix, Aciphex, and Prevacid, which decrease *gastric* (stomach) acid secretion.

Viral infections

Viral respiratory infections, such as the common cold or flu, can aggravate airway inflammation and trigger asthma symptoms. Asthmatic children under age 10 are particularly prone to asthma symptoms precipitated by *rhinovirus infections* (upper respiratory infections, usually referred to as the common cold).

Rhinovirus infections cause bronchial hyperreactivity and promote allergic inflammation, leading to increased asthma symptoms. For infants and toddlers, viral infections of all types are the most frequent cause of severe asthma episodes because infants and younger children have smaller airways that are often more susceptible to bronchial obstruction. These infections are also the most frequent cause of episodes in adults, especially those with nonallergic (intrinsic) asthma.

Inform your doctor whenever you experience flu or cold symptoms. As comforting as you may find chicken soup when you're sniffly and sneezy, you may require early and aggressive medication therapy to keep the virus from adversely affecting your asthma.

Consider the following measures when dealing with viral infections:

✔ If your have persistent asthma, ask your doctor about receiving an annual flu vaccine to reduce the risk of suffering from an influenza respiratory infection that could aggravate your asthma symptoms.

✔ New prescription antiviral medications, such as zanamivir by inhalation (Relenza) and oseltamivir phosphate by oral tablet (Tamiflu), can stop the flu dead in its tracks and get you back on your feet sooner if you take these drugs within the first two days of developing flu symptoms. Common flu symptoms include high fever, muscle aches, fatigue, and increased respiratory symptoms. Using these antiviral products can reduce the respiratory complications that accompany influenza infections, making these medications especially beneficial if you have asthma. However, these medications are only for influenza and aren't effective against the common cold.

✔ If your young child or infant experiences repeated viral infections that cause coughing and wheezing episodes, and your family medical history includes *atopy* (the genetic susceptibility for the immune system to produce antibodies to common allergens, which leads to allergy symptoms), make sure your doctor evaluates your child for the possibility of asthma. (See Chapter 18 for more information about asthma and children.)

What to do about the flu

Antiviral medications can help you avoid coming down with influenza even when you've had a flu shot. Flu vaccines consist of the World Health Organization's (WHO) best guess of the viruses from the preceding year that may cause the flu during next year's winter season. However, the WHO's predictions aren't always accurate. As a result, a flu shot may not fully protect you against the viral strains that cause the current year's flu epidemic, thus making antiviral medications extremely beneficial.

Chapter 6

Understanding Asthma and the Role of Allergies

*I*n terms of germs, the world can still be a rough place. Despite major advances during the past 100 years in fighting infectious diseases and providing effective medical care, viruses, bacteria, fungi, and other potentially harmful agents remain constant threats to your health. That's why your body's defense network is so important to your well-being.

Your frontline defense against potentially infectious intruders is your skin. (Your mucous membranes, as well as your stomach's highly acidic digestive juices, your gut's beneficial bacteria, and certain nonspecific cells, also act as immediate defenders against uninvited guests.) The second, far more complex and fundamental defense apparatus in your body — and one of the most important keys to the survival of the human species — is your immune system.

Because numerous immune system processes can play important roles as underlying factors in asthma and allergy (as well as in many other diseases), doctors frequently need to apply their understanding of *immunology* (the science of immunity) when evaluating and treating asthma. I devote this chapter to explaining the immunologic basis of allergic asthma and other allergic reactions so that you can have a better understanding of what may be at the root of your ailment and to review with you what your physician considers when diagnosing and treating your condition.

Protecting Your Health: How Your Immune System Works

Your immune system's most basic function is to distinguish between your body (self) and potentially harmful (non-self) agents. Your immune system performs the following functions to protect you:

- ✔ **Recognizes foreign (therefore, potentially harmful) microorganisms, their products, and toxins, all known generally as** *antigens.* These substances can stimulate a response from your immune system and react with an antibody or a sensitized *T-cell* (a specialized immune system cell involved in cell-mediated immunity, as I explain in "Reacting to allergen exposures," later in this chapter). Allergens, which usually consist of proteins, are particular types of antigens, which initiate an allergic response that often triggers respiratory symptoms in asthma patients.

- ✔ **Identifies self-antigens.** These antigens are usually damaged and improperly functioning cells in your body. Malignant cells that can develop into tumor-causing cancerous cells are an example of self-antigens.

- ✔ **Assists in removing antigens from your body.** Specialized immune system cells recognize, surround, and destroy these intruders through a complicated series of immunological processes.

The immune system's defense is vital to the survival of all animals. If your immune system functions properly, its protective function is an underlying, ongoing, and generally imperceptible aspect of your everyday existence.

Your immune system can work as a double-edged sword, however. In some cases, it deploys its defensive functions too zealously while trying to protect your body against any type of perceived threat. In such cases, rather than preventing infections, your immune system can actually instigate certain types of health problems, including

- ✔ **Autoimmune disorders:** These disorders include serious diseases such as rheumatic fever, a rare complication of an inadequately treated strep infection of the upper respiratory tract (strep throat), in which the immune system can attack heart tissue cells that cross-react with *Streptococcus* bacterial antigens. This kind of complication is why taking the full course of antibiotic therapy your doctor prescribes for strep throat is important and that you return to your doctor's office for a repeat throat culture to make sure that your infection has completely resolved. (For more information on cross-reactivity, see Chapter 11.)

In other cases, the immune system (for reasons doctors are still working to discover) loses its ability to differentiate between certain self and non-self substances. This inability to distinguish can cause diseases such as systemic lupus erythematous, psoriasis, rheumatoid arthritis, and some forms of diabetes, when your immune system perceives otherwise functional and vital cells in your body as antigens and turns its firepower on them.

✔ **Rejection of organ transplants:** Doctors usually try to find a close genetic match between patient and organ donors to reduce the risk of the patient's immune system rejecting the donated organ. In many cases, however, physicians still need to administer drugs to suppress the patient's immune system and prevent organ rejection. This suppression of the immune system can then increase the risk of opportunistic infections, potentially harming the patient.

✔ **Allergic conditions:** If you have asthma or allergies, you almost certainly have an immune system that works too well or overreacts. Doctors use the term *hypersensitivity* to refer to allergies because your immune system is overly sensitive to substances such as pollens, animal dander, and other types of allergens that offer no real threat to your health. With hypersensitivity, your immune system acts sort of like an alarm system that summons a SWAT team regardless of whether a cat burglar or just a cat is intruding on your property.

Classifying Immune System Components and Disorders

Your immune system consists of several related processes. Think of these processes as a civil defense network of arsenals, supply lines, logistical support, and command and control centers for the cells that actually defend your body. The most important organ and tissue components of your immune system include the following:

✔ **Bone marrow:** In your bone marrow, stem cells (early, nonspecific types of cells) originate, developing into *B-cells* (specialized types of plasma cells) that subsequently secrete distinct forms of plasma proteins, known as *antibodies.* These antibodies are divided into the following five classes of *immunoglobulins* (identified by the prefix Ig):

• **IgG:** The major component of gamma globulin used for treating certain types of immune deficiencies, IgG antibodies account for at least three-quarters of your body's antibodies. IgG antibodies along with IgM antibodies and your white blood cells defend you against bacterial infections. IgG antibodies also play an important role in preventing allergens from initiating an allergic reaction. As a response to *immunotherapy* (allergy shots), the production of IgG antibodies is believed to work by competing with IgE for antigen by binding to mast cells, thus preventing the subsequent release of chemical mediators of inflammation that produce asthma and allergy symptoms. (See "Reacting to allergen exposures," later in this chapter, for more information.)

- **IgM:** About 5 percent of your antibodies belong to this class, which plays a role in the primary immune response and also enhances the role of IgG antibodies.

- **IgA:** The primary antibody in your mucous membrane surfaces, IgA antibodies reside in your saliva, tears, and in the secretions of the mucosal surfaces of your respiratory bronchi, gastrointestinal, and genital tracts, where these antibodies protect against infection. They're also present in mother's milk, thus providing antibody protection for breastfed newborns.

- **IgD:** This antibody class, which binds to the antigen at cell surface contact, seems to exist in very small quantities and plays a nonspecific role in the immune process.

- **IgE:** Although present in only minute quantities in your body, IgE antibodies (also known as *reaginic antibodies*) are key players in allergic reactions. Although everyone produces IgE antibodies, most allergy sufferers have an inherited tendency to overproduce these agents. IgE antibodies can induce other cells, particularly mast cells and *basophils* (special sentinel cells, as I explain in "Reacting to allergen exposures," later in this chapter), to start a complex chain reaction that culminates in your allergy symptoms.

  Mast cell surfaces have special IgE receptor sites. Two allergen-specific IgE antibodies linking to an allergen (such as pollen, animal dander, molds, dust mite allergens, insect sting venom, and certain foods and drugs) on the mast cell surface can trigger a Type I allergic reaction (see "Classifying Abnormal Immune Responses," later in this chapter).

✔ **Thymus:** Secretions of special hormones (such as thymosin) from this gland are vital for regulating your immune system's functions. The thymus also helps "educate" (encode) certain T-cells, which then play a key role in developing antibodies against antigens.

✔ **Lymph nodes:** The lymphatic system provides drainage for your immune system. Your lymph nodes filter out material that comes from an infection. If you seem to have, for example, strep throat, your doctor checks for swollen lymph nodes downstream from the infected area (under your throat) as an indication of infection.

TECHNICAL STUFF

Inflaming you for a good reason

You may wonder why you're equipped with IgE antibodies if they're so problematic. This seemingly bothersome immunoglobulin is actually a significant part of the reason the human species has made it this far. During prehistoric days, in addition to the challenges of hunting and gathering daily meals (and trying not to become another animal's chow in the process), humans also had to contend with all sorts of infectious agents, especially parasites.

The potent inflammatory action triggered when a parasite-specific antigen would bind with cell-bound IgE antibodies probably ensured that parasitic infections couldn't affect enough humans to endanger the species. In fact, IgE antibodies remain important players in the immune responses of some people in less-developed regions of the world, where parasites continue to pose threats to human health — but where rates of asthma and allergies are much lower than in the more developed world. Occasionally, I see patients who have recently arrived from less-developed countries and who have highly elevated IgE and *eosinophil* (specialized white blood cells that play an important role in the inflammatory process) levels in their blood tests. In those cases, I rule out parasitic infections before moving on to a more likely diagnosis of an allergic condition. However, because parasites are such an extremely rare problem in the U.S. population, elevated IgE and eosinophil levels are almost always a sign that I'm dealing with an allergic patient.

In most modern-day humans, IgE antibodies play a role similar to that of fat cells. In prehistoric days, humans needed fat cells to store food and stave off hunger when their hunting and gathering was less than productive. Now human fat cells turn into love handles, and IgE antibodies trigger allergies.

Some researchers have hypothesized that exposure to key types of infections during childhood leads the immune system to function properly and focus primarily on developing antibodies against harmful agents that enter the body. However, for reasons that are currently the subject of intense scientific inquiry and debate, the vast majority of asthma and allergy sufferers have an immune system that also works overtime to protect the body against mostly harmless allergens.

According to some studies, attempts to provide near-antiseptic environments for infants and young children may partially be to blame for this type of overzealous immune system and the resulting high incidence of asthma and various allergies in the most developed parts of the world. One of the main arguments of this so-called "hygiene hypothesis" is that without a real threat to our health (such as infectious diseases) during our early years — and the widespread use nowadays of immunizations, antibiotic therapy, and better hygiene — the "bored" immune system fixates on any foreign protein, however innocent, which enters the body. As a result, the body's immune system produces antibodies intended to destroy that relatively harmless invader the next time the immune system detects its presence.

✔ **Spleen:** This organ filters and processes antigens in your blood.

✔ **Lymphoid tissues:** These important immune system participants, which include your tonsils, adenoids, appendix, and parts of your intestines, help process antigens.

Protecting and serving in many ways

Your immune system's protective mechanisms consist of four basic components. Think of these components as separate armed forces branches that use different but related means to accomplish the immune system's overall defense mission. The four basic components are

✔ **Humoral immunity:** This component (which isn't a vaccine against stand-up comedians) acts similarly to an internal air force, using *B-cells* (see "Classifying Immune System Components and Disorders," earlier in this chapter) to produce and deploy antibodies (the immune system's equivalent of high-tech weaponry). This component provides your body with its primary defense mechanism against bacterial infection and also plays a major role in developing allergies in people with a family history of *atopy* (the genetic susceptibility that can predispose the immune system to develop hypersensitivities and produce antibodies to otherwise harmless allergens).

✔ **Cell-mediated immunity:** This component uses *T-cells* (see "Protecting Your Health: How Your Immune System Works," earlier in this chapter) and related cell products (sort of like the army, battling in the trenches), rather than antibodies, to directly protect you against viruses, fungi, intracellular organisms, and tumor antigens.

✔ **Phagocytic immunity:** The function of this component is similar to a mop-up squad (or vultures and other scavengers), because it uses so-called *scavenger cells* (macrophages) that circulate throughout your body, looking for debris to clean up. This form of immunity doesn't play a significant role in the allergic process.

✔ **Complement:** This term describes a composite system of plasma and cell membrane proteins that interact with one another, as well as with antibodies, and serve as important mediators in your civil defense system, protecting the homefront like the Department of Homeland Security. Diseases associated with complement deficiency vary depending on which component of the complement system is lacking. Some people may have an increased susceptibility to infection, some may experience a rheumatic disorder (such as lupus erythematous or rheumatoid arthritis), and some may have hereditary *angioedema* (deep swellings) that occur without hives and can potentially cause life-threatening symptoms.

Distinguishing between immune deficiencies and allergic conditions

Years ago, when I mentioned immune deficiency, people needed an extensive explanation of the subject. Now I spend most of my time clarifying that immunodeficiency isn't synonymous with AIDS (Acquired Immunodeficiency Syndrome), but rather that AIDS represents just one out of a whole multitude of immune-deficiency diseases.

If your doctor advises testing for immune deficiency, she isn't necessarily ordering an HIV test. (Remember, HIV is the virus that causes AIDS.) Instead, your physician is most likely ordering immune-deficiency tests to rule out other types of diseases.

Although allergic conditions are almost always synonymous with an overactive immune system, rare cases exist in which people with IgA deficiencies, who have recurring infections, may also have allergic conditions. However, immune deficiencies of any type are very rare when compared to the overall incidence of allergic disorders.

Keep in mind the following important points about immunodeficiencies and allergic conditions:

- ✔ In most cases, if you have allergies and a medical history of recurring infections, your over-responsive immune system is actually swamping your system with excess mucus that gets infected and indirectly causing your infections such as sinusitis or bronchitis.

- ✔ In more than 20 years of treating patients for recurring infections, I've seen only a handful of patients with immune deficiencies. In the vast majority of cases, I found that these patients actually had allergies.

- ✔ If you have a bacterial infection such as sinusitis or bronchitis, your physician should evaluate whether your infection is a complication of *allergic rhinitis* (hay fever) and/or asthma before checking for much less common immune deficiencies.

- ✔ Doctors can rule out the vast majority of immune-deficiency syndromes by using simple blood tests that measure your blood count and antibody levels. For this reason, I strongly advise against indiscriminately receiving gamma-globulin therapy (see the "Classifying Immune System Components and Disorders" section, earlier in this chapter) unless you first have an immune work-up that reveals a significant deficiency requiring this kind of treatment.

Immunizing and immunology

You often hear that life is a constant learning process. This statement is especially true for your immune system. In fact, your immune system is a seemingly limitless learning machine. It constantly memorizes countless antigens and remembers these encounters, allowing your defenses to react to future exposures.

The memory chips of any computer that you use in your lifetime pale in comparison to your immune system's virtual total recall. Through the *humoral component* (see "Protecting and serving in many ways," earlier in this chapter), your immune system can recognize hundreds of trillions of antigens and produce specific antibodies against each and every one of these substances. Compare this feat to remembering the name, looks, and characteristics of every single person, animal, and plant that you encounter throughout your lifetime (which could come in handy at your high school reunion).

Memorizing menaces to your health

Your immune system's phenomenal capacity to memorize explains how having a particular viral infection usually enables you to acquire immunity to that specific virus for the future. Your immune system usually recognizes the antigen on subsequent exposure, thus triggering a rapid response from its specialized mechanisms and cells, which neutralize and dispose of the offending virus before it can adversely affect you.

Many ancient cultures recognized that people who survived infectious diseases were usually immunized against catching the same ailment again. In fact, ancient Chinese and Egyptian doctors practiced limited forms of immunization.

Fooling your immune system for your own good

Immunization tricks your immune system into thinking that you've actually had a full-blown infection, without risking the potentially life-threatening consequences that a disease such as polio can cause. Your immune system's reaction to the perceived infection ensures that if you ever receive exposure to that same virus, your defensive mechanisms will respond rapidly and effectively, thus protecting your health.

Vaccines developed thanks to advances in immunology are the main reason that parents in the United States and many other parts of the world no longer need to worry about their children succumbing to a summer epidemic of polio. Other diseases that medical science has successfully brought under control as a result of immunizations include smallpox, diphtheria, *pertussis* (whooping cough), tetanus, chickenpox, measles, German measles (rubella), and mumps, as well as some forms of hepatitis and meningitis.

In fact, stimulating your immune system into producing a protective immune response against allergens is the underlying basis of *immunotherapy* (allergy shots), as I explain later in this chapter.

Classifying Abnormal Immune Responses

As I mention earlier in this chapter, your immune system can cause you trouble when it malfunctions, either because of a deficiency or by doing its job too well. Scientists refer to these abnormal responses according to four distinct classifications of reactions.

Although allergic responses can involve aspects of all four types of these mechanisms, Types I and IV, which process and memorize previous antigen encounters, are the most important in the vast majority of allergic conditions.

IgE-mediated reactions (Type 1)

IgE-mediated reactions (Type I) result in immediate allergic reactions. Also known as *immediate hypersensitivity,* they often result from an insect sting or the injection of a drug such as penicillin in people who have extreme sensitivities to these triggers. The most dramatic and dangerous Type I reaction is anaphylaxis (see Chapter 1).

Allergic asthma, allergic rhinitis, and certain types of drug allergies are other examples. Because of the sudden onset of the allergic reaction, allergy skin testing (see Chapter 11) can provide quick results in identifying the triggers in many cases. For a more in-depth explanation of Type I reactions, see "Developing an Immediate Hypersensitivity," later in this chapter.

Cytotoxic reactions (Type 11)

Cytotoxic reactions (Type II) involve the destruction of cells, such as the reactions that result when red blood cells break down. This mechanism can potentially lead to anemia and fewer platelets, a situation that decreases your blood's ability to clot.

Certain drugs, such as penicillin, sulfonamides, and quinidine, can trigger cytotoxic reactions. Type II reactions play a role in Rh-factor anemia and jaundice in newborns and are also the way a patient's body may reject an organ transplant.

Immune complex reactions (Type III)

Manifestations of *immune complex reactions (Type III)* include fever, skin rash, hives, swollen, tender lymph nodes, and aching or painful joints. These types of reactions are among the ones that physicians usually refer to as *serum sickness.* Typically, these symptoms appear one to three weeks after taking final doses of drugs such as penicillin, sulfonamides, thiouracil, and phenytoin.

Type III reactions also play a role in the development of autoimmune disorders, such as systemic lupus erythematous, rheumatoid arthritis, some forms of diabetes, and certain types of kidney disease.

Cell-mediated reactions (Type IV)

Allergic contact dermatitis is one of the primary examples of *cell-mediated reactions (Type IV),* a localized, non-systemic reaction. Doctors also use the term *delayed hypersensitivity* to describe this process, in which contact with an allergen results in an allergic reaction hours or even days later. (For example, if you have allergic contact dermatitis, you may not realize that you've contacted poison ivy until you're driving home from your weekend camping trip.)

Although the delayed reaction is rarely life-threatening, in some cases it may take longer to subside or disappear than reactions involving atopic conditions, such as immediate hypersensitivity (see "IgE-mediated reactions [Type I]," at the beginning of this section).

Developing an Immediate Hypersensitivity

Type I allergic reactions involve numerous complex processes, with many players taking part in various ways. This section explains the roles that the most important cells and chemicals play in developing your sensitivities and triggering your reactions.

Setting the stage for allergic reactions

Significant cell participants in Type I reactions include the following:

✔ **Mast cells:** These connective-tissue cells play a pivotal role in allergic disease processes. Mast cells are primarily located near blood vessels and mucus-producing cells in the tissues that line various parts of your body. With allergies, doctors concern themselves with your mast cells' actions in the lining of your eyes, ears, nose, sinuses, throat, the airways of your lungs, your skin, and your gastrointestinal (GI) tract.

✔ **Basophils:** These cells live in your bloodstream near the surfaces of tissues and are important players in late-phase reactions. (See "Reacting to allergen exposures," later in this chapter, for more information.)

Mast cells and basophils are among the first cells that antigens encounter when entering your body. These sentinel cells are coated with numerous IgE receptor sites that can accommodate IgE antibodies that are specific to various allergens (corresponding, for example, to different pollens and animal dander).

These cells also contain potent chemical mediators of inflammation that are released when IgE and a specific allergen cross-link and activate them, resulting in the inflammation that leads to allergic symptoms.

✔ **Eosinophils:** Other mediators, including those from mast cells, attract these white blood cells to the site of an allergic reaction and generate an array of inflammatory mediators, including enzymes that can cause tissue damage. Eosinophils also play prominent roles in late-phase reactions that affect some people with asthma, particularly with symptoms of chest congestion that can occur hours after an initial episode of asthma. (See "Reacting to allergen exposures," later in this chapter.) If you have uncontrolled asthma, the chronic inflammatory process may lead to *airway remodeling* — the replacement of healthy tissue with scar tissue — and can potentially cause irreversible loss of lung function.

Preventing this type of serious lung damage is one of the main goals of treating asthma early and aggressively, particularly with inhaled corticosteroids. (See Chapter 15 for an extensive survey of asthma-controller medications.) Because eosinophils tend to increase in the bloodstream of patients with allergic asthma, your doctor may order a complete blood count (CBC) including a peripheral eosinophil count when diagnosing your condition.

Histamine (see Chapter 1) and leukotrienes (see Chapter 15) are just two of the potent chemical mediators of inflammation released from mast cells and basophils during allergic reactions. This multitude of mediators can induce the following actions in your body:

✔ Attract other inflammatory cells to the area to amplify the inflammatory reaction.

✔ Cause tissue damage, often with accompanying pain and discomfort.

✔ Constrict the smooth muscles of your respiratory airways.

- ✔ Dilate your blood vessels, leading to increased fluid leakage, which increases inflammatory action.

- ✔ Increase mucus secretions, resulting in a runny nose, watery eyes, cough, and chest congestion, depending on where the trigger causes the allergic reaction.

- ✔ Promote the production of IgE and activate the eosinophils, thus supporting allergic inflammation.

Reacting to allergen exposures

This section shows you how the players I describe in the preceding section interact. A typical sequence of reactions in an IgE response (immediate hypersensitivity) consists of the following steps:

1. **Your immune system receives exposure to an allergen.**

   Allergen exposures can result from the following occurrences:

   - **Inhaling:** Inhalant allergens (or *aeroallergens*) such as pollens, molds, dust mite allergens, and animal dander often pass through your nose and/or your mouth, putting the allergens in contact with immune cells lining your nose, mouth, throat, and airways of the lungs. Common symptoms of these exposures include runny nose, sneezing, watery eyes, stuffy nose, postnasal drip, coughing, chest tightness, wheezing, and shortness of breath.

   - **Ingesting:** You may swallow allergens, such as those contained in peanuts, shellfish, eggs, milk, or in drugs such as penicillin. These exposures can trigger oral symptoms such as itching and swelling of the tongue, lips, and throat; GI tract symptoms such as nausea, stomach cramps, vomiting, and diarrhea; skin reactions such as hives and angioedema; and respiratory symptoms such as coughing, wheezing, and shortness of breath.

   - **Injecting:** Medical syringes and insect stingers are vehicles for injecting allergens. Injections can cause particularly severe reactions because allergens go directly into your bloodstream, which can spread the allergens rapidly to organs throughout your body. Penicillin shots are the most dramatic (and often severe) examples of drug-related anaphylaxis in people with penicillin hypersensitivities. The venom from stinging insects can also cause potentially life-threatening reactions.

   - **Touching (direct contact):** Direct contact exposures typically involve Type IV delayed hypersensitivity responses, including reactions to poison ivy, nickel, and latex, among numerous others. Symptoms from direct contact usually result in localized, topical reactions such as skin rashes.

2. Your body develops an IgE antibody response to the allergen.

If you have an atopic predisposition for developing allergies, scavenger cells (macrophages) that usually rid your body of foreign proteins (such as allergens) act as antigen- (allergen-) presenting cells. This setup triggers T-cells to recruit B-cells that develop into plasma cells. This process culminates in the production of specific IgE antibodies designed against the allergen (see Figure 6-1).

3. Allergens bind to specific IgE antibodies attached to the surface of mast cells or basophils.

The first time you're exposed to the allergen, you don't typically experience a reaction. However, you produce specific IgE antibodies that bind to receptor sites on mast cells. Thus your immune system is *sensitized,* and further exposure to that allergen initiates an allergic response.

4. You're re-exposed to the allergen.

The allergen attaches to two specific IgE antibodies on the mast cell surface.

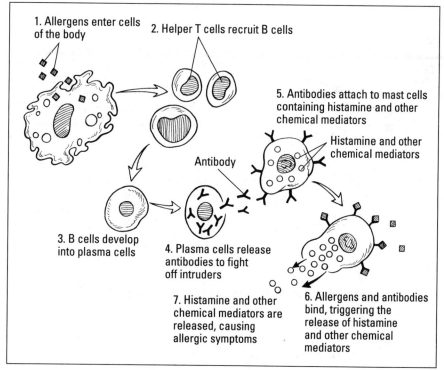

Figure 6-1:
The allergic inflammatory response is a complex process involving many types of cells.

1. Allergens enter cells of the body

2. Helper T cells recruit B cells

5. Antibodies attach to mast cells containing histamine and other chemical mediators

Histamine and other chemical mediators

Antibody

3. B cells develop into plasma cells

4. Plasma cells release antibodies to fight off intruders

7. Histamine and other chemical mediators are released, causing allergic symptoms

6. Allergens and antibodies bind, triggering the release of histamine and other chemical mediators

5. **The allergen cross-links to two specific IgE antibodies on the mast cell surface. This activates the mast cell to release its potent chemical mediators of inflammation, which affect various organs and trigger your allergic symptoms.**

In some cases, particularly with reactions to insect stings and penicillin, you may think that your allergic reaction was the result of just a single exposure. In most instances, however, you received a prior, sensitizing exposure, perhaps in one of the following ways:

- With regard to insect stings, you may have been stung as a child. If that experience wasn't traumatic and resulted only in a minor, localized reaction, you may have forgotten about it.

- Your first exposure to penicillin allergens may be even less memorable: The cow's milk or beef that you eat can include this antibiotic from the animal's feed.

Doing it one more time: The late-phase reaction

WARNING!

The allergic response consists of two phases involving inflammatory cells and powerful chemical substances. The immediate, early-phase reaction occurs within one hour of allergen exposure. An additional, late-phase reaction can occur in some people anywhere from three to eight hours after the early-phase reaction. The chemicals from the mast cells call eosinophils to action, to stage a second, rallying effort against the allergen, hours after you think you've recovered from asthma symptoms or an allergic episode. In some cases, this late-phase reaction can actually be more severe than the initial reaction.

Because antihistamines and quick-relief bronchodilators are only effective for dealing with early-phase reactions, your doctor may need to prescribe corticosteroids to control late-phase symptoms. Immunotherapy is a unique form of treatment that helps decrease both early- and late-phase reactions to allergen exposures, as I explain in "Reaping the Benefits of Immunology," later in this chapter.

Becoming hyperresponsive

Typically, if you're chronically exposed to an allergen — for instance, animal dander — you may find that during ragweed season, your symptoms appear to become more bothersome even at lower levels of exposure than you have experienced previously. By increasing your *allergen load* (your total level of exposure, at any one time, to any combination of allergens that trigger your allergies — see Chapter 10), other allergens and irritants may be more likely to also cause problems for you. In this case, eliminating animal dander from your home could result in fewer asthma and/or allergy symptoms during ragweed season.

Conversely, although your friend's cat may not be an issue for you most of the year, Fluffy's dander may trigger your asthma and/or allergic rhinitis symptoms during ragweed season. That's because exposure to the pollen causes you to develop a lower threshold for allergy symptoms (making you *hyperresponsive*) when exposed to this friendly feline.

Reacting nonspecifically

Another reaction complication that occurs from chronic allergen exposure is an increase in nonspecific reactivity. *Nonspecific reactivity* develops when your nasal passages and breathing airways become so inflamed and sensitized by repeated, constant exposure to triggering allergens that nonallergic irritants also cause reactions. Nonspecific irritants often include

- ✔ Tobacco smoke (from cigarettes, cigars, pipes)
- ✔ Fumes and scents from household cleaners, strongly scented soaps, and perfumes and colognes; from glues, solvents, and aerosols; and from unvented gas, oil, or kerosene stoves
- ✔ Smoke from wood-burning appliances or fireplaces
- ✔ Air pollution
- ✔ Gases, from chemicals found primarily in the workplace

Although the reactions triggered by irritants aren't IgE-mediated, they still increase injury to already sensitive areas. If you're continuously exposed to allergens and irritants, a vicious cycle can develop. The irritants compound the damage that allergic reactions cause, thus aggravating your affected areas further and increasing their sensitivities, resulting in more symptoms and further injury to your airways.

Reaping the Benefits of Immunology

Immunology provides great benefits for treating asthma and other allergic conditions, enabling doctors to modify your immune system's reactions to triggers of airway disease with immunotherapy (allergy shots). The immunologic response that results from immunotherapy promotes immune system actions that protect rather than damage your body, as I explain in Chapter 11.

Immunotherapy is the most effective way, in most cases, to treat the underlying causes of allergic ailments such as allergic asthma, allergic rhinitis (and allergic conjunctivitis), and allergies to insect stings.

Enhancing your future with immunology

The advances that medical science has made with immunology during the last century are among the greatest human achievements in the history of mankind, producing medical miracles that would've seemed like sheer fantasy 100 years ago. The continued progress in our understanding of immunology can enable medical researchers to find far more effective ways of preventing infectious diseases. Immunologic research has already helped control some forms of cancer with the use of interferons, anti-tumor antibody therapy, and other immunologic interventions.

In the quest for more effective medications to control asthma and other allergic disease symptoms, immunology has been the key to developing a new and innovative medication, based on using a high-tech antibody known as *recombinant human monoclonal antibody* (rhuMab), which is an anti-IgE antibody. The first drug in this class, omalizumab/ rhuMAb-E25 (Xolair) — recently approved by the FDA — binds immunologically with circulating IgE. This process prevents the binding of IgE to mast cells, thus blocking the initiation of the allergic reaction. (I discuss IgE antibodies more extensively in Chapter 17.)

The study of immunology matters a great deal to the whole human race. Physicians and scientists must continue to advance their knowledge about the immune system and unlock its secrets. The 21st century will see the development of vaccines for many serious diseases such as herpes; respiratory syncytial virus (RSV) infections, which cause bronchiolitis in infants (see Chapter 18); and the worldwide scourge of AIDS. Likewise, the 21st century will also result in the development of more effective forms of immunotherapy for allergies. Immunologic research may one day even produce a vaccine against allergies and asthma. (If that happens, and my patients no longer need my care, maybe I could fulfill my fantasy of trying out for a spot on the Senior Golf Tour.)

Chapter 7

Hay Fever and Asthma: The United Airway

*H*ay fever (known medically as *allergic rhinitis*) is the most common allergic disease in the United States and often coexists with asthma. As many as 45 million Americans may suffer from some form of hay fever, including 10 to 30 percent of all adults and up to 40 percent of all children. That's a lot of sneezing fits, runny noses, clogged sinuses, and itchy, watery eyes.

Hay fever affects so many people that the estimated costs of medical treatment, absenteeism, and lost productivity from this type of allergy are perhaps as high as $11 billion annually in the United States. U.S. schoolchildren with hay fever miss the equivalent of 1.5 million school days per year and are at an increased risk of

- ✔ Experiencing developmental delays (such as hearing and speech difficulties)

- ✔ Suffering from poor school performance (due to drowsiness and irritability)

- ✔ Developing learning disabilities (due to poor focus and concentration)

- ✔ Having emotional and behavioral problems

Rhinoids, rhinitis, and rhinos: It's all Greek to your nose

Rhinitis is the medical term for inflammation of the nasal mucous membranes. The word derives from *rhin,* the ancient Greek for nose — hence the rhinoceros with horns *(keros)* on its nose — but has no relation to the Rhine, although your nose may run like a river during allergy season.

The second part of the term, *itis,* means swelling or inflammation, as in *tonsillitis* (an inflammation of the tonsils) or *appendicitis* (an inflammation of the appendix), and of course — you guessed it — *rhinitis,* an inflamed nose. Here's some more nosy terminology that you can use to impress your friends and to better understand your doctor:

- **Rhinology:** The anatomy, pathology, and physiology of the nose

- **Rhinoscopy:** An examination of nasal passages

- **Rhinovirus:** A virus that causes respiratory disorders such as the common cold

- **Rhinopharyngitis:** An inflammation that affects the mucous membranes of the nose and throat

- **Rhinorrhea:** Runny nose

- **Rhinosinusitis:** An inflammation of the nose *and* sinuses

Although the effects of hay fever are rarely life-threatening (even though some people sometimes feel as if they could die when symptoms take hold), hay fever can still be a debilitating disease with serious consequences if you don't treat and manage it appropriately — especially if you have asthma. That's because the allergic reactions associated with hay fever are among the most serious and frequent triggers of respiratory symptoms in the vast majority of asthma patients. Your respiratory tract is what I like to call the *united airway,* and treating your nose is often essential in treating the underlying inflammation that characterizes asthma.

Catching Up with Your Runny Nose

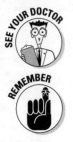

Although often called hay fever, allergic rhinitis itself doesn't cause a fever. If you do run a temperature while experiencing symptoms that resemble hay fever, you may actually be suffering from a viral or bacterial infection, such as sinusitis (see Chapter 2), influenza (flu), or pneumonia.

In order to effectively and appropriately manage hay fever, I strongly advise you to consider the following factors:

✔ **You're in it for the long-term:** This disease usually recurs persistently and indefinitely after you have become sensitized to the allergens (see Chapter 6) that trigger hay fever symptoms.

✔ **You need a healthy nose:** Because your nose is such a vital part of your respiratory system, your nasal health is vital to your overall wellness. Lack of treatment or ineffective or inappropriate management of hay fever can lead to complications such as nasal polyps (outgrowths of the nasal lining), sinusitis (inflammation of the sinuses; see Chapter 13), recurrent ear infections (potentially causing hearing loss; see Chapter 13), aggravation of bronchial symptoms, dental and facial abnormalities, poor speech development in children, and disruption of normal sleep patterns resulting in daytime fatigue.

Not only does your nose hold up your sunglasses, but it also provides other beneficial functions:

- Your nose helps to warm and humidify the air you breathe in.

- The interior of your nose acts to filter and cleanse the air you breathe in, through the action of the *cilia* (tiny hair-like projections of certain types of cells that sweep mucus through the nose).

- Your nose is also critical for your sense of smell and the quality of your voice. For example, when your nose is stuffy or congested, your voice often sounds different (often referred to as *nasal voice*).

✔ **You need to know why you're blowing your nose:** A proper diagnosis of your hay fever condition requires a review of your medical history, a physical examination, observation, analysis, and, in some cases, skin testing to identify the allergens involved, all to help determine the most effective course of treatment.

✔ **You need to avoid allergic triggers:** In many cases, the most effective and least expensive method of managing your hay fever is to avoid the allergens that trigger your symptoms. Although you may not be able to completely avoid all the allergens that cause your symptoms, partial avoidance may provide you with enough relief to substantially improve your quality of life (see Chapter 10 for avoidance information).

✔ **You should be cautious when using medications:** If you suffer from hay fever, you may resort to common first-generation, over-the-counter (OTC) antihistamines, decongestants, and nasal sprays to relieve your symptoms. However, many of these medications often produce significant side effects, including drowsiness (seriously limiting the safe use of these antihistamines), impaired vision, hypertension, nausea, gastric distress, constipation, insomnia, and irritability — and that's the short list. Besides creating more havoc in your life than allergic rhinitis already provides, these side effects can also be potentially dangerous. Overusing OTC decongestant nasal sprays can also lead to a condition known as *nasal rebound.* (See Chapter 12 for more on nasal rebound.)

Rose fever and other nose misnomers

Roses, like hay, receive a bad rap. Because these flowers tend to bloom in spring and summer when levels of wind-borne tree and grass pollens are usually at their peak, some hay fever sufferers mistakenly blame roses for causing allergy symptoms (hence the term *rose fever*). However, insects pollinate the most attractive, colorful plants — including roses. In contrast to lighter tree, weed, and grass pollen and mold spores, the pollen that these plants produce is a sticky, heavier pollen that's much less likely to become wind-borne.

In fact, among the more than 700 species of North American trees, only about 10 percent release pollens that trigger symptoms of allergic rhinitis. Please note, however, that if you're a gardener and/or a florist who maintains a consistently high exposure to many types of flowers (not just roses), you can become sensitized to pollen from flowering plants, resulting in a form of occupational allergic rhinitis.

✔ **Your doctor can prescribe new and improved medication:** In cases where avoidance doesn't provide you with sufficient relief, newer and safer prescription drugs — including second-generation nonsedating and less-sedating antihistamines and nasal sprays — are often effective and produce fewer side effects than their OTC counterparts. However, these prescription drugs are effective only if you follow your doctor's instructions and take them properly.

Classifying Types of Hay Fever

Hay fever is a common and nonspecific term for many varied types of allergic rhinitis, and it's often used in a general manner when discussing nasal inflammatory disorders, as well as for selling hay fever medications. Because the term *hay fever* describes so many different nasal inflammatory disorders, you may not be aware that allergists make distinctions between the different forms of allergic rhinitis. Allergists group these forms according to the various types and patterns of exposure.

The three principal classifications of hay fever are: seasonal allergic rhinitis; perennial allergic rhinitis, including perennial allergic rhinitis with seasonal *exacerbation* (worsening); and occupational allergic rhinitis.

Seasonal allergic rhinitis

Seasonal allergic rhinitis is the most common form of allergic rhinitis, with symptoms occurring at specific times of the year when particular pollen and/ or mold spore allergens are in the air. Hay fever symptoms can vary from year to year, however, due to climatic conditions and regional differences that affect the quality and quantity of pollen and mold spores in the environment. Hay fever symptoms can also vary because of the timing and types of exposure that you experience to these substances.

The levels of wind-borne tree, grass, and weed pollens are usually at their peak in the United States and Canada during the following times of year:

- ✔ **Late winter (warmer climates) to late spring:** Tree pollens.
- ✔ **Late spring to early summer:** Grass pollens.
- ✔ **Mid-summer to fall:** Weed pollens, especially ragweed, which accounts for up to three-quarters of seasonal allergic rhinitis cases in the United States. The presence of weed pollen may continue in warmer climates through December, in the absence of an early frost.

Wind-borne mold spores are present at various levels for most of the year, but they tend to cause a significant problem mostly during the late summer and fall. For more details on what's blowin' in the wind, turn to Chapter 10.

Perennial allergic rhinitis

Perennial allergic rhinitis is usually the result of your immune system becoming sensitized to a triggering agent or combination of agents that are constantly present in the environment, whether in the home, outdoors, at work or school, or other locations that you frequent. The symptoms involved in this condition can be just as severe as the symptoms of seasonal allergic rhinitis.

A season for all allergies

The term *allergy season* usually denotes the period from mid-spring to early summer, when a high concentration of airborne pollens and mold spores affects a significant number of sensitized people. Similarly, the period from late summer to fall, when weed pollens proliferate, is often termed *ragweed season*. However, no matter what the time of year, if enough allergenic pollen is present, it's going to be someone's allergy season. Allergists often use the term *pollination season* instead of *allergy season* to designate a period of time when significant amounts of tree, grass, or weed pollens are in the air.

We're not just making hay

The term *hay fever* is actually a misnomer, stemming from 19th-century studies of English farmers who mistakenly blamed spring hay cutting as the cause of nasal inflammatory ailments. Likewise, people in the 19th century referred to any ailment as a fever. In 1871, Charles H. Blackley identified airborne pollen from various plants — especially grasses — that depend on wind for cross-pollination as the primary cause of hay fever. The term "grass grief" didn't catch on, however, so we continue to use *hay fever* as a generic term for what doctors call *allergic rhinitis* — usually for the most common variety, *seasonal allergic rhinitis.*

During allergy or ragweed season, or at other times of the year when significant quantities of allergenic material are present, if you already have perennial allergic rhinitis, you may also experience a seasonal worsening of your allergies, resulting in even more disabling symptoms. Doctors refer to this condition as *perennial allergic rhinitis with seasonal exacerbation* (worsening). In some cases, consistent and long-term exposure to multiple allergens can also lead to *chronic allergic rhinitis,* which means that your allergy symptoms are severe on a constant basis.

Occupational allergic rhinitis

Occupational allergic rhinitis is more difficult to diagnose and treat because it often involves various combinations of a multitude of potential triggering agents and irritants found in many workplaces and occupations. Also, this specific type of hay fever often affects people with occupational asthma. (I provide details on occupational asthma in Chapter 5.) Your doctor should determine the following factors in the course of diagnosing occupational allergic rhinitis:

✔ Do your symptoms primarily occur at work? Or, if already present elsewhere, do your symptoms worsen while in the workplace?

✔ Do your symptoms disappear or improve after you leave work — at the end of the day; during weekends or vacations; when your work location changes; or if you take a new job?

✔ Do any of your colleagues and coworkers experience similar allergic symptoms?

What Makes Noses Run?

In addition to wind-borne grass, weed, and tree pollens and mold spores, other allergic and nonallergic rhinitis triggers found in indoor environments include

- Dust mite allergens

- Indoor mold growths

- Animal dander, saliva, and urine from warm-blooded pets such as dogs and cats

- Waste and remains of pests, such as mice, rats, and cockroaches

- Allergens found in workplaces, schools, or other indoor or enclosed locations that you frequent

- Allergenic substances, such as fibers, latex, wood dust, various chemicals, and many other items

As I explain in Chapter 6, many substances that don't trigger an allergic response from your body's immune system can still intensify allergy or asthma conditions. Allergists refer to these substances as *irritants.* Common types of irritants include tobacco smoke, aerosols, glue, household cleaners, perfumes and scents, and strongly scented soaps. In some cases, changes in weather conditions can trigger symptoms of rhinitis in susceptible individuals.

Getting a Medical Evaluation

I strongly advise anyone who experiences significant hay fever symptoms — especially if you have asthma — to consult a physician to determine whether those symptoms are the result of a form of allergic rhinitis, a nonallergic type of rhinitis, a sinus infection, or a respiratory disease. A proper diagnosis is critical for the effective and appropriate management of any of these conditions.

Understanding that sneezy, itchy, and runny feeling

Many allergic rhinitis sufferers mistakenly assume that they have lingering colds that afflict them every spring (or whenever the weather changes).

However, even though viral infections such as the common cold and flu may follow cyclical patterns, the frequency of these illnesses usually isn't as consistent or as constant as seasonal, perennial, or occupational allergic rhinitis. Symptoms associated with these forms of allergic rhinitis may often include

- Runny nose with clear, watery discharge
- Nasal congestion (stuffy nose)
- Sneezing
- Postnasal drip (nasal discharge down the back of your throat)
- Itchy, watery eyes (allergic conjunctivitis)
- Itchy nose, ears, and throat
- Persistent irritation of the mucous membranes of the eyes, middle ear, nose, and sinuses (in chronic cases)

Approximately half of all patients with allergic rhinitis experience additional clinical symptoms due to a *late-phase reaction* (see Chapter 6), occurring three to ten hours after allergen exposure, which typically leads to persistent symptoms, especially nasal congestion. The late-phase reaction is also implicated in *nonspecific reactivity* (increased sensitivity) of the nasal lining to nonallergic irritants (see Chapter 6).

Allergic rhinitis usually does *not* cause symptoms such as fever, sore throat, green or yellow thickened nasal drainage, achy muscles or joints, or tooth or eye pain. If you're experiencing these types of symptoms, the source of your ailment may be a type of viral or bacterial infection or the result of some physical factor, such as injury. Your doctor should evaluate your condition.

If you have a deviated (crooked) septum (the *septum* is the bony cartilage between your nostrils), it can block one or both sides of your nose, leading to a runny or congested nose. Because the resulting symptoms resemble allergic rhinitis, examination of your septum should be part of your physical examination. Surgical correction of a deviated septum may be necessary to relieve severe nasal airway obstruction.

Seeing red: Allergic conjunctivitis

Symptoms such as redness over your eyeballs and the underside of your eyelids, as well as swollen, itchy, and tearing eyes, are characteristic of what doctors refer to as *allergic conjunctivitis*. This ailment often coexists with allergic rhinitis, and most of the same allergens as those involved with allergic rhinitis can trigger seasonal or perennial outbreaks of this conjunctivitis.

Telltale signs: Salutes, shiners, and creases

The symptoms of allergic rhinitis that I list in this chapter often produce a distinctive combination of gestures and facial features, particularly in children and adolescents. If you or someone close to you seems to suffer from allergic rhinitis, keep these sufferer-specific characteristics in mind. These physical signs are often so unique that I can usually tell, when looking in the waiting room, who are the likely allergic rhinitis sufferers. When my children were younger, I noticed similar traits among their friends who had allergies as well. The following gestures and facial formations are characteristics that you and your doctor should look for to help diagnose your specific condition:

✔ **Allergic salute:** As tempting as it may be to consider this gesture a sign of respect for your doctor, the allergic salute actually describes the way that most people use the palm of their hand to rub and raise the tip of their nose to relieve nasal itching and congestion (and possibly to wipe away some mucus).

✔ **Allergic shiner:** Allergic rhinitis symptoms can really beat up some patients. Dark circles under the eyes, due to the swelling and discoloration caused by congestion of small blood vessels beneath the skin in this area, can give you the appearance of having gone a few rounds with Mike Tyson.

✔ **Allergic (adenoidal) face:** Allergic rhinitis may cause swelling of the *adenoids* (lymph tissue that lines the back of the throat and extends behind the nose), resulting in a sort of tired and droopy appearance.

✔ **Nasal crease:** This line across the bridge of the nose is usually the result — particularly in children — of rubbing the nose (allergic salute) to relieve nasal congestion and itching.

✔ **Mouth breathing:** Cases of allergic rhinitis in which severe nasal congestion occurs can result in chronic mouth breathing, leading to the development of a high, arched palate, an elevated upper lip, and an overbite. (This symptom is one of the main reasons why so many teens with allergic rhinitis wind up at the orthodontist.)

All that drips isn't allergic

Many people think that runny, congested noses and sneezing are always the result of an allergic reaction. However, be aware that rhinitis also comes in nonallergic flavors, such as the following types:

✔ **Infectious:** Upper respiratory viral ailments such as the common cold are often the cause of acute or chronic nasal distress.

✔ **Hormonal:** Women may experience severe nasal congestion while taking birth control pills, as well as during ovulation or during pregnancy — most notably from the second month to the full term. In pregnancy cases, congested nose symptoms usually disappear after delivery.

✔ **Emotional:** Women and men may experience runny and congested noses during sexual arousal. Other intensely emotional situations (such as laughing or crying) can also provoke your nose to run or congest.

✔ **Vasomotor:** The most typical examples of this form of nonallergic rhinitis are the nasal congestion, runny nose, and sneezing that can occur as a result of sudden weather or temperature changes (for example, a blast of cold air). Exposure to bright lights or irritants, such as tobacco smoke, perfume, bleach, paint fumes, newsprint, automotive emissions, and solvents, can also trigger vasomotor rhinitis.

✔ **Drug-induced:** Anti-hypertensives (medications for high blood pressure), as well as aspirin and nonsteroidal anti-inflammatory drugs (NSAIDs) like ibuprofen, can also induce symptoms of a runny or congested nose. Overusing OTC nasal decongestant sprays (Afrin, Neo-Synephrine) can lead to chronic drug-induced nasal congestion (due to nasal rebound from the medication), a condition that doctors describe as *rhinitis medicamentosa*. Abused illegal drugs, such as cocaine, can also produce rhinitis symptoms.

✔ **Gustatory:** Hot, spicy foods — especially those with serious peppers — can provoke watery eyes, runny noses, and sneezing (and temporarily clear sinuses in the process — whew!). Beer, wine, and other types of alcoholic drinks can also produce these sorts of symptoms in some people. This type of immediate, localized nonallergic reaction to certain types of cuisine and alcoholic beverages isn't the same as the more complex allergic process that occurs with a food allergy, as I explain in Chapter 8.

In order to effectively diagnose your condition, a physician must review your medical history, as well as your family's history of allergies, and perform a physical examination. If your family doctor suspects a form of allergic rhinitis, he will probably refer you to a specialist, such as an allergist (someone like me) or an otolaryngologist (an ear, nose, and throat doctor), in the following situations:

✔ If clarification and identification of the triggers of your condition are needed

✔ If the management of your allergic or nonallergic rhinitis isn't resulting in a substantial improvement of your condition, due to inadequate treatment and/or adverse reactions to medications

✔ If you need to find out how to avoid allergens and irritants that may be triggering your symptoms (see Chapter 10)

✔ If your rhinitis or side effects of medications for the condition impair your abilities to perform in your career or occupation (especially in operating an airplane or motor vehicle)

✔ If the disease has a significant adverse effect on your quality of life by affecting your comfort and well-being

✔ If rhinitis complications develop, such as sinusitis, *otitis* (ear inflammation), and facial signs (see the "Telltale signs: Salutes, shiners, and creases" sidebar, in this chapter)

✔ If you have coexisting conditions such as recurring or chronic sinusitis (see Chapter 13), asthma (see Chapter 2) or another respiratory condition, otitis (see Chapter 13), or nasal polyps

✔ If your doctor needs to prescribe oral (systemic) corticosteroids (see Chapter 12) to control your symptoms

✔ If your symptoms last more than three months

✔ If your medication costs are a financial hardship

Knowing what the doctor's looking for

In addition to performing a general observation to check for the hallmarks of allergic rhinitis (see the sidebar "Telltale signs: Salutes, shiners, and creases," in this chapter), your doctor will most likely examine the following areas:

✔ The front of your nose, to check for an allergic crease and the condition of your *septum* (the "great divide" of cartilage between your nostrils).

✔ Your nasal passages, to check for swelling of the nasal *turbinates* (protruding tissues that line the interior of the nose — see Figure 7-1), nasal *polyps* (pale, round or pear-shaped, smooth, gelatinous outgrowths of the nasal lining), congestion, and the character, color, and amount of secretions from your nose.

✔ The inside of your mouth and the back of your throat for redness, swelling, enlarged or diseased tonsils, and to check drainage from the nasal cavity. In addition, your doctor may check for the presence of a high arched palate and/or *malocclusion* (misalignment of jaw and teeth, due to mouth breathing and tongue thrusting).

✔ Your neck and face, to check for lumps and sensitive, painful, or numb areas.

✔ Your eyes and ears, for signs of inflammation and/or infection.

✔ If indicated, further examination may include checking your vocal cords, adenoids, sinuses, and *Eustachian tubes* (the connection between your middle ear, nose, and throat that causes your ears to pop when descending in an airplane).

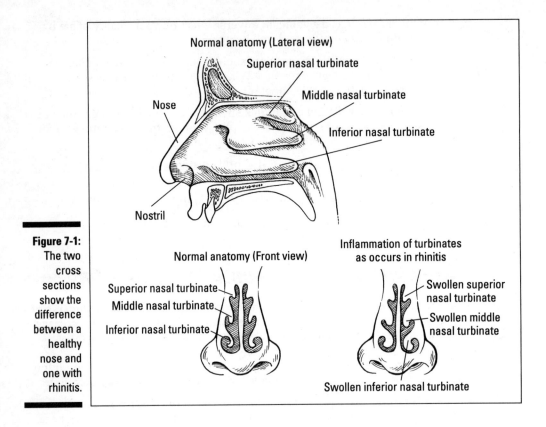

In addition to evaluating your physiological condition, your physician also attempts to determine

- ✔ The pattern, frequency, and seasonal variations of the allergic reactions that you experience.

- ✔ The types of allergens and irritants to which you may be exposed at home, work, school, friends' and relatives' homes, and other locations that you frequent, such as malls, theaters, restaurants, and even modes of transport, such as vehicles, trains, boats, and airplanes.

Doing your part

You can also keep track of when and where your allergic symptoms occur in order to help with the diagnostic process. For example, you may experience mild but manageable hay fever symptoms when visiting friends who have dogs and cats. However, you may find that, on occasion, your symptoms from those visits are more severe.

Skin tests: The gold standard

Your doctor may also need to conduct allergy skin tests to confirm and identify the specific allergens that trigger your condition. In some cases, skin testing can also indicate your level of sensitivity to the allergens that bother you. A skin test procedure generally involves the doctor placing a drop of a suspected allergen on your skin and then using a device that pricks, punctures, or scratches the area to see whether the allergen produces a reaction. If you're allergic to that specific allergen, your skin reacts in a way that resembles a mosquito bite or hive. If you're on pins and needles to gather more information about skin tests, see Chapter 11.

If you can track the times and dates of your allergic episodes, you can greatly help your doctor in determining whether the presence of seasonal allergens such as ragweed may worsen your condition by increasing your allergen load (see Chapter 10).

Managing Rhinitis

Three basic approaches exist for treating and managing allergies, including forms of allergic rhinitis.

Avoiding allergens

Benjamin Franklin once advised, "An ounce of prevention is worth a pound of cure." Eliminating (or at least lessening) your exposure to allergens and irritants can often result in less severe symptoms and less need for medication. In Chapter 10, I give you more detailed advice on what allergens and irritants to avoid and how to avoid them, especially in your home and bedroom, where most people spend the greater parts of their lives.

Treating with medications

Pharmacotherapy is the term doctors use for treating patients with medications. This form of therapy is particularly important in allergic diseases, because complete avoidance of allergens can be difficult. Therefore, your doctor may also recommend or prescribe one or more medications to help manage your condition, depending on the nature and severity of your symptoms, occupation, age, and other factors that your physician may assess. I provide an in-depth analysis of these products and their recommended uses and side effects in Chapter 12.

Treating the cause of your allergies

If your doctor concludes that avoidance and drug therapies don't provide effective results, and if the severity of your symptoms or the nature of your occupation warrants it, your doctor may advise you to consider *immunotherapy,* otherwise known as *desensitization, hyposensitization,* or just plain-old *allergy shots.* Immunotherapy treatment for allergic rhinitis generally requires at least three years of injections. (For an in-depth discussion of immunotherapy, turn to Chapter 11.)

Considering special cases

Certain groups of hay fever patients require more specialized treatment and consideration. These groups include

- ✔ **Children:** Oral antihistamines and mast cell stabilizer sprays (nasal cromolyn, such as Nasalcrom) are currently the first medication options for younger patients who experience allergic rhinitis symptoms. Your family doctor may also consider prescription nasal corticosteroid sprays (Flonase, Rhinocort AQ).

- ✔ **Elderly people:** Doctors generally advise that elderly patients use nonsedating antihistamines, which produce fewer significant side effects, instead of first-generation OTC antihistamine products (see Chapter 12 for details about allergic rhinitis medications). In addition, nasal corticosteroids are often recommended for elderly patients. Doctors often warn patients (usually in the elderly age group) with insomnia, prostate problems, hypertension, and heart conditions to avoid taking oral decongestants because the medications can possibly aggravate their preexisting medical problems.

- ✔ **Pregnant women:** Physicians often consider mast cell stabilizer sprays (nasal cromolyn, such as Nasalcrom) as the first medication option for the relief of allergic rhinitis symptoms among pregnant women. During the first trimester of pregnancy, your doctor may advise you to avoid oral decongestants. However, after the first trimester of pregnancy, your doctor may recommend antihistamines such as chlorpheniramine (Chlor-Trimeton), loratadine (Claritin), cetirizine (Zyrtec), and/or nasal corticosteroids such as budesonide (Rhinocort AQ).

✔ **Athletes:** Your doctor needs to make sure that any recommended or prescribed OTC or prescription product isn't on any sports federation's list of banned substances. The U.S. Olympic Committee (USOC) and the International Olympic Committee ban the use of all oral and nasal decongestants and oral corticosteroids. In addition, some international sports federations also ban the use of oral antihistamines. Using other nasal products may require written approval by governing sports bodies. Obviously, whether the use of a product is governed or not, if you're an athlete, you need to avoid any medication that may adversely affect your performance or give you an unfair competitive advantage.

Chapter 8

Food Allergies and Asthma

● ●

In This Chapter

▶ Categorizing adverse food reactions

▶ Investigating allergic and nonallergic food hypersensitivities

▶ Understanding how food intolerance differs from food hypersensitivity

▶ Getting medical attention for severe food reactions

▶ Preventing allergic food reactions

● ●

*I*f the food you eat bites you back with fits of wheezing, outbreaks of eczema, gastric distress, or other symptoms (perhaps even including life-threatening bouts of anaphylactic shock), you're not alone. Adverse food reactions affect at least one in four Americans at some point in their lives. Food allergies can even trigger asthma symptoms that, in some cases, cause life-threatening respiratory symptoms in certain susceptible asthmatics.

However, not all food ingredients that can cause adverse reactions are triggers of *food hypersensitivity* (the more precise term for *food allergy*). Even though 40 percent of Americans believe that their unfortunate gastronomical experiences result from allergies to certain foods, most cases involve various forms of food intolerance, food poisoning, and other types of nonallergic conditions.

Types of Adverse Food Reactions

Because the range of adverse food reactions can include a constellation of nasal, respiratory, skin, gastrointestinal, and oral symptoms occurring separately or in combination, doctors usually classify these reactions according to the mechanisms that the reactions involve.

The following list summarizes the two main classifications of adverse food reactions:

✔ **Food hypersensitivity:** These reactions occur when your immune system responds to specific proteins in certain foods. The reactions can include allergic mechanisms involving IgE antibodies (see Chapter 1) as well as nonallergic mechanisms.

  • Allergic food hypersensitivities include gastrointestinal (GI) tract allergies, hives and other allergic skin reactions, and even *anaphylaxis* (a severe, abrupt reaction that affects many organs of the body simultaneously and can potentially be life-threatening).

  • Nonallergic food hypersensitivities (sometimes referred to as *non-IgE food reactions*) include syndromes such as food-induced enterocolitis, colitis, and malabsorption, as well as celiac disease, dermatitis herpetiformis, and pulmonary hypersensitivity. I discuss these medical conditions in greater detail in "Nonallergic (Non-IgE) Food Hypersensitivities," later in this chapter.

✔ **Food intolerance:** These types of reactions result from nonallergic, non-immunologic responses to offending substances in various foods. Forms of food intolerance include

  • Lactose intolerance

  • Pharmacologic food reactions

  • Metabolic food reactions

  • Food additive reactions

  • Food poisoning

  • Toxic reactions

Although allergic reactions to food can be severe (and should be appropriately diagnosed and managed), the actual number of adults in the United States who suffer from true food hypersensitivities is closer to 1 percent of the population. However, food allergies may affect as many as 6 percent of infants and children, with allergic reactions to peanuts topping the list of triggers of severe, even life-threatening respiratory symptoms in some children with asthma. According to one recent study of life-threatening asthma attacks, half of the children hospitalized in these cases had food hypersensitivities, especially to peanuts.

Allergic Food Hypersensitivities

In the case of *IgE-mediated food hypersensitivity,* commonly known as a *food allergy,* your immune system cooks up specific IgE antibodies (see Chapter 1) against specific allergens. The level of exposure required for your immune system to be sensitized to a particular food varies, depending on the allergens involved. The major food allergens that have been identified are mostly proteins, often found in the following foods:

- ✔ Peanuts (the leading cause of severe allergic food reactions), soybeans, peas, lentils, beans and other legumes, and foods containing these products as ingredients. Because a wide variety of foods include peanuts and soybean products as ingredients, these legumes often act as hidden triggers of food allergies. See the section "Anaphylaxis and allergic food reations," later in this chapter, for more information on peanut issues. Likewise, you can find details on uncovering hidden allergenic ingredients in many common foods in "Avoiding Adverse Food Reactions," later in this chapter.

- ✔ Shellfish, such as shrimp, lobster, crab, clams, and oysters.

- ✔ Fish — both freshwater and saltwater.

- ✔ Tree nuts, including almonds, Brazil nuts, cashews, hazelnuts, and walnuts.

- ✔ Eggs, especially egg whites, which contain the predominant allergenic proteins, ovalbumin, and ovomucoid. The yolk is less allergenic than the egg white.

- ✔ Cow's milk and products that contain milk protein fractions, such as *casein* (80 percent of the protein in cow's milk) and whey, which includes lactalbumin and lactoglobulin.

- ✔ Wheat, an important ingredient in bran, malt, wheat flour, graham flour, wheat germ, and wheat starch. Corn, rice, barley, oats, and other grains and cereals are less common food allergy triggers.

Of these culprits, the products that trigger allergic food reactions in children most frequently are milk, eggs, peanuts, tree nuts, fish, soy, and wheat. In adults, the likeliest causes of allergic food reactions include fish, shellfish, peanuts, and tree nuts.

Although most children lose their sensitivity to milk and eggs by age 3, food allergies involving peanuts, fish, shellfish, and tree nuts can last a lifetime.

Additives and allergies

Allergic mechanisms may or may not play a part in some adverse food reactions commonly associated with food additives. When additives are in the picture, identifying a suspected food allergen can get complicated, because finding out whether the food itself or the additive causes the problem is often difficult.

Additives, such as sulfites, are often used as antioxidants to preserve wine, dried fruit, shrimp, and potatoes. These additives have been implicated in cases of allergic food hypersensitivities, including potentially life-threatening *bronchospasm* (constriction of the airways) and asthma symptoms, especially in severe asthmatics who require long-term treatment with oral corticosteroids. (See Chapter 15 for information on long-term asthma therapy and these types of medications.)

Exposure to sulfites, when used in salad bars and in the guacamole served in some restaurants, can trigger asthma symptoms in susceptible asthmatics when they inhale the sulfite fumes from treated foods. These antioxidant additives are sometimes used to prevent discoloration and to keep greens looking perky. That's why some salad bar lettuce — which may sit out for hours during the day — doesn't seem to wilt, unlike the salads most of us prepare at home.

The U.S. Food and Drug Administration (FDA) prohibits using sulfites on fresh fruits and vegetables meant to be eaten raw (like with a salad bar) and requires manufacturers to label products that contain sulfites. However, precut or peeled potato products used in some restaurants to make common side dishes (such as french fries and hash browns) may still contain sulfites. Therefore, if you have asthma, always ask questions about the food served in restaurants.

You may need to actually speak with the people preparing your food, such as the chef, or perhaps with a restaurant manager who has precise information on what are the various dishes' ingredients. Your food server may not have many of those details. If you're unable to determine whether or not sulfites are being used in certain dishes, you may want to avoid ordering those items altogether.

Doctors often need to be detectives to determine the causes of adverse food reactions. For example, if you experience an adverse food reaction to a hot dog, your doctor must determine whether your reaction is because of allergens in the meat, or whether you're suffering from hot dog headache due to nitrites used to retard meat spoilage, or even whether you're reacting to an added food dye that creates the pink coloring.

Other, less obvious sources of food allergens may possibly cause adverse reactions in a smaller number of susceptible individuals. These much less frequently problematic food allergens (listed in family groupings to keep it all in the family) include the following:

- ✔ **Goosefoot family:** Spinach, beets, Swiss chard, pigweed
- ✔ **Gourd family:** Watermelon, honeydew, cantaloupe, other melons, pumpkins, squash

- ✔ **Lily family:** Onions, leeks, garlic, asparagus
- ✔ **Mustard family:** Broccoli, cabbage, cauliflower, horseradish, turnip, radish, mustard
- ✔ **Nightshade family:** Tomatoes, potatoes, eggplant, bell pepper, red pepper
- ✔ **Plum family:** Apricots, cherries, peaches, almonds, plums

How allergic food hypersensitivities develop

Atopy, the genetic predisposition to develop allergies, is a significant factor in the development of food allergies. An infant's immune system can begin responding to food allergens soon after birth.

As I explain in Chapter 1, your inherited tendency to develop allergies can express itself in other allergic conditions also, such as *allergic rhinitis* (hay fever, see Chapter 7) and *atopic dermatitis* (eczema). The predisposition toward allergies passes between generations, but the specific allergies themselves may not. Therefore, Mom may be allergic to lobster, Junior may break out in hives after eating peanuts, and baby Betty may get congested after drinking cow's milk formula.

The severity of your symptoms may also depend on your sensitivity level to particular food allergens and the quantities of these foods you consume. In some cases, ingesting small amounts of these foods may not trigger adverse reactions.

Gastrointestinal tract allergies

Allergic reactions involving the digestive system can develop within a few minutes to several hours after ingesting food allergens, and they frequently result in abdominal pain, vomiting, and diarrhea. The most significant classifications of gastrointestinal (GI) allergies include

- ✔ **Gastrointestinal food hypersensitivity reaction:** This reaction generally occurs with other atopic conditions, such as allergic rhinitis and atopic dermatitis, and can cause nausea, stomach pain, vomiting, and, in some cases, diarrhea. In rare cases, a widespread systemic reaction such as anaphylaxis can also result. (See "Anaphylaxis and allergic food reactions," later in this chapter.)

✔ **Cow's milk allergy:** More than 2 percent of infants develop allergies to the proteins casein and whey (including lactalbumin and lactoglobulin) in cow's milk, resulting in adverse reactions (such as colic, vomiting, and diarrhea) even to minute amounts of these proteins. This reaction isn't the same as the more familiar syndrome known as *lactose intolerance,* which is a nonallergic, nonimmunologic response rather than an IgE-mediated reaction.

✔ **Allergic eosinophilic gastroenteropathy:** This rare condition can cause nausea and vomiting following meals, abdominal pain, and diarrhea. If not managed effectively, this type of allergy can result in *malabsorption* (poor absorption of food nutrients) and malnutrition, leading potentially to stunted or slowed growth in infants and weight loss in adults.

✔ **Oral allergy syndrome:** If you have allergic rhinitis, you may also experience oral allergy symptoms after consuming certain fresh fruits and raw vegetables. This cross-reactivity syndrome can occur if you're sensitive to ragweed pollen (with bananas and melons such as cantaloupe, honeydew, and watermelon), birch pollen (with apples, carrots, potatoes, hazelnuts, and members of the plum family), and mugwort pollen (with celery, apples, and kiwi fruit). Your symptoms may include severe itching and swelling of the lips, tongue, and palate, as well as blistering of the throat and the mouth's mucus lining.

Because these fruits and vegetables seem to trigger reactions only in their raw state, you may be able to consume these foods in cooked or frozen forms. However, make sure that you check with your doctor before you cook up that vegetable stir-fry or cool off with a melon sorbet.

Hives and other food-related skin reactions

Allergic food hypersensitivities involving IgE antibodies can also trigger skin reactions in people whose atopic predisposition shows up through skin conditions. These conditions include

✔ *Atopic dermatitis* **(eczema):** Eggs, milk, peanuts, tree nuts, soybean, and wheat can contribute to outbreaks in more than one-third of children affected by this skin condition.

✔ *Urticaria* **(hives):** These itchy welts can erupt from various types of reactions to many foods including peanuts, tree nuts, milk, eggs, fish, shellfish, soybeans, and fruits, as well as food additives such as sodium benzoates, sulfites, and food dyes. Skin contact with raw meats, fish, vegetables, and fruit can also trigger hives. Allergic-food hypersensitivities are more likely to act as triggers of *rapid-onset urticaria* (a particularly quick and severe eruption of hives) in children than in adults. Food-related exercise-induced anaphylaxis, which I discuss later in this chapter, can also trigger hives and angioedema.

> ✔ *Angioedema:* Also known as *deep swellings,* this condition results in deeper tissue inflammation and skin swelling, and is more likely to produce painful and burning sensations rather than itching. Angioedema can erupt as a reaction to the same food allergens that trigger hives.

In severe cases of hives and angioedema, symptoms can also include swelling of the tongue, throat, airway, and difficulty swallowing, as well as fainting. If angioedema affects your face, the swelling may potentially lead to breathing difficulties. If you experience swelling of your airway, get emergency care immediately.

Anaphylaxis and allergic food reactions

The most extreme of all allergic food symptoms is *anaphylaxis.* This abrupt, systemic allergic reaction, often caused by the same foods that trigger hives and angioedema, affects several organs simultaneously and can quickly turn life-threatening. In recent years, the incidence of this severe, and sometimes fatal, reaction has been rising at an alarming rate among asthmatics, with most of these episodes due to accidental ingestion of peanuts, tree nuts, or seafood.

What is particularly disturbing is the fact that so many of these known high-risk patients are aware of their diagnosis but still don't carry appropriate emergency medication, such as an epinephrine kit, when they experience their anaphylactic reaction, or don't receive immediate, potentially life-saving emergency care in time.

As I explain in the "Preparing for emergency treatment for anaphylaxis" section, if you're an asthma patient or susceptible to food allergy-related anaphylactic reactions, keep emergency medication with you at all times. Wear a MedicAlert bracelet, especially for children in school.

Generalized urticaria (Total body hives)

Generalized urticaria (widespread hives occurring simultaneously over much of your body surface area) can often be the initial symptom of impending anaphylaxis and can result in a sudden swelling *(angioedema)* of the lips, eyelids, tongue, and windpipe *(laryngeal edema),* as well as wheezing and dizziness. This particularly dangerous reaction can quickly progress to anaphylaxis, leading to shock, hypotension, *arrhythmia* (irregular heartbeat), and even cardiorespiratory arrest. In rare cases, this type of reaction can be fatal.

Common triggers of total body hives include foods such as peanuts and shellfish (in people who have extreme hypersensitivities to these foods), severe allergic reactions to medications such as penicillin and related compounds, generalized hypersensitivity to latex, and/or extreme sensitivities to insect stings, including those of honeybees, yellow jackets, wasps, hornets, and fire ants.

Food-dependent exercise-induced anaphylaxis

Food-dependent exercise-induced anaphylaxis, a variant of exercise-induced anaphylaxis — which I explain in Chapter 9 — can occur when you exercise within three to four hours after eating a particular food. Two forms of this condition exist.

✔ You may develop anaphylaxis if you ingest particular foods, especially celery, shellfish, wheat, fruit, milk, or fish, prior to exercise. If you experience this reaction and you can identify the specific foods that trigger your episodes, your doctor may advise allergy skin testing (see Chapter 11) to confirm your sensitivity to the suspected foods.

✔ You may develop anaphylaxis while exercising, regardless of the type of food you've consumed.

Avoiding peanut problems in children

As a parent of a peanut-allergic child, you need to pay close attention to products that may contain peanuts, because they can potentially cause life-threatening anaphylactic reactions in children (as well as adults) who are extremely allergic to this food.

Keep these important points in mind about peanuts and children:

✔ Many foods contain peanuts as a not-so-obvious added ingredient. Therefore, examine all food labels for peanut ingredients and carefully select menu items when dining out with a child who is allergic to peanuts. (See "Avoiding Adverse Food Reactions," later in this chapter, for more information on foods that contain peanuts.) You may want to pack your child's lunch to reduce the risk of your child unknowingly consuming foods with minute traces of peanuts in school lunches.

✔ Because so many foods include peanuts as ingredients, instruct your young child not only to avoid peanuts but also never to accept foods — particularly snacks and candy bars — from others, especially playmates and young siblings.

✔ Because the peanut food allergy issue has received widespread media attention, some airlines are introducing peanut-free flights. If you suffer from food allergies of any kind, however, ask questions about the food on your flight, even if the airline claims that no peanuts or peanut ingredients are in the snacks or meals.

✔ A child who has a peanut hypersensitivity should wear a MedicAlert bracelet, especially at school. Also, ask your family doctor about supplying your child's school with an emergency epinephrine kit. Make sure school personnel know how and when to administer this medication.

Preparing for emergency treatment for anaphylaxis

If you're prone to anaphylaxis, carry injectable epinephrine with you at all times and receive emergency care as soon as possible after an attack occurs. Make sure you have an emergency plan in place that includes the following items:

- ✔ Medications your doctor has prescribed for you in the event of an anaphylactic reaction
- ✔ A list of your symptoms
- ✔ A written treatment plan prepared by your physician
- ✔ Your physician's name and contact information

If you're treated for anaphylaxis, don't be surprised if you continue to be observed in the emergency room for several hours after responding to initial rescue therapy. Unfortunately, in a few cases, patients who have responded well to initial anaphylaxis treatment have been immediately discharged from the emergency room but within a few hours have experienced a severe late-phase, or second reaction, known as *biphasic anaphylaxis.*

Ask your doctor whether an emergency epinephrine kit, such as an EpiPen (or EpiPen Jr. for children under 66 pounds), with an injectable dose of epinephrine, is advisable for you or your child. Parents and caregivers of children under 30 pounds (about 14 kilograms), who are too small for the dose of a pre-loaded EpiPen Jr., should be taught how to properly administer the correct dose of epinephrine by syringe to their infant or young child. Wear a MedicAlert bracelet or necklace in case you're unable to speak during a reaction. The appendix provides more information on how to obtain these items.

Managing and preventing anaphylaxis

Food hypersensitivity is a leading cause of anaphylaxis. Current estimates are that as many as 125 people in the United States die each year from food-induced anaphylactic reactions. As you may expect, the most effective long-term method for preventing food-induced anaphylactic reactions is to avoid eating foods that trigger the reaction. I provide more details on avoiding food allergens and establishing a safe diet in "Avoiding Adverse Food Reactions," later in this chapter.

If your child suffers from food-induced anaphylaxis, notify babysitters, relatives, other children's parents, daycare workers, teachers, and other school personnel of your child's sensitivities.

Nonallergic (Non-IgE) Food Hypersensitivities

You can also have food hypersensitivity from immune system reactions that don't involve the production of IgE antibodies. The most significant nonallergic food reactions include the following:

✔ **Food-induced enterocolitis syndrome:** This condition primarily occurs in infants between 1 and 3 months of age. Characteristic symptoms include prolonged vomiting and diarrhea, often resulting in dehydration. Triggers are usually the proteins in formulas that contain cow's milk or soy substitutes. Occasionally, breastfed infants may also suffer from this syndrome, presumably as the result of a protein ingested by the mother and transferred to the infant in maternal milk. Similar symptoms can occur in older children and adults in response to eggs, rice, wheat, and peanuts. However, most children outgrow this type of hypersensitivity by their third birthday.

✔ **Food-induced colitis:** Cow's milk and soy protein hypersensitivity have been implicated in this disorder, which can occur in the first few months of life and is usually diagnosed through the presence of blood in the stools, either seen by the naked eye or hidden *(occult),* of children who otherwise appear healthy. This condition often diminishes after 6 months to 2 years if children avoid the implicated food allergens.

Feeding a hypoallergenic formula to your baby may help overcome food-induced colitis.

✔ *Malabsorption syndrome:* This condition involves hypersensitivities to proteins in foods such as cow's milk, soy, wheat and other cereal grains, and eggs. Symptoms include diarrhea, vomiting, and weight loss or failure to gain weight.

✔ *Celiac disease:* This condition is a more serious form of malabsorption syndrome, and it can cause intestinal inflammation. Symptoms range from diarrhea and abdominal cramping to anemia and osteoporosis. Celiac disease only seems to occur in people who inherit an atopic predisposition. Affected individuals develop a hypersensitivity to a component of gluten called *gliadin,* which you find in wheat, oats, rye, and barley. If you suffer from this syndrome, however, you're not necessarily doomed to a life without pasta and pancakes. Resourceful sufferers of celiac disease have come up with many gluten-free products, ranging from beer to pretzels.

✔ *Dermatitis herpetiformis:* This condition is a non-IgE-mediated food hypersensitivity to gluten that produces skin eruptions in addition to causing intestinal inflammation. Typical symptoms include a chronic, itchy rash that appears primarily on the elbows, knees, and buttocks, although the disease can affect other areas as well.

✔ ***Pulmonary hypersensitivity:*** This rare condition, induced by cow's milk, primarily affects young children. Characteristic symptoms include a chronic cough, wheezing, and severe anemia. Removing the offending dairy products from the diet can substantially alleviate symptoms.

Understanding the Differences between Food Allergy and Food Intolerance

As I explain earlier in this chapter, many adverse food reactions don't involve an immune system response. These types of direct, nonimmunologic reactions are considered signs and symptoms of food intolerance and include the conditions that I explain in the following sections.

Lactose intolerance

If you're lactose intolerant, odds are your body doesn't produce sufficient amounts of the lactase enzyme in order for you to properly digest cow's milk. If you drink milk or consume foods with high milk content, you may experience stomach cramps, bloating, nausea, gas, and diarrhea.

Avoiding cow's milk and cow's milk products or adding the lactase enzyme to those foods are the standard ways of managing lactose intolerance. In contrast with the cow's-milk allergy (which I mention earlier in "Allergic Food Hypersensitivities"), you may be able to consume small quantities of cow's milk without suffering an adverse reaction.

Metabolic food reactions

In some cases, eating average or normal amounts of particular foods (especially fatty foods) may disrupt your digestive system. These disruptions, called *metabolic food reactions,* may be caused by

✔ Medications (for example, antibiotics) you're taking for illnesses

✔ A disease or condition (such as a gastrointestinal virus) that may affect your digestive system

✔ Malnutrition (for example, due to vitamin or enzyme deficiency)

Always remember to ask your doctor if any medication you're taking might disrupt your digestive system.

Pharmacologic food reactions

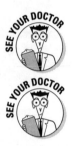

More serious forms of metabolic food reactions can result if you combine certain foods and drugs that don't mix well. Beware of the following potentially dangerous combinations:

- ✔ Grapefruit juice, which is usually harmless, sometimes causes harmful interactions when taken with calcium channel blockers, such as Procardia.

  If you have a heart condition, ask your doctor about possible interactions between grapefruit juice and any over-the-counter (OTC) or prescription antihistamines you may take.

- ✔ If you take blood-thinning drugs such as Coumadin, check with your doctor before eating foods rich in vitamin K like broccoli, spinach, and turnip greens, because they can reduce the medications' effectiveness.

- ✔ A harmful potassium buildup can occur if you overindulge on bananas while taking ACE inhibitors, such as Capoten and Vasotec.

- ✔ Avoid foods high in tyramine, such as cheese and sausage, if you take MAO inhibitors, because the combination can cause a potentially fatal rise in blood pressure. Tyramine may also aggravate or trigger migraine headaches.

- ✔ The caffeine in coffee, tea, and colas can interact badly with ulcer medications such as Tagamet, Zantac, and Pepcid AC. If your doctor prescribes theophylline for your asthma, reduce your caffeine intake, because caffeine can worsen side effects, such as GI irritation, headache, jitteriness, and sleeplessness.

Food additive reactions

Doctors associate many types of food additives with adverse food reactions. The most frequently implicated food additives are

- ✔ **Monosodium glutamate (MSG):** When consumed in large quantities, this flavor enhancer reportedly causes burning sensations, facial pressure, chest pain, headache, and, in rare cases, severe asthma symptoms. Although many sufferers associate these types of reactions with eating Chinese or other types of Asian foods, no conclusive studies have determined a clear link between consuming MSG and adverse food reactions. In any event, with the recent increase of MSG-free restaurants in many parts of the United States, you should have no trouble finding a place to chow down on chow mein without suffering ill effects.

✔ **Tartrazine (yellow dye No. 5):** This and other food dyes can aggravate chronic hives and may actually be an ingredient in the very same children's syrups used to treat allergic symptoms such as hives — another good reason to always check medication labels.

✔ **Sulfites:** Commonly found in processed foods and almost always in wines, sulfites can produce respiratory difficulties. In some cases, sulfites can also trigger potentially life-threatening airway constriction and asthma symptoms in some individuals (see the sidebar "Additives and allergies," earlier in this chapter).

Food poisoning

Food poisoning can result from bacterial contamination of improperly prepared or handled foods, especially meats or salads. You've probably heard of bacterial bad guys such as salmonella, E. coli, listeria, and staphylococcus enterotoxin. These bacteria are the usual suspects in outbreaks of food poisoning. Food poisoning symptoms typically include nausea, vomiting, and diarrhea and can often mimic the flu. In rare cases, food-poisoning reactions can be fatal if not treated in time.

Researchers believe that many cases of illness mistakenly diagnosed as the 24-hour flu bug are actually the result of ingesting tainted foods. A particular reaction from spoiled fish, known as *scombroidosis,* can mimic food allergy due to the release of histamine-like chemicals. Itching, hives, and even shortness of breath can occur depending on the amount of spoiled fish a person has eaten.

If many people develop similar symptoms after eating the same meal (the potato salad that sat in the sun all afternoon at the family picnic, for example), food poisoning is the likely cause of all those urgent trips to the restroom.

If you experience severe gastric distress that seems related to food poisoning, make sure you drink enough liquid to avoid dehydration, which is one of the most serious adverse effects. If your condition doesn't improve within 24 hours, seek medical attention.

Diagnosing Adverse Food Reactions

In order to diagnose your adverse food reactions, your physician should take a detailed medical history and conduct a physical examination. Your doctor may also ask you about the specific details of your reaction to figure out what may cause your reactions.

Keeping a food diary

A detailed food diary, in which you record everything you consume (even those midnight snacks) and describe your reactions, can help your doctor diagnose your condition.

A well-kept food diary can assist you in telling your doctor about the following items:

- ✔ The timing of your reactions. For example, do they occur immediately after you've consumed a food or liquid, and if not, how long afterward?
- ✔ The amount of food that seems to trigger a reaction.
- ✔ Where and how the food was prepared.
- ✔ The duration and severity of your symptoms.
- ✔ Any activities, especially exercise, associated with your reactions.

Considering atopic causes

As part of the physical examination, your doctor should also look for signs of atopic diseases, including

- ✔ Dry, scaly skin, which can indicate eczema
- ✔ Dark circles under your eyes, which may indicate hay fever
- ✔ Wheezing and coughing, which can signal asthma symptoms

Eliminating possible food culprits

In some cases, your doctor may advise an *elimination diet* for you as a way of confirming what triggers your adverse reactions. This process involves eliminating suspected foods from your diet, one at a time, under your doctor's supervision. If your symptoms significantly improve, your doctor may then gradually reintroduce the likeliest food suspect to determine whether it's the source of your woes.

Only undertake an elimination diet under your physician's direction. You don't want to deprive yourself of foods that may not cause your symptoms and are vital for your overall health. Your doctor may also advise an elimination diet in order to prepare you for an oral food challenge, which I describe in the following section.

Testing for food allergens

If your doctor can't readily identify the cause of your reactions, he or she may also recommend confirming a suspected food allergen with the allergy tests that I describe in the following sections.

Skin testing

Skin testing involves using specific food extracts to evaluate your sensitivity to suspected allergens. Only a qualified specialist, such as an allergist, should perform skin testing. Skin testing for food allergens isn't always recommended.

In some cases, your doctor may not advise skin testing because a positive reaction may involve unacceptable risks of inducing anaphylactic shock, particularly if you're highly sensitized to certain foods, such as peanuts.

In general, prick-puncture tests are the only skin tests that your doctor needs to administer when attempting to identify suspected food allergens. (See Chapter 11 for more about prick-puncture tests.)

Oral food challenges

Oral food challenges involve actually ingesting — under medical supervision — minute quantities of food that contain suspected allergens.

To ensure the most accurate diagnosis, your doctor should administer an oral food challenge while you're symptom-free, usually as a result of a food elimination diet. Depending on the severity of your adverse food reactions and the type of food allergen that your physician suspects as the cause, your doctor may choose to administer one or more of the following types of oral food challenges:

- ✔ **Open challenge:** In this type of test, your doctor informs you of what type of food you're ingesting.

- ✔ **Single-blind challenge:** With this test, your doctor doesn't inform you of what you're eating. However, your doctor or the clinician administering the test knows the ingredients.

- ✔ **Double-blind, placebo-controlled oral food challenge (DBPCOFC):** This elaborate procedure is the gold standard for identifying food allergens. Neither you nor your doctor (nor the clinician who administers the test) knows the contents of the test. A third party, such as a nurse or a lab technician, prepares the opaque capsule for testing. In most cases, your doctor schedules a DBPCOFC so you can fast for a prescribed amount of time beforehand. You also need to stop taking antihistamines (based on your doctor's advice) prior to the challenge, because these drugs can interfere with the accuracy. The initial dose of the suspected food in this test is usually half of the minimum quantity that your doctor estimates as the trigger for your reaction. After the test, the technician identifies the capsule's contents to help your doctor make the proper diagnosis.

Take this challenge only in a facility equipped to treat potentially severe reactions. If your history of adverse food reactions is life-threatening, your doctor will most likely advise you that an oral food challenge is too risky.

Radioallergensorbent testing (RAST)

Your doctor may recommend *radioallergensorbent testing,* a type of blood test that measures levels of food-specific IgE antibodies in your blood, if skin testing or oral food challenges seem too risky. Most allergists rarely use RAST because it isn't as accurate as skin testing and may result in an incomplete profile of your allergies. For more information on this test, see Chapter 11.

Avoiding Adverse Food Reactions

After your doctor determines the source of your adverse food reactions, the most effective long-term approach to managing your condition and preventing further reactions is strict avoidance of the implicated food. That may seem like an obvious solution. However, you may need to become an expert at reading ingredient listings when you buy groceries. In some cases, food allergens and other types of precipitants may hide under arcane names in food labels. Hidden ingredients in many processed and packaged foods may also be sources of problematic allergens.

For updates and information on food allergens and related issues and to find out how to decipher ingredients listed on food labels, contact The Food Allergy & Anaphylaxis Network at 800-929-4040 or visit the organization's Web site at www.foodallergy.org.

Make sure that your family, friends, and colleagues all understand what causes your adverse food reactions. You can then minimize the chances of erupting in hives at the Thanksgiving meal or during that crucial dinner with your boss and the company's new clients.

If you have a life-threatening food allergy, you may need to avoid certain restaurants. In many cases, food servers don't have enough information about the ingredients in the establishment's menu to guarantee you an allergen-free meal, although some restaurants actually do offer dishes without common food allergens. However, double-check all the ingredients in the menu item with the chef or restaurant manager. In particular, inquire whether the restaurant prepares allergen-free meals using surfaces, cookware, fryers, and utensils that are separated from the other items in the kitchen.

If effective management of your adverse food reactions involves excluding common food groups from your diet for long periods, consider professional dietary advice in order to prevent nutritional deficiency or malnutrition.

Chapter 9

Asthma and Exercise

· ·

In This Chapter

▶ Knowing how exercise can trigger asthma symptoms

▶ Maintaining fitness with asthma

▶ Making the connection between asthma and athletes

· ·

*Y*ou don't have to sit on life's sidelines just because you have asthma, even though most asthmatics are susceptible, in varying degrees, to symptoms of *exercise-induced asthma* (EIA — also known as *exercise-induced bronchospasm* or EIB). As I explain in this chapter, you can effectively manage EIA through appropriate use of medications that your doctor prescribes and by also integrating a suitable warm-up and cool-down routine into your exercise regimen.

Understanding EIA

Typically, EIA symptoms start minutes after you begin vigorous activity, when the airways in your lungs become narrow and constricted. These respiratory symptoms usually reach their peak of severity between five and ten minutes after you stop exercising. In many cases, the symptoms can spontaneously resolve (without the use of a short-acting inhaled bronchodilator) within 30 minutes.

Exercises that involve breathing cold, dry air, such as running outdoors or skiing, are more likely to trigger EIA than activities that involve breathing warmer, humidified air, such as swimming in a heated pool. However, a few studies have also cautioned that chlorine and other chemicals used in heated and non-heated pools seem to also act as EIA triggers in some asthmatics.

Although EIA usually relates to outside activities, using home-exercise equipment or simply running upstairs can precipitate an asthma episode in some people. If you have an increased sensitivity for EIA, make sure that your doctor knows so that he can evaluate and treat your condition.

Keeping Fit Despite EIA

Although EIA symptoms occur frequently in asthmatics when they exert themselves vigorously, for certain individuals, physical activity may be the only trigger that precipitates respiratory symptoms such as coughing, wheezing, and shortness of breath. Occasionally, patients mistakenly attribute their EIA symptoms to just "being out of shape," rather than seeking a proper medical diagnosis.

However, if you're experiencing respiratory symptoms connected to exercise and other types of intensive physical activities, make sure that you get a proper diagnosis. Although EIA episodes usually last for only a few minutes, they can still be frightening for many people and, as a result, could unnecessarily limit your physical activities.

Diagnosing EIA

Properly diagnosing and treating EIA usually means that you can enjoy an active lifestyle. Doctors can often prescribe medications to prevent or at least substantially reduce your EIA symptoms, thus allowing you to participate in many types of exercise and sports in spite of your asthma.

Receiving appropriate treatment for EIA is also essential for your well-being because so many people in the United States and other developed countries simply don't get enough exercise. According to a recent report by the Centers for Disease Control and Prevention (CDC), adult asthmatics in the United States are even less likely on average to meet national recommendations for physical activity than nonasthmatics.

I'm not suggesting you run a marathon tomorrow, but as I emphasize in many other parts of this book, staying in good physical shape can only help in managing your asthma (and any other ailment) successfully. So don't let your susceptibility to EIA keep you from getting the exercise you need. Rather, consult with your doctor to find effective ways of managing your condition that can also allow you to stay in shape.

Keeping a record of your activities and noting when you experience asthma symptoms and what steps you normally take to relieve them can assist your doctor in developing the most effective treatment program. Because certain drugs are more effective in preventing and controlling EIA, *when* you take your prescribed medication is often just as important as *what* you take. Work with your doctor to determine the best time to take your prescribed medication in order to ensure that it provides maximum relief.

Controlling EIA with medications

In many cases, competitive athletes with asthma or EIA use inhaled cortico-steroids daily to control their airway inflammation. Many competitive athletes also add a long-acting inhaled beta$_2$-adrenergic bronchodilator daily, such as salmeterol (Serevent, Serevent Diskus) or formoterol (Foradil), and/or a short-acting inhaled beta$_2$-adrenergic bronchodilator, such as albuterol (Proventil, Ventolin), prior to exercise or athletic events.

To prevent EIA, your doctor may recommend that you inhale your dose of pre-scribed short-acting beta$_2$-adrenergic bronchodilator 15 to 30 minutes before you begin to exert yourself. The long-acting bronchodilators salmeterol — available in dry-powder inhaler (DPI) formulation as Serevent Diskus or as Serevent MDI in a metered-dose inhaler (MDI) — and formoterol, available only as a DPI as Foradil Aerolizer, may be prescribed for use 30 minutes before exercising. Doctors usually prescribe these medications as part of combination therapy with inhaled corticosteroids. (See Chapter 14 for the differences between DPIs and MDIs.)

Other long-term controller drugs that doctors also prescribe to treat EIA symptoms include cromolyn (Intal) and nedocromil (Tilade), which are both inhaled mast cell stabilizers (see Chapter 15). These products are also usu-ally best taken 15 to 30 minutes before exercising. Recent studies have shown that when taken regularly, montelukast (Singulair), a leukotriene inhibitor (also see Chapter 15), may also be an effective long-term, preventive treat-ment for EIA.

Athletes and EIA

According to recent studies of respiratory conditions, Olympic-level competi-tors as a group are most likely to experience EIA episodes. Research indicates that hard breathing by these competitors during sports events and intensive workouts may be an important factor in triggering their respiratory symptoms.

Breathing competitively: Nose versus mouth

Another reason for athletes being at increased risk for EIA is due to the fact that all people — not just Olympic champions — switch from nose breathing to mouth breathing when they're strenuously exerting themselves. As I explain more extensively in Chapter 7, one of your nose's most important functions is to protect your airways from particulate matter in the air. Your nose acts to filter and cleanse the air you inhale, through *cilia* (tiny hair-like projections of certain types of cells that sweep mucus through the nose).

However, filtering isn't in your mouth's job description. Therefore, when you're seriously exerting yourself and gulping in air through your mouth, you're also increasing the chances of inhaling allergens and irritants that can more easily get into the airways of your lungs and potentially trigger more serious reactions.

Because your body needs all the oxygen it can get when you're vigorously working out and/or competing, breathing through your mouth can virtually be a reflex, which is all the more reason to make sure that you're taking medications to prevent or at least reduce the severity of EIA symptoms.

Contrary to popular myth, sports federations such as the National Collegiate Athletic Association (NCAA) or the U.S. Olympic Committee haven't banned the use of inhaled corticosteroids that athletes take on a regular basis to control asthma symptoms. (The steroids that various sports committees ban are actually male hormones that some athletes take by tablet or injection to build muscle mass.) However, some common over-the-counter (OTC) medications, such as pseudoephedrine (Sudafed), are banned due to their stimulant effects. Check with your sports federation before taking any medication, including OTC products.

Warming up and cooling down to prevent EIA

Many doctors also advise some type of warm-up and cool-down routine (even if you don't have asthma) when engaging in exercise or sports-related activity. Consult with your physician to determine the type of pre- and post-exercise routine that's most beneficial for you. After you've determined the warm-up and cool-down plan, incorporate that routine into your asthma management plan.

As long as you stick to your asthma management plan, asthma shouldn't prevent you from enjoying or even excelling at a wide range of physical activities. Consider the examples of Jackie Joyner-Kersee and other Olympic champions who also suffer from asthma. (See Chapter 22 for more famous folks with asthma — the list may surprise you!)

Part III
Treating Your Asthma

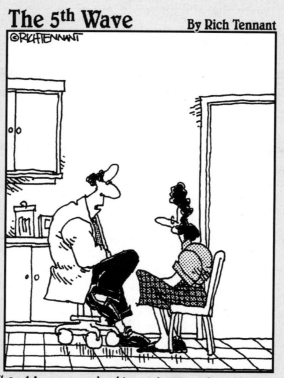

The 5th Wave — By Rich Tennant

"Sudden perspiration, shallow breathing, and a rapid heart rate are all signs of an asthma attack. The fact that these symptoms only occur when the pool boy is working in your backyard, however, raises some questions."

In this part . . .

Asthma is a multifaceted, chronic, inflammatory airway disease of the lungs that causes breathing problems. It requires proper diagnosis, early and aggressive treatment, and effective long-term management. That's what Part III of this book is all about. In particular, Chapter 10 looks at how to avoid those allergens that bother you the most. Chapter 11 discusses testing for allergies and *immunotherapy* (allergy shots). Chapters 12 and 13 examine what you and your doctor can do to relieve your nasal allergies and treat any complications.

Chapter 10

Avoiding Allergens That Cause Respiratory Symptoms

In This Chapter

▶ Understanding what you're breathing

▶ Reading pollen counts: News you can use

▶ Minding mites and other dusty denizens

▶ Knowing how your home affects your health

▶ Identifying allergens and irritants in your environment

▶ Eliminating, controlling, and avoiding allergens and irritants in your home

Something's in the air — and it may be affecting your asthma. Under normal circumstances, breathing is a reflex you don't even think about — as long as nothing in the air interferes with the process. However, unless you live in a bubble, every time you breathe in, you inhale more than just oxygen into your nose and lungs.

In fact, the air that most people breathe is full of many types of airborne particles that are too small for the naked eye to see. In addition to pollutants and other airborne materials, these particles include allergenic substances, known as *aeroallergens,* that can trigger allergic reactions and significantly affect the well-being of people with asthma or allergies. The inhaled aeroallergens that trigger allergic reactions are known as *inhalant allergens.*

The following common inhalant allergens are the most frequent triggers of *allergic rhinitis* (also known as hay fever; see Chapter 7) and asthma. (See Chapter 5 for further information on what these allergens do to people with asthma.)

✔ Pollens produced by wind-pollinated plants, such as ragweed

✔ Wind-borne mold spores

✔ Household dust, which can contain various types of allergenic substances, such as dust mite allergen, dander, and other allergenic materials from household pets and pests, allergenic fibers, and indoor mold spores

In this chapter, I give you the lowdown on these common inhalant allergens and explain the dangers of each in detail. I also discuss ways you can avoid or at least limit your exposure to these allergens.

Pollens

Pollens can trigger allergic rhinitis and asthma symptoms. Plants that depend on wind rather than insects for *pollination* — grasses, trees, and weeds — produce pollens. These plants release their wind-borne pollens in huge quantities to reproduce. For example, ragweed plants may release up to 1 million pollen granules in a day, and the massive amounts of pollen granules that some trees release can resemble clouds.

Pollens are such universal features of life on our planet that pollen samples from excavation sites enable archaeologists and botanists to reconstruct what the natural environments of ancient times probably were like.

Pollen particulars

Seed-bearing plants reproduce by pollination, which involves the transfer of pollen granules — the plants' sperm cells — from male parts of a plant to receptive female reproductive sites. When pollen granules reach female sites, they produce pollen tubes that carry the sperm cells close to the female reproductive cells. (See, technical stuff can sometimes be exciting!)

A variety of means, including insects, animals, and the wind, provide transportation for pollen granules. Wind-borne pollens that trigger allergic rhinitis symptoms come from three classifications of plants:

- ✔ **Grasses:** The grasses that cause most grass-induced allergic rhinitis are widespread throughout North America and were imported from Europe to feed animals and create lawns. By contrast, the many native grasses of North America produce little pollen. I provide more details on these grasses in the "Allergens in the grass" section, later in this chapter.

- ✔ **Weeds:** The most important weeds that trigger symptoms of allergic rhinitis are those of the tribe *Ambrosieae,* known as *ragweeds.*

- ✔ **Trees:** Most trees that release symptom-causing pollens are *angiosperms* (which means "flowering seeds," and yet these trees don't actually flower), such as willows, poplars, beeches, or oaks. Similarly, pollens from a few *gymnosperms* (naked seeds), such as pines, spruces, firs, junipers, cypresses, hemlocks, and cedars, also can trigger symptoms of allergic rhinitis.

Dead wood

Although you may experience respiratory symptoms when exposed to the pollen of certain grasses, weeds, or trees, that doesn't actually mean you're allergic to the pollinating plants themselves. When you're allergic to oak pollen, you're not allergic to the actual oak tree. You're only allergic to the pollen granules produced by the tree. Therefore, even though oak pollen may trigger your asthma symptoms, you nevertheless can use furniture made from the wood of the tree. That antique oak desk in your study won't trigger your allergies — it stopped pollinating a long time ago.

Although these plant groups account for most cases of pollen-induced allergic rhinitis, only a small percentage of the members of each group has been shown to produce allergenic pollen.

Blowin' in the wind

Wind pollination has worked well for certain plants for millions of years, enabling many of them to survive and flourish in environments that don't provide many insect or animal pollinators. The much younger species of man (*Homo sapiens* — you and me) has also flourished in these areas, with the result that we're often in the pollen path of wind-pollinating plants. Instead of wind-borne pollen granules reaching their intended targets, they often end up in your eyes, nose, throat, and lungs, causing allergic reactions in susceptible individuals.

Pollens (and molds) for all seasons

Most wind-pollinating plants in the United States and Canada release their pollens at specific times during the year that can be classified into five pollen seasons. Whenever your respiratory symptoms begin or worsen during one of these seasons, the predominance of particular pollens during that particular time of year may be the cause of the allergic reactions that complicate your asthma. Here's the type of pollen (or molds) that may affect you in each of the five pollen seasons:

- ✔ When your symptoms get worse during spring, the probable cause is tree pollen.

- ✔ In late spring and early summer, grass pollen is the likely culprit.

- ✔ From late summer to autumn, weed pollen, especially from ragweed, may cause you problems.

- ✔ Especially during the summer and fall but also throughout the year — except during snow cover — mold spores, particularly those of airborne molds, may trigger your allergies.

✔ In winter, wind-borne pollens rarely are a factor in most parts of the United States and Canada. However, in the warmer southern regions of the United States that don't experience prolonged periods of freezing temperatures (such as southern California), pollinating plants and molds still release allergy-triggering pollen and mold spores whenever there's no snow cover.

When your allergic rhinitis symptoms follow a seasonal pattern, such as those I just listed, consult your doctor to find out whether specific pollens are the problem. You may also want to ask your doctor for information on the major aeroallergens for the area 50 to 100 miles around where you live and work.

Non-natives

A list of local allergenic plants can serve as a good starting point for figuring out what plants may be affecting your allergies. However, knowing about non-native plants in your environment also is useful. Non-native plants in your environment often include trees and grasses — some of which may also produce allergenic pollen — that may have been planted around your community for decorative purposes.

Counting your pollens

Many newspapers and television and radio news programs regularly report *pollen counts*. The pollen count is the measurement of the total number of granules of a kind of particular pollen per cubic meter of air per day. Pollen counters rate the resulting numbers according to five categories, ranging from absent to very high.

Take my pollen, please!

Plants that are the main culprits in allergic rhinitis depend on wind pollination because they're not pretty or colorful enough to attract insects or other animals to do the pollinating. Most flowers that appeal to people — and to insects and other animals — produce heavier pollens that stick to the insects or animals that carry it to female plant reproductive sites, so you're far less likely to acquire sensitivities to pollen from roses or other attractive, colorful plants, unless you experience constant, close contact with flowers. When you experience allergy symptoms after stopping to smell the roses, pollens from nearby grasses, weeds, or trees may cause your reaction.

Go west, young pollen!

When I was a boy growing up in New York, I remember my doctor telling patients with asthma and allergies to move to Arizona because of the area's dry climate and sparse plant population. Through the years, plenty of folks have indeed moved to Arizona (and not just because of my doctor). Many of Arizona's new residents decided to plant non-native ornamental plants, such as mulberry trees, to spruce up the desert scenery. Mulberry trees thrive in the hot, dry climate and produce clouds of allergenic pollen. As a result, Phoenix and other cities in the state are now major allergy centers. In fact, some of the busiest allergists in the United States practice in Arizona.

Running the numbers

Bear in mind that the severity of symptoms triggered by pollens depends not only on the actual pollen count but also on the particular pollen being measured. In addition, the proximity of the collection station to the particular pollen being reported usually affects the actual count; moreover, each region of the world has its own predominant allergy-producing pollens. Table 10-1 provides the generally accepted guidelines for interpreting pollen counts for ragweed, which is the most closely followed type of pollen count in many parts of the United States and Canada.

Table 10-1	Ragweed Pollen Count Guidelines	
Category	*Pollen Grains Per Cubic Meter Per Day**	*Degree of Symptoms*
Absent	0	No symptoms.
Low	0–10	Symptoms may only affect people with extreme sensitivities to these pollens.
Moderate	10–50	Many people who are sensitive to these pollens experience symptoms at this rating.
High	50–500	Most people with any sensitivity to these pollens experience symptoms.
Very High	More than 500	Almost anyone with any sensitivity at all to these pollens experiences symptoms. If you're extremely sensitive to ragweed pollen, your symptoms can be severe at this level.

These figures are averages.

Here are some other factors to keep in mind when reading a pollen count:

✔ Today's pollen count was collected yesterday and usually reflects what was in the air 24 hours ago.

✔ Rain can clear pollen out of the air temporarily. However, short thunderstorms — the kind that are characteristic of late spring and summer in parts of North America — can actually spread pollen granules farther.

✔ Hot weather increases pollination, whereas (you probably figured this one out already) cooler temperatures reduce the amount of pollen that plants produce.

✔ Pollen grains typically are at their highest concentrations from mid-morning to early afternoon.

✔ Because they're wind-borne, many pollen granules travel great distances, so the plants in your backyard or your neighbor's garden may not be what's triggering your allergies. Chopping down the olive tree in front of your house may have little, if any, effect on your allergies.

Quality, not quantity

Not all pollens are equal. Studies show that a little pollen from grasses such as Bermuda and bluegrass or trees such as oak and elm can go a long way in triggering allergies. On the other hand, your allergic rhinitis symptoms usually are triggered only by much higher and direct exposures to pine and eucalyptus pollen. These pollens are large and heavy and don't disperse widely in the wind. Similarly, a moderate ragweed pollen count usually has far more effect than even a high English plantain count, depending especially on your sensitivity to those pollens. So knowing the types of pollens that are blowing in the wind, and how much of those pollens are actually in the wind, is important.

Consider the following tips to help you minimize problems during those high pollen–count days:

✔ Whenever your community reports high counts for pollens to which you are allergic, you can take steps to avoid or reduce your exposure to those pollens. For details on how, see the "Pollen-proofing" section, later in this chapter.

✔ If complete or significant avoidance isn't practical or possible, you can use pollen counts to help you determine (based on your doctor's advice) when to take medication to prevent the onset of symptoms or at least keep them from interfering dramatically with your life. For an extensive survey of allergic rhinitis medication, see Chapter 12.

> ✔ The most important pollen levels for you to consider are the ones that trigger your allergies. Many people react differently to different levels of airborne pollen, and pollens vary between regions. However, you need to be concerned when pollen counts reach the moderate range, because that's generally when many people with allergies start to experience symptoms.

Contact the National Allergy Bureau (NAB) of the American Academy of Allergy, Asthma, and Immunology (AAAAI) for more information about the pollens and molds in your area. Check out the NAB Web site at `www.aaaai.org/nab` or call 414-272-6071. I list additional information on organizations and health agencies that can provide you with more extensive local pollen surveys in the appendix.

Allergens in the grass

Grass pollens are the most common cause of allergies in the world. Although only a small percentage of the more than 1,000 species of grasses in North America actually produce pollen that triggers asthma symptoms and allergic reactions, these particular species are widespread throughout the continent and release huge amounts of pollen granules into the air. Most of these allergy-triggering grasses are non-native plants that were imported to grow feed for farm animals and for planting lawns.

Wind-pollinated grasses release vast amounts of pollen granules during the late spring pollen season. The most significant allergy-symptom provoking grasses are Bermuda grass, bluegrass, orchard grass, ryegrass, timothy, and fescue. Of those grasses, Bermuda grass may be the most significant allergy trigger. Bermuda grass releases pollen almost year-round and abounds throughout the southern United States, where it's cultivated for ornamental purposes and as animal feed. Other grasses, such as rye, timothy, blue, and orchard, share allergens in common, so an allergy to pollen from one of these grasses may also indicate sensitivity to allergens from one or more of these other grasses.

Wheezy weeds

Weeds are plants, too. Many people just don't consider them to be desirable plants. For the sake of allergies, however, when I refer to *weeds,* I mean the small, wild, annual plants of no agricultural value or decorative interest. The wind-pollinated weeds that release allergenic pollen don't produce very attractive or conspicuous flowers. The most significant of these wind-pollinated weeds, in terms of allergic triggers, include ragweed, mugwort, Russian thistle, pigweed, sagebrush, and English plantain.

Ragweed to starboard, Captain!

Is that seasickness or allergies? Ragweed pollen has such a broad range that it has been detected 400 miles out to sea. So if you're on the ocean during ragweed season, I suggest taking your medication with you. (Make sure it's non-drowsy, especially when you're at the helm.)

Ragweed is a significant trigger of asthma symptoms and is the most common cause of allergic rhinitis reactions in North America. Many people who are sensitive to ragweed may also experience cross-reactivity to cocklebur.

In the United States, from the mid-Atlantic to northern parts of the Midwest, where ragweed is most highly concentrated, pollination usually begins around August 15 and generally lasts through October (and/or until a first frost), depending on climate conditions. Ragweeds are early risers, with most plants releasing pollen between 6 and 11 a.m. Hot and humid weather usually leads to an increased release of pollen.

Although ragweed pollen is most prevalent east of the Mississippi River, you can find related weed pollens, such as those produced by marsh elder and cocklebur, throughout most parts of North America.

Can't sneeze the forest for the trees

Of the 700 species of trees that are native to North America, only 65 produce pollen that triggers allergic rhinitis. The pollination season for most of these species usually runs from the end of winter or the beginning of spring until early summer.

Pollens from these types of trees have much shorter ranges than the pollens that wind-pollinating grasses and weeds release. As a result, in most cities and towns, weed and grass pollens are far more likely to affect you than tree pollens. However, in the southeastern United States, the spring tree season is a major problem, with high peaks of pollination over a prolonged period of time.

Trees that produce the most allergenic pollen in North America include elms; willows and poplars; birches; beeches, oaks, and chestnuts; maples and box elders; hickories; mountain cedars; and ashes and olives.

Molds

Talk about moldies and oldies: Molds are some of the oldest and most common organisms on the planet, and they're widespread in most homes. Think of molds as microscopic fungi or mushrooms. You've probably encountered various forms of mold at home, from splotches on your shower door to the greenish growth on that tomato you forgot way in the back of your fridge last year (hope your mom doesn't find out).

As far back as 1726, mold spores were suspected of being a source of respiratory symptoms. Throughout the United States and Canada, mold spores are some of the most common inhalant allergens, outdoors and indoors, and can be significant triggers of asthma, allergic rhinitis, and other respiratory ailments.

Mold counts usually are much higher than pollen counts and usually rise to peak levels during summer months. Outdoor mold spores are present almost year-round unless prolonged snow cover occurs. This mold-spore propensity is in contrast to pollens, which are released by plants, usually only during distinct seasons. However, at any time, mold counts can suddenly and dramatically rise within a short period and then drop down to previous levels just as abruptly. Because molds also thrive indoors, you may be exposed to mold spores continuously throughout the year.

Outdoor molds grow on field crops such as corn, wheat, soybeans, and on decaying organic matter such as compost, hay, piles of leaves, and grass cuttings, and types of foods, including tomatoes, sweet corn, melons, bananas, and mushrooms.

Spreading spores

As is true of grasses, weeds, and trees, only a few forms of molds produce allergens that trigger asthma and allergic rhinitis symptoms. Airborne mold spores occur almost everywhere on the planet except at the North and South poles. So unless you're a polar bear or a penguin, odds are that you receive some degree of exposure to mold particles, regardless of where you are. These molds include

- **Cladosporium:** These species produce some of the most abundant windborne spores in the world and flourish almost everywhere, except in the coldest regions.
- **Alternaria:** These outdoor molds are among the most prominent causes of allergy symptoms in sensitized people.

✔ **Aspergillus:** A medically important indoor mold, found in agricultural areas, crawl spaces of homes, and even outdoor air throughout North America. A variety of allergic respiratory diseases associated with exposure to aspergillus are recognized, including allergic asthma (see Chapter 5), hypersensitivity pneumonitis (*farmer's lung*), and a serious respiratory disease known as allergic bronchopulmonary aspergillosis (ABPA).

Moldy matters

Here are some factors that can help you determine whether mold spores are triggering your respiratory symptoms:

✔ You experience asthma and allergic rhinitis symptoms most of the year, rather than during specific seasons.

✔ Your symptoms worsen during summer months, even when pollen allergens aren't present to any significant degree.

✔ Your asthma and/or allergies worsen near croplands, especially around grains and overgrown fields, or during or immediately following gardening.

House Dust

House dust may be the most prevalent of all triggers of respiratory symptoms in your life. Recent studies show that the major inhalant allergens found in house dust can be the most important risk factors in triggering asthma attacks.

Let me reassure you: Dust isn't dirt, and it isn't an indication of poor housekeeping. I'm a clean freak, so I keep my house immaculate. However, whenever I go away for a week, I invariably return to find a coating of dust on most surfaces, even though I sealed up the place and nobody has been to visit. Household dust is inescapable because it's a normal breakdown product of fibers and other materials found throughout your indoor environment.

Common components of house dust include

✔ Dust mite allergens

✔ Animal dander

✔ Insect fragments

✔ Fibers such as acrylic, rayon, nylon, cotton, and other materials

✔ Wood and paper particles

✔ Hair and skin flakes

✔ Tobacco ash

✔ Particles of salt, sugar, other spices, and minerals

✔ Plant pollen and fungal spores

Dust mites

The most potent allergen in house dust comes from the house dust mite (*Dermatophagoides pteronyssinus* and/or *Dermatophagoides farinae,* depending on where you live). Check out Figure 10-1 to see a dust mite. These tiny, eight-legged microscopic spider relatives live in house dust where they feed on dead skin flakes that warm-blooded creatures such as humans constantly shed (hence the scientific name *dermatophagoides,* meaning skin-eater; but don't worry — dust mites don't eat living skin) at rates of up to 1.5 grams per day — that's a lot of dust mite chow.

The fecal matter (or waste, to put it more delicately) that they produce, at the average rate of 20 particles per day, is the most prevalent form of house dust allergens and often causes respiratory problems in humans.

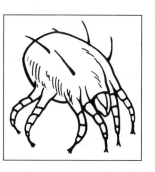

Figure 10-1: Dust mites are among the most abundant sources of allergic triggers.

Eighty percent of patients with allergies test positive for sensitivity to the dust mite allergen. Because dust mites usually are as snug as bugs in a rug, people rarely come into direct contact with the live creatures themselves — just with their waste or decomposing bodies, which also can be a significant source of house dust allergens. Dust mites thrive in dark, warm, and humid environments such as mattresses, pillows, box springs, rugs, towels, upholstered furniture, drapes, and stuffed toys.

Mattresses and box springs usually provide the greatest concentration of human skin flakes for these creatures, which is why the average bed contains 2 million dust mites. As a result, your asthma and/or allergy symptoms may worsen in bed or while napping on your upholstered couch, because you inhale significant amounts of dust mite allergens while sleeping. That's why many of the steps that I recommend for your home in the section about "Avoidance and Allergy-Proofing," later in this chapter, focus on your bedroom.

If you wonder about the seriousness of dust mite infestations, consider this study: Dust mites were stained with a dye and then released on a couch in a home. (The family gave informed consent for the experiment.) By the next day, the dust mites had infested the family car, and some of the creatures also were found on the clothes of family members who sat on the couch. Within ten days, marked dust mites were recovered from every room in the house.

In another experiment, dust mites in an infested rug were killed and the rug was cut into pieces and stored at different combinations of temperature and humidity. Almost two years later, the allergens from the dead mites were as potent as they originally were.

What else is in my house dust?

Dander from household pets is another major trigger of respiratory symptoms. Although you may not have pets of your own, whenever you're in contact with other pet owners, dander from their animals can get on your hands or clothes, which you then introduce into your home. In addition, the urine from household pests, such as mice and rats, can be significant triggers of asthma symptoms and allergic reactions. Furthermore, recent studies increasingly show that allergens in cockroach debris and waste can contribute to asthma attacks, especially in children.

Dust gets in your eyes . . . or nose, throat, and lungs

The following is a list of symptoms that you can use to determine whether inhalant allergens in house dust trigger your respiratory symptoms:

- ✔ You experience asthma and/or allergy symptoms as a result of dusting, making beds, or changing blankets and bed linens.

- ✔ Your symptoms seem to occur year-round rather than seasonally.

- ✔ Your symptoms are worse when you're indoors.

- ✔ Your symptoms are worse when you awaken in bed in the morning.

Avoidance and Allergy-Proofing

In the first part of this chapter, I tell you about the most important and prevalent triggers of respiratory symptoms that affect most asthma patients. In the rest of the chapter, I discuss various steps you can take to avoid those triggers. Using these methods usually helps you improve your life with asthma.

Avoiding — or at least significantly decreasing your exposure to — substances in your environment that trigger your asthma attacks and allergic reactions often helps relieve your symptoms and thus improves your overall health. These avoidance measures also can reduce the need for medication or shots, thereby saving you much time and money.

Why avoidance matters

You've probably heard the joke about the patient who complains, "Doc, it hurts when I do this," to which the doctor replies, "Then stop doing that." (For more great doctor jokes, come to one of my book signings.) Silly as that joke seems, the doctor's advice exemplifies the basic concept of avoidance. Depending on your sensitivity, avoid the substances or levels of exposure to the substances that trigger (that's why such substances are called *triggers*) an allergic reaction.

Avoidance seems simple enough. In real life, however, the trick is figuring out — short of living in a bubble — the practical and effective steps you can take to minimize your contact with allergy triggers.

Developing an avoidance checklist

Environmental control measures are vital components of any allergist's treatment plan. Every practicing allergist focuses on helping you create and implement an effective avoidance strategy for you, your spouse, your child, or other people with asthma who live with you. The plan that you and your allergist develop will likely include these general steps:

1. **Identifying asthma and allergy triggers in your environment, especially indoor allergens and irritants.**

2. **Recognizing situations in which you may come into contact with those allergy triggers.**

3. **Discovering how to avoid allergens or minimizing contact with them.**

4. **Allergy-proofing your home.**

Taking time for terminology

In case you're also allergic to jargon, the following list explains common technical terms that allergists use when discussing avoidance and allergy-proofing:

- ✔ **Allergen load:** Your total level of exposure, at any given time, to any combination of allergens that trigger your allergies.

- ✔ **Allergic threshold:** Your level of sensitivity to an allergen. A low allergic threshold means that your sensitivity to an allergen is high — even a small exposure to the substance can trigger your symptoms. A high allergic threshold means that your body requires a higher concentration of allergens to trigger symptoms. Your threshold level, however, can decrease when you're exposed too often to large quantities of an allergen or to a combination of allergens.

- ✔ **Allergy trigger:** A normally harmless substance, such as pollen, dust, animal dander, insect stings, and certain foods and drugs, that can provoke an abnormal response by your immune system whenever you're sensitized to that substance. Doctors usually refer to these substances as *allergens*.

- ✔ **Cross-reactivity:** Your immune system is an expert at recognizing related allergens in seemingly unrelated sources. Therefore, if you're exposed to related allergens within a short time, your allergen load can exceed your allergic threshold, thereby triggering allergic reactions and asthma symptoms.

- ✔ **Desensitization:** In the context of avoidance and allergy-proofing, *desensitizing* describes the active process of removing, shielding, or reducing the sources of allergens in your environment. Your allergist may advise you to desensitize your home, focusing especially on the bedroom of any person with asthma. *Desensitization* also refers to a form of treatment in which an allergist injects small amounts of an allergen extract under your skin so that your body can discover how not to react to the substance (see Chapter 11).

- ✔ **HEPA:** HEPA stands for high efficiency particulate arrester — an air filtration process developed for hospital operating rooms and other locations that require a sterilized environment. HEPA filters absorb and contain 99.97 percent of all particles larger than 0.3 microns ($\frac{1}{300}$th the width of a human hair). When the unit truly operates at that level, only 3 of 10,000 particles manage to sneak back into the room. Vacuum cleaners and air purifiers with ULPA (see definition later in this list) and HEPA filters are vital tools for desensitizing and allergy-proofing your indoor environment.

- ✔ **HVAC:** Heating, ventilation, and air-conditioning systems — your home's lungs. The quality of air that you breathe indoors is largely dependent on the condition of these systems and the air that flows into and out of your environment through them.

> ✔ **ULPA:** Ultra low penetration air is even more thorough than the HEPA process. This filtration system is designed to absorb and contain 99.99 percent of all particles larger than 0.12 microns.

Knowing your limits

Avoidance measures rarely require the complete elimination of all asthma and allergy triggers and irritants in your environment. In many cases, you may need only to limit your exposure to certain triggers to prevent or alleviate your respiratory symptoms.

Think of your allergic threshold as a cup and the allergy triggers in your environment as liquid pouring into that cup. Overflowing your small cup (low allergic threshold) may require only a small amount of liquid (allergens), thereby triggering an allergic reaction. A larger cup — a higher threshold — can accommodate more liquid without overflowing (without triggering an allergic reaction). Knowing your limit is the key to mastering your threshold.

Another important concept to bear in mind when considering avoidance is imagining a scale balancing your allergic threshold on one side with allergen load on the other. You won't set off your allergies unless your level of exposure to allergen triggers overloads your allergic threshold. Keep in mind, however, that your scales can tip not only from excessive exposure to a single allergen but also from exposure to small amounts of a variety of allergens.

Crossing the line

Cross-reactivity also is an important factor in causing allergic reactions and asthma symptoms. It can contribute toward overloading your allergic threshold. For example, when you have sensitivity to ragweed, you may also be sensitive to allergens in melons — honeydew, cantaloupe, and watermelon.

This phenomenon occurs because, in some individuals, an allergenic cross-reactivity that exists between certain food proteins and nonfood protein sources can look similar to your immune systems. As a result, in addition to ragweed allergy symptoms during ragweed season, you may also experience itching and swelling of your mouth and lips when eating melons, even though these fruits may not present a problem for you during the rest of the year. Some people also experience cross-reactivity reactions between latex and — of all things — bananas, avocados, papaya, kiwi, and chestnuts.

The Great Indoors

Early on, our human ancestors realized that getting out of the elements and into some type of shelter was a key aspect of surviving the dangers and challenges of the prehistoric world. For the most part, humans have become indoor creatures, progressing from cave and tree dwellings to suburbs, malls, and tightly sealed office buildings. In their dwellings, most people have the means of shielding themselves from the adversities of weather and climate and they're safe (for the most part) from predators. Safety from their own kind is, of course, another story.

One of the downsides of modern structures is that indoor environments — at home, work, school, and even in cars and other enclosed means of transportation — can often contain far more significant sources of asthma and allergy triggers than outdoor environments. Irritants and allergens can concentrate in most enclosures, and because people spend so much time indoors, that's where they often experience the most significant exposure to allergy triggers.

Energy-conservation building codes adopted in the United States since the 1970s have worsened the concentration of allergens within structures, because airborne particles that contain allergens and irritants often remain trapped indoors. Although I'm certainly in favor of energy-efficient structures (especially when I see my utility bill), you need to ensure that the air you breathe inside — especially at home — is as safe as possible.

Indoor air pollution: Every breath you take can hurt you

If you have asthma and/or allergic rhinitis, you may focus your attention solely on pollen counts, air pollution, and other elements of the outdoor environment as the prime sources for allergens and irritants that trigger your symptoms and reactions. You may also assume that indoor air is cleaner and safer than the air that you breathe outside. However, according to Environmental Protection Agency studies, indoor air can actually contain as much as 70 times the pollution of outdoor air.

According to the American Lung Association, most people spend 90 percent of their time indoors, spending 60 percent of that time at home. Therefore, indoor air pollution is a serious concern for everyone, particularly because studies show that it can cause or aggravate asthma and allergies.

Allergens on the barbie?

The issue of outdoor and indoor exposure to allergens and irritants is similar to the difference between barbecuing outside or inside. When you cook outside, smoke dissipates. Yes, smoke contributes to overall air pollution, but that's another story. This backyard barbecue process is similar to the way outdoor air dilutes the effects of pollutants and allergens.

If you're crazy enough to bring your grill inside, seal all the windows and doors, turn off the ventilation, and then fire up the coals, smoke would fill your house within two minutes. Now, imagine that smoke as indoor allergens and irritants. All too frequently, many people breathe this polluted air in their indoor environments. The allergy-proofing steps I provide in the next section show you how to avoid and control indoor air pollution.

Allergy-Proofing Begins at Home

Allergen avoidance begins at home. Although I certainly advise you to avoid or limit exposure to allergens and irritants outside, at work, at school, or in other indoor locations, avoidance therapy actually can have the most beneficial impact in your home. Even when you're exposed to allergy triggers outside your home, reducing your exposure to those allergens and irritants at home may prevent your allergen threshold from overloading.

On average, most people spend a third of their lives in the bedroom — much of that time in bed. As a result, the bedroom is the most important single area of your home. After allergy-proofing your bedroom, try using it as much as possible to ensure that you give your allergies a rest.

In and around your home, the most common and important sources of allergens that you need to focus on when allergy-proofing are

- Dust and dust mites
- Pets
- Mold
- Pollen

Controlling irritants at home also is vital to successful avoidance therapy. Although these substances don't trigger allergic responses by your body's immune system (as is the case with allergens), they often worsen existing asthma or allergy conditions.

Tobacco smoke is the most significant irritant found in the home that aggravates allergy and asthma reactions. Other important irritants, in alphabetical order, include

✔ Aerosols, paints, and smoke from wood-burning stoves

✔ Glue

✔ Household cleaners

✔ Perfumes and scents

✔ Scented soaps

The basics of allergy-proofing are illustrated in Figure 10-2 and explained in more detail in the sections that follow.

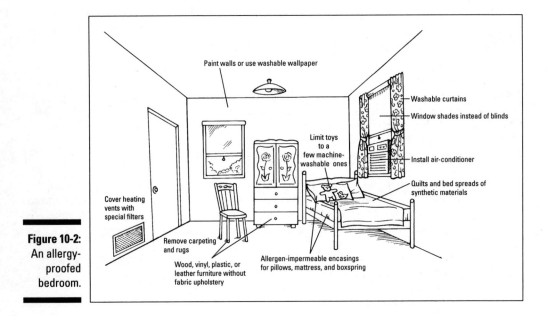

Figure 10-2: An allergy-proofed bedroom.

Controlling the dust in your house

Studies show that the average six-room home in the United States collects 40 pounds of dust each year. House dust is one of the most prevalent asthma and allergy triggers in any home, and unfortunately, it's everywhere. Think of house dust as one of life's inevitabilities — along with death and taxes.

Ridding your house of dust mites

Allergy-proofing your bedroom and home likely involves dealing with dust mites more than with any other allergy trigger, because these microscopic creatures produce the single largest component of house dust that triggers respiratory symptoms in asthma patients. Although you've probably never seen them, dust mites are a fact of life — they're bound to follow almost any-place you settle.

Controlling dust mites in the bedroom

Few of us ever go to bed alone. Dust mites thrive in dark and humid environments such as mattresses, pillows, and box springs. In fact, the average bed contains 2 million dust mites, which means that you may breathe in significant amounts of dust mite allergens while you sleep. Dust mites also survive well in blankets, carpets, towels, upholstered furniture, drapery, and children's stuffed toys.

Although eradication of these natural inhabitants of your home is virtually impossible — the females lay 20 to 50 eggs every three weeks — you can take practical and effective steps to minimize exposure to dust mite allergens.

In my experience, taking the measures I describe with the following household items often results in a significant decrease in respiratory symptoms and medication requirements for patients with asthma and allergies. (The appendix provides more information about obtaining the items I mention in this list.)

✔ **Beds:** Encase all pillows, mattresses, and box springs in special allergen-impermeable casings, and mount all beds on bed frames. Wash all bed linens in hot water (at least 130 degrees) every two weeks. Only use pillows, blankets, quilts, and bedspreads made of synthetic materials. Avoid down-filled (feather) comforters and pillows.

✔ **Temperature and climate control:** Don't locate your bedroom in a warm (more than 72 degrees), humid area. Likewise, use air conditioners or dehumidifiers to keep the humidity in your home below 50 percent. You may want to use a humidity gauge to monitor humidity levels.

✔ **Carpets and drapes:** Whenever possible, go for the bare look in your home — remove carpeting and thick rugs. Bare surfaces such as hardwood, linoleum, or tile floors are inhospitable to dust mites and are also much easier to clean, thereby minimizing dust buildup. If you can't remove your carpeting and rugs, treat them with products that deactivate dust mite allergens. I also recommend washable curtains or window shades rather than heavy draperies or blinds.

✔ **Housekeeping:** Vacuum thoroughly, at least once a week, with a HEPA or ULPA vacuum cleaner (see the "Taking time for terminology" section, earlier in this chapter). When you have allergies, wear a dust mask when cleaning or engaging in any activity that stirs up dust, and consider cleaning your furniture with a tannic acid solution.

✔ **Ventilation:** Use HEPA air cleaners to keep the indoor air throughout your home as pure as possible. (See the "Taking time for terminology" section, earlier in this chapter.) Cover any heating vents with special vent filters to clean the air before it enters your rooms.

✔ **Decorations and furnishings:** Use furniture made of wood, vinyl, plastic, and leather throughout your home rather than furniture made of upholstery. Likewise, make your bedroom as uncluttered and wipeable as possible. Avoid shelves, pennants, posters, photos or pictures, heavy cushions, and other dust collectors. Limit the clothes, books, and other personal objects in your bedroom to the essentials, and make sure that you shut the ones you keep in closets or drawers when not in use.

If your child has allergies or asthma, don't turn his or her bedroom into a stuffed animal zoo. Instead, try limiting those types of toys to a few machine-washable ones. Keep your child's stuffed animals and toys in the closet or in a closed chest, container, or drawer when not in use.

Regulating pet dander

Pets are cherished members of many households. However, *dander* (skin flakes) from these animals is a significant source of allergy triggers for many people. All warm-blooded household pets, regardless of hair length, produce proteins in their dander and saliva that can trigger allergies. Dead skin cells in their dander can even serve as a food supply for dust mites. Cat dander residue can linger at significant exposure levels in carpets for up to 20 weeks and in mattresses for years, even after you remove the animal.

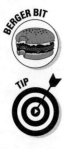

I usually advise people with asthma or allergies not to introduce new pets into their homes. If you already have a pet, I realize that removing this member of the family can be a very emotional issue for you and other household members, even though Fluffy or Fido's dander may be triggering your respiratory symptoms or those of your children.

If finding a new home for your pet isn't likely, I advise the following measures:

✔ Keeping your pet outdoors whenever possible.

If keeping your pet outdoors isn't possible, by all means, try to keep the pet out of the patient's bedroom. Also consider running a HEPA filter 24 hours a day in the bedroom and keeping the door closed.

✔ Making sure that anyone who touches your pet washes his or her hands before contacting the patient or entering the patient's bedroom.

✔ Washing your pet with water once a week. Doing so may remove surface allergens and possibly reduce the amount of dander that can stick to other household members' clothes and bodies (thereby reaching the patient's bedroom). Although it may take some training (and a few scratch marks), even cats can get used to baths.

Controlling mold in your abode

Molds release fungal spores into the air. Theses spores settle on organic matter and grow into new mold clusters. When inhaled by sensitized individuals, these airborne spores can trigger allergic symptoms. Airborne mold spores are more numerous than pollen grains, and unlike pollen, they don't have a limited season. In many parts of the United States and Canada, mold spores may be present until the first snow cover.

Outdoor mold spores can enter your home through the air, by blowing in open windows and doors, and through vents. Indoor molds can grow year-round, and they thrive in dark, humid areas of the home, such as basements and bathrooms. Molds also grow under carpets and in pillows, mattresses, air conditioners, garbage containers, and refrigerators. The older your home, the larger the amount of mold that grows there.

Limiting your exposure to mold spores is a key part of allergy-proofing your home. I advise the following steps for controlling molds in and around your home:

✔ Avoiding damp areas of your home, such as an unfinished basement or a room with a water leak. Or use a dehumidifier to lower humidity in those areas to 35 percent to 40 percent.

✔ Making sure your clothes dryer vents to the outside.

✔ Ventilating your bathroom well, especially after showers or bathing. Use mold-killing and mold-preventing solutions behind the toilet, around the sink, shower, bathtub, washing machine, and refrigerator, and in other areas of your home where water or moisture collect.

✔ Cleaning any visible mold from the walls, floors, and ceiling by using a nonchlorine bleach.

✔ Taking out the trash and cleaning your garbage container regularly to prevent mold growth.

✔ Drying out damp footwear and clothing in which mold can breed. Don't hang clothes outside, where they can become landing areas for mold spores.

✔ Limiting the number of indoor plants or removing them altogether, because mold may grow in potting soil. Dried flowers may also contain mold, so avoid them, too.

If you have allergies or asthma, avoid exposure to outdoor molds around your home. These molds proliferate in fallen leaves, compost, cut grass, fertilizer, hay, and barns. Whenever you must work in your yard, wear a well-fitting breathing mask. Cut back any heavy vegetation around your home to enable the structure to breathe and to prevent dampness and mold growth.

Pollen-proofing

Allergic rhinitis is perhaps the best-known allergy of all. Many people associate this type of allergy primarily with outdoor exposure to pollen. However, you may also experience significant levels of pollen at home, and these exposures also can trigger allergic rhinitis symptoms.

Most pollens are wind-borne; they often blow indoors (typically through open windows and doors) and trigger allergic symptoms, such as allergic rhinitis, within your home and not just outdoors. Wind-pollinated trees, grasses, and weeds produce pollen during various times of the year. (See the "Counting your pollens" section, earlier in this chapter, for details about pollen counts and contact information for the National Allergy Bureau so that you can obtain its reports on local pollen and mold conditions.)

Take the following steps, especially during periods of high pollination, to avoid excessive exposure to pollen:

✔ Avoiding intense outdoor activities, such as exercise or strenuous work, during the early morning and late afternoon hours when pollen counts are highest. Whenever you need to work outside, wear a pollen and dust mask.

✔ Closing windows and running a HEPA or ULPA air purifier.

✔ Cleaning and replacing your air conditioner filters regularly.

✔ Washing your hair before going to bed to avoid getting pollen on your pillow.

✔ Using a clothes dryer rather than hanging the wash outside where it acts as a filter trap for pollen. You may like the idea of fresh, air-dried laundry, but your target organs (see Chapter 1) won't enjoy the allergic reactions that all the fresh pollen triggers — especially when you hang sheets and pillowcases out on the line.

To find out more about other allergy-control products, such as pillow, mattress, and box spring encasings that are often recommended, turn to the appendix at the back of the book.

Chapter 11

Getting Allergy Tested and Allergy Shots

....

....

*D*epending on the severity and nature of your asthma and allergies (such as allergic rhinitis, or *hay fever*) and the degree of your exposure to allergens that trigger your respiratory symptoms, avoidance measures and *pharmacotherapy* (treatment with medications) may not be all that you require for effectively managing your condition. You may also need to identify and address root causes of your condition instead of simply treating your symptoms. As a result, your doctor may refer you to an allergist for skin tests and possible immunotherapy.

Doctors use skin tests to confirm that your symptoms result from allergies instead of some other cause. Doctors also use skin tests to identify, if possible, the specific allergens that trigger your asthma symptoms and allergic symptoms and reactions. Later in this chapter, I explain the two most common types of allergy skin testing that doctors use.

Meanwhile, *immunotherapy* is also known as *allergy shots, desensitization, hyposensitization,* or *allergy vaccination.* The advisability of this treatment depends on whether skin testing provides clear evidence that you're allergic to specific allergens, what those allergens are, and how they correlate with your medical history.

This chapter takes a closer look at both of these specialized diagnostic and treatment procedures, so you know what to expect.

Diagnosing with Skin Tests

Allergists consider skin tests the most reliable and precise method for diagnosing allergies.

Doctors use skin tests to determine whether a minute dose of a suspected allergen — which an allergist or clinic staff member administers in solution form on or just below your skin — produces a small-scale, localized positive response known as a *wheal and erythema (flare) reaction.* A wheal and erythema reaction is a reddened and small-scale swelling of your skin that resembles a mosquito bite, hive, or bump at the site of the allergen test. A positive reaction confirms that you have sensitivity to the administered allergen but may also indicate your specific sensitivity level to that allergen.

After completion of the skin tests, you should remain under observation for at least 30 minutes. If the tests produce a positive reaction, your allergist or test administrator examines and measures the resulting wheal and erythema. Clinicians use these measurements to help determine your level of sensitivity to the specific allergen that was administered. If your physician concludes that you need immunotherapy, knowing your level of sensitivity to the allergen often is important in determining a safe starting dosage for your first series of allergy shots.

Pins and needles

Most allergists use two types of skin tests to evaluate allergic ailments:

- **Prick-puncture:** Sometimes referred to as a *scratch test,* clinicians perform this test on the surface of your back or on your forearm.

- **Intracutaneous:** Allergists perform this test, also known as *intradermal testing,* only when the prick-puncture test fails to produce a significant positive result. The intracutaneous test involves a series of small injections of allergen solution in rows just below the surface of the skin on your arm or forearm.

For both prick-puncture and intracutaneous tests, a positive reaction usually appears within 20 minutes. With either test, you needn't worry about someone turning you into a pincushion or sticking you with a giant syringe. The intracutaneous test uses only very fine needles just beneath the surface of the skin and, like the prick-puncture test (on the surface of the skin), produces minimal discomfort.

Skin tests and antihistamines: Not a good mix

After carefully reviewing your condition and history, if your doctor advises skin testing, you probably need to discontinue using your antihistamine medications (and other products in certain cases, but usually not your asthma drugs) for several days prior to the test. The presence of these drugs in your body can interfere with the skin test results. However, it's unlikely that you'll need to stop most of your other medications.

Never abruptly stop taking your asthma medications without first checking with your doctor. Fortunately, most asthma medications don't interfere with allergy skin testing.

The following list offers some general guidelines about discontinuing various common products; however, your allergist can provide you with more exact instructions, based on the specific medications that you take.

- Discontinue older, sedating, first-generation, over-the-counter (OTC) antihistamines such as Benadryl, Chlor-Trimeton, Dimetapp, Tavist-1, and similar products for 48 to 72 hours before your skin test.

- You may need to stop using newer, nonsedating, second-generation antihistamines, such as Allegra, Clarinex (and its OTC precursor, Claritin), Zyrtec, or Seldane, for as long as two to four days prior to testing. Likewise, studies show that Hismanal can interfere when taken up to three months prior to having skin tests. Therefore, you and your physician need to plan accordingly whenever you take Hismanal and anticipate taking a skin test. (Seldane and Hismanal no longer are available in the United States but still are sold in Canada and other countries; see Chapter 12.)

- Make sure your allergist knows if you're taking beta-blockers (Inderal, Tenormin) or monoamine oxidase inhibitors (Nardil, Parnate), because special precautions must be taken when administering skin tests to patients who take these drugs. They sometimes can render epinephrine ineffective. *Epinephrine* is a rescue medication that doctors use for emergency treatment in cases when rare, severe allergic reactions occur following skin testing.

- Because some of them have antihistamine effects, certain antidepressants also can interfere with skin tests. If you're taking antidepressants, such as trycyclic antidepressants (Elavil or Sinequan), check with the doctor who prescribed them to find out whether you can safely stop taking those products for a brief period or whether substituting another antidepressant (such as Prozac or Paxil) that doesn't have antihistaminic properties is possible. If discontinuing these drugs to undergo skin testing is permitted, you may need to stop taking them for three to five days prior to your test.

Don't ever stop taking any prescribed medication (for any medical condition) without first checking with your physician.

✔ Skin conditions such as contact dermatitis, eczema, psoriasis, or lesions (irritations) in the skin test area also can interfere with your test results. Make sure that your doctor knows about any such conditions before you undergo any skin testing.

Starting from scratch: Prick-puncture procedures

Allergists consider prick-puncture tests the most convenient and cost effective screening method for detecting *specific IgE antibodies*, which are produced by your immune system (see Chapter 6 for an extensive discussion about the immune system) in response to a wide variety of inhalant and food allergens.

When performing a prick-puncture test, an allergist or other qualified medical professional first places a drop of a suspected allergen (in solution form) on your back or your forearm. The test administrator then uses a device that pricks, punctures, or scratches the area to see whether the allergen produces a reaction. The device merely scrapes the skin, without drawing blood.

Alternatively, multiple prick-puncture tests can be administered simultaneously with a *Multi-Test* — a sterile, disposable multiple skin test applicator with eight heads. This procedure uses an applicator that has a specific allergen extract on each of its eight applicator heads and is applied directly to the patient's skin, as shown in Figure 11-1.

Figure 11-1:
A multiple skin test applicator can be used to administer prick-puncture skin tests.

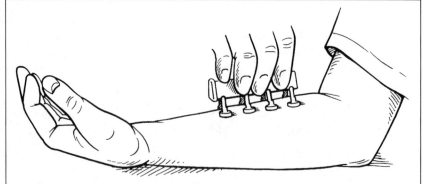

You may have to undergo as many as 70 prick-puncture tests to conclusively identify inhalant allergens. The number of tests you receive varies according to factors such as the area where you live, work, or go to school, and the types of allergen exposure that you receive. In many cases, your doctor requires fewer tests.

The number of prick-puncture tests that your doctor may need to administer to determine your specific food allergies varies from 20 to 80. However, only a few selected foods (milk, eggs, peanuts, tree nuts, fish, shellfish, soy, and wheat) account for the vast majority of cases of allergic food reactions. By first taking a detailed medical history, in many cases your doctor may need to perform only a few carefully chosen food allergen skin tests to confirm a likely diagnosis of *food hypersensitivity,* or food allergy (see Chapter 8).

Some food allergies, such as peanut hypersensitivity, can trigger serious reactions. Whenever a patient tells me, "Doctor, anytime I eat anything that has peanuts in it, I nearly die," I take his or her word for it. If you suffer from specific severe food allergy reactions, I strongly advise against skin tests — and never recommend intracutaneous tests — because the resulting positive reaction can produce serious or even life-threatening results. Before you have any kind of skin test, always tell your doctor about any serious food reactions that you may have experienced in the past.

Getting under your skin: Intracutaneous testing

If your prick-puncture tests are inconclusive, your doctor may need to perform up to 40 intracutaneous tests — rarely that many in the case of suspected food allergies — to produce a significant positive reaction and confirm the diagnosis of an allergy.

Because intracutaneous tests involve injecting an allergen extract just below the surface of your skin, the risk — although small — of a widespread systemic reaction exists. Rarely should an intracutaneous test be done for a particular allergen without a prior prick-puncture test for that same allergen. The type of adverse reaction that can result from administering a particular allergen usually is far less serious with a prick-puncture test, and it alerts your allergist to the potential danger of performing an intracutaneous test with that allergen.

Because of a variety of factors, including the types of allergen extracts that your allergist administers, delayed reactions can occur with prick-puncture tests but occur more often following intracutaneous tests. The characteristic signs of these reactions include swollen, reddened, numb bumps at the skin test site.

Delayed reactions can develop three to ten hours after your test and may continue for up to 12 hours thereafter. The bumps usually disappear 24 to 48 hours later. These delayed reactions, which are known as *late-phase skin reactions,* aren't a sign of immediate hypersensitivity (which I explain in Chapter 6), and allergists often tell their patients to ignore these late reactions.

Skin test side effects

Skin testing occasionally produces adverse side effects in ultrasensitive individuals, but only rarely. As you'd expect, adverse reactions occur far less frequently with prick-puncture tests than with more invasive intracutaneous tests. These side effects can range from large local reactions on the skin to systemic reactions, such as sneezing, coughing, tightness of the chest, swelling of the throat, itchy eyes, and postnasal drip.

In very rare cases, death from *anaphylaxis,* a life-threatening reaction that affects many organs simultaneously, has occurred following a skin test. For that reason, medical facilities where doctors perform skin tests need to have appropriate emergency equipment and drugs on hand in the unlikely event that using these items becomes necessary.

Blood testing for allergies

Although most allergists consider skin tests the gold standard for diagnosing allergies, they may not work for every patient. Your allergist may advise diagnosing your allergic condition with a blood test known as *radioallergensorbent testing* (RAST) or Enzyme-Linked Immunosorbent Assay (ELISA). Your doctor may advise you to have a blood test instead of a skin test for the following reasons:

✔ Your prescribing physician advises you not to discontinue medications such as antihistamines and antidepressants that can interfere with skin test results.

✔ You suffer from a severe skin condition such as widespread eczema or psoriasis (over a large part of your body), and your doctor is unable to find a suitable skin site for testing.

✔ If your sensitivity level to suspected allergens is so high that any administration of those allergens may result in potentially serious side effects (for example, a history of life-threatening reactions to the ingestion of peanuts), then avoid allergy skin testing.

✔ When problematic behavioral, physical, or mental conditions prevent you from cooperating with the skin-testing process.

Because RAST can require only one blood sample to analyze many allergens, this method may seem more convenient than skin testing. However, other than the exceptions I list earlier in this section, most allergists rarely use RAST, because it isn't as accurate as skin testing and can result in an incomplete profile of your allergies. In addition, RAST is more expensive and time-consuming, because a laboratory must analyze blood samples and report test results, which often takes at least two days. If your results return inconclusive, your allergist must perform the test again and wait for new results. In comparison, skin testing usually provides results on the spot within 15 to 30 minutes.

Reviewing Immunotherapy

Immunotherapy (also known as *allergy shots, desensitization, hyposensitization,* or *allergy vaccination*) currently is the most effective form of treating the underlying immunologic mechanism (see Chapter 6) that causes allergic conditions such as allergic rhinitis, allergic conjunctivitis, allergic asthma, and allergies to insect stings. However, immunotherapy, at present, doesn't provide a safe and effective treatment for food allergies.

Seeing how immunotherapy works

How exactly does immunotherapy work? The following information may help you understand it better:

- **Decreasing production of IgE antibodies.** IgE antibodies are the agents that bind with allergens at receptor sites on the surfaces of mast cells, thus initiating the release of potent chemical mediators of inflammation such as histamine and leukotrienes. These chemicals trigger allergic reactions and asthma symptoms. (See Chapter 6 for an extensive explanation of the complex immune system responses involved in asthma and allergies, such as allergic rhinitis.)

- **Initiating the production of other allergen-specific IgG antibodies.** *Allergen-specific IgG antibodies* also are known as *blocking antibodies.* Immunotherapy can stimulate your body to produce blocking antibodies, which compete with mast-cell bound IgE for antigen, thus preventing the initial sensitization, activation, and subsequent release of potent chemical mediators of inflammation from these cells. To find out more about the cast of Ig (immunoglobulin) antibodies and other characters involved in the complex immune system responses that result in allergy and asthma symptoms, turn to Chapter 6 (especially if you're a budding immunologist).

✔ **Stabilizing the actual mast cells (and basophils).** Doing so means that even if IgE antibodies and allergens cross-link on the surface of these cells, your potential allergic reaction is usually less severe, because the release of potent chemical mediators of inflammation is reduced. In addition, immunotherapy can result in decreasing the actual number of mast cells (and basophils) in the affected areas. This reduction in activation and numbers of these cells also results in suppressing the inflammatory late-phase allergic response following allergen exposure (see Chapter 6).

Deciding whether immunotherapy makes sense for you

Immunotherapy may be appropriate for treating your allergies and thus can help you manage your asthma more effectively depending on the following factors:

✔ Effectively avoiding allergens that trigger your asthma symptoms and allergic reactions is impractical, or even impossible, because the life you lead inevitably results in allergen exposure.

✔ Your respiratory symptoms are consistently severe or debilitating.

✔ Managing your asthma and/or allergies requires prohibitively expensive courses of medication, which produce side effects that adversely affect your overall health and quality of life. If the health and financial costs of multiple allergy drugs outweigh their benefits, immunotherapy may make more sense for you.

✔ Allergy testing provides conclusive evidence of specific IgE antibodies, thus enabling your allergist to identify the particular allergens that trigger your symptoms.

✔ You haven't experienced serious adverse side effects (as a result of skin testing) to the allergens that your doctor will use in your subsequent course of immunotherapy.

✔ You can make the commitment to see the therapy process through. Immunotherapy isn't a quick fix, and it requires a significant investment of your time.

If you suffer from an unstable heart condition and you take beta-blockers such as Inderal, if you have high blood pressure and take angiotensin converting enzyme (ACE) inhibitors (Capoten, Vasotec), or if you take monoamine oxidase (MAO) inhibitors (Nardil, Parnate), don't consider immunotherapy unless your physician advises you that the benefits of starting immunotherapy outweigh the risks of discontinuing those medications.

Getting shots

Injections, or shots, are the most effective and reliable method of administering specially prepared, diluted allergen extracts that allergists use when providing immunotherapy treatment. If needles give you nightmares, relax. Allergy shots are much less painful or traumatic than deep intramuscular shots often needed to effectively administer immunizations or certain medications (such as cortisone or penicillin). That's because doctors usually administer allergy shots with the same type of fine needle they use in intracutaneous testing, thus causing minimal discomfort.

BERGER BIT

I'm often amazed at how well kids handle allergy shots after getting over their initial fears about that first shot. After the first shot, allergy shots aren't usually a problem for most children, especially when they notice that their respiratory symptoms are starting to improve. I don't claim that kids love getting allergy shots (or going to the doctor for anything besides a lollipop), but they usually quickly discover that receiving these injections beats not being able to breathe properly.

Allergens that doctors commonly use in immunotherapy treatments for allergic asthma, allergic rhinitis, and allergic conjunctivitis include extracts of inhalant allergens from tree, grass, and weed pollens; mold spores; dust mites; and sometimes animal danders.

In preparing your allergen extract (serum or vaccine), your doctor includes only those allergens for which you previously have demonstrated sensitivity in your skin testing. If your skin tests show sensitivity to multiple allergens (you're sensitive to many grass and weed pollens, for example), your allergist may mix all the different grass extracts into one vial and all the different weed extracts into another vial. Preparing the serum in such combinations ensures that you receive only one shot for each group of extracts, thus reducing the number of injections that you need for effective therapy.

Your allergist may even determine that mixing doses of all your allergens into a single shot on a particular visit is an option for you based on:

✔ Your allergic sensitivity

✔ The volume of extract that needs to be administered

✔ The types of allergen extracts he uses for your therapy

In some cases, for your comfort, it may be preferable to split the required dose of your allergy shot into two or more separate injections.

Although this treatment can greatly reduce your allergy symptoms, immunotherapy isn't considered a guaranteed permanent cure for asthma and allergies (see Chapters 1 and 6). You likewise still need to continue practicing avoidance measures while receiving immunotherapy, because doing so can significantly enhance the effectiveness of your treatment.

Immunotherapy can significantly improve your respiratory symptoms, thus reducing your need for allergy medication, which, in turn, makes this treatment the closest thing to a currently available cure for allergies and the respiratory symptoms they trigger. However, always tell your allergist:

- Whenever you're considering taking medications — including OTC drugs — for allergies or nonallergic conditions.

- About any changes in your medical condition, even if the changes may not seem directly connected to your allergies.

   Pregnancy, which I mention in the nearby sidebar, is an example of a change in medical condition that you need to report to your allergist.

Your adherence is key for an effective immunotherapy program. Follow and maintain the shot schedule (see the next section) that your allergist prescribes as closely as possible. However, avoid shots under the following circumstances:

- **Exercise:** Make sure that you don't engage in strenuous physical activity for at least one hour before and two hours after your allergy shots. Exercising at these times can increase your risk of experiencing a serious adverse reaction because exercise increases your blood circulation, potentially resulting in a rapid absorption of the allergen from the shot and possibly even causing a severe reaction.

- **Illness:** If you run a fever, tell your allergist. Receiving an allergy shot while you're ill isn't a good idea because your fever symptoms can make detecting an adverse reaction to the shots difficult.

- **Immunizations:** Try to avoid scheduling any immunizations on the same day as your allergy shots because potential adverse effects from the immunization can make a reaction from an allergy shot difficult to identify. If you do get an immunization shot on the day of your scheduled allergy shots, let your allergist know; she may advise you to not get your allergy shots that same day.

Shot schedules

The most effective way of administering immunotherapy is by providing *perennial therapy,* which involves receiving shots of allergen extracts year-round. Studies show that perennial therapy provides the longest and most successful reduction of your level of sensitivity to specific allergens.

Pregnancy and immunotherapy

If you become pregnant while receiving immunotherapy, you'll be glad to know that your allergy shots are safe during pregnancy. In fact, your allergist may advise you to continue receiving immunotherapy, possibly at a reduced dosage, to minimize any risk of reactions to allergy shots and to continue to provide relief from your respiratory symptoms.

If you stop treatment, you can run the risk of experiencing worsening symptoms. This worsening can lead in turn to increased needs for medication that may not be desirable during your pregnancy. However, if you're already pregnant and are considering whether or not to start a course of immunotherapy, your allergist may advise you to delay beginning this form of treatment until after delivery.

A typical course of perennial immunotherapy may follow these steps:

✔ Your allergist begins your therapy by administering shots once or twice a week, starting with a very small amount of a diluted dose of allergen extracts.

✔ Your allergist gradually increases your allergen dosage by increasing the amount and concentration of the extract week by week until you reach the maintenance dose in about three to six months. The *maintenance dose* refers to a predetermined amount of maximal concentration or the highest strength that you can tolerate without producing adverse reactions.

✔ After reaching your maintenance dose, allergy symptom relief usually begins. When relief starts, you can continue receiving shots at the maintenance dose level. Likewise, your allergist may extend the interval between your shots from one week to as many as four, depending on your response to the treatment and the levels of exposure that you encounter in your environment.

Every time you receive your allergy shots, expect to wait at least 20 minutes afterwards in your allergist's office so that a medical staff member can inspect and evaluate the areas of skin around your shots and monitor you for any early signs of anaphylaxis. Another benefit of staying in your allergist's office after your shot: In the rare event that you experience a severe reaction, qualified medical personnel can immediately provide emergency assistance.

A long-term relationship

For inhalant allergens, an effective immunotherapy program usually requires shots for at least three to five years. In many cases, if your sensitivity to allergens improves during the course of immunotherapy, you can maintain your level of allergy improvement for several years (or even life-long in some cases) after discontinuing the shots.

However, in some cases, withdrawing from immunotherapy results in the reappearance of allergic symptoms. Therefore, your allergist needs to evaluate the specifics of your individual case when considering the possibility of discontinuing immunotherapy.

Considering side effects

The possibility — however small — of anaphylactic reactions exists any time your allergist injects allergenic proteins into your body. In some unfortunate cases, people have died after receiving their allergy shots. Therefore, although the odds of a serious reaction to allergy shots are far less than those of getting into a bad car crash on the way to your allergist's office, take as many precautions as possible. After receiving an allergy shot, immediately tell your doctor or nurse if you're experiencing any of the following signs of serious adverse side effects:

- ✔ Itchiness of the feet, hands, groin area, and underarms
- ✔ Large-scale skin reactions, such as hives or flushing
- ✔ Upper and lower respiratory symptoms, such as sneezing, coughing, tightness of the chest, a swollen or itchy throat, itchy eyes, postnasal drip, difficulty swallowing, and a hoarse voice
- ✔ Nausea, diarrhea, and stomach cramps
- ✔ Dizziness, fainting, or a severe drop in blood pressure

Because the threat of severe adverse reactions exists, I strongly advise against giving yourself allergy shots at home. Although practices vary in different areas, the vast majority of my colleagues insist that patients receive their allergy shots only in an appropriate medical facility because of this small chance of adverse, life-threatening reactions.

Looking at Future Forms of Immunotherapy

New forms of immunotherapy treatment are just around the corner. The most promising therapies include

- ✔ **Nasal sprays:** Nasal sprays that are under development may provide a less needle-dependent form of administering allergen extracts to patients.

✓ **Sublingual-swallow immunotherapy.** This form of allergy treatment, known as *SLIT,* currently is used in some European countries mainly for pollen allergies. The therapy involves holding drops of allergen extract under the tongue for as long as two minutes before swallowing. Although studies show that SLIT can be effective in reducing symptoms of certain pollen-triggered allergic reactions, patients often need to hold as many as 20 drops (1 ml) under their tongues before swallowing, and that can be challenging for some people. And, unlike allergy shots, which usually require a visit to your doctor's office, SLIT is intended more as a self-administered therapy, meaning patients can take their doses at home. This raises issues of compliance, because patients may not always be able to adhere on their own to the proper way of taking these drops.

✓ **Solid/tablet forms of SLIT:** Researchers currently are developing a solid form of SLIT, which would consist of a disintegrating tablet that gradually dissolves under the tongue and insures that patients consistently receive an exact dose of prescribed allergen extracts.

✓ **Anti-IgE antibodies:** The agent in this medication named Xolair (recently approved by the FDA) is a high-tech antibody known as *recombinant human monoclonal antibody.* Researchers designed this drug to bind to the part of the IgE antibody that otherwise would bind with the IgE receptor site on mast cells, thus preventing the activation of these cells and subsequent allergic reaction (see Chapter 6 for more information about the immune system). In my opinion, this drug not only improves asthma and allergic rhinitis treatment but may also include the potential to block many types of allergic reactions that science hasn't had much success in controlling adequately — for example, severe allergic food reactions.

Chapter 12

Relieving Your Nasal Allergies

*M*any people with asthma also have *allergic rhinitis* (hay fever). Extensive studies over the last 30 years have shown that patients with allergic asthma usually are more successful in managing their respiratory condition if they take effective measures to control their allergic rhinitis symptoms.

The multiple allergens, which commonly trigger the allergic reactions that induce symptoms of allergic rhinitis, also often aggravate or worsen the respiratory symptoms associated with asthma. Remember, your airways, from your nasal passages down to the smallest bronchioles in your lungs, form a continuum.

You can take avoidance measures and allergy-proof your home and office to significantly improve your quality of life by decreasing your exposure to the substances that trigger your allergic reactions and, in most cases, your asthma episodes. (See Chapter 10 for more on allergy-proofing and avoidance measures.) However, because allergens, such as pollens, molds, and dust, are everywhere, complete avoidance can be difficult, if not impossible.

Fortunately, medications are available. If used properly — based on your physician's advice — medications can prevent or relieve your allergic reactions. In this chapter, I explain how the most common nasal allergy medications work, what potential side effects they have, and how you can make smart choices to control your allergic reactions. Effectively treating those reactions is often the single most important factor in reducing — and in some cases even eliminating — many common respiratory symptoms, thus improving your asthma and your overall quality of life.

Getting Familiar with Pharmacology

The many drugs available for treating nasal allergies have various uses and characteristics. Some allergy medications are designed for one specific purpose, while others have more flexible uses. In general, nasal allergy medications fall into three categories of usage:

- ✓ **Preventive:** If used properly, these types of medications can keep your nasal symptoms from developing. For people who have chronic symptoms of rhinitis, allergic or nonallergic (see Chapter 7), the most effective approach is to use antihistamines (oral or nasal) and nasal corticosteroid medications preventively (see the "Using Nasal Corticosteroids" section, later in this chapter).

- ✓ **Stabilizing:** These drugs can often stop a reaction that's already in process before your immune system can release potent chemical mediators of inflammation, such as histamine and leukotrienes (see Chapter 6), that produce noticeable symptoms.

- ✓ **Relief:** Most of the commonly available over-the-counter (OTC) oral antihistamines and decongestants fall into this category. Most people use them to relieve the symptoms of rhinitis after symptoms have occurred. As I explain in this chapter, you're usually not taking full advantage of medications, such as antihistamines and nasal corticosteroid sprays, if you only use them after your symptoms have started.

Whether prescribed or purchased OTC, a few basic types of drugs are used to treat nasal allergies, including the following:

- ✓ Antihistamines (available in various forms OTC and by prescription)

- ✓ Antihistamine nasal sprays (available by prescription only)

- ✓ Decongestants (available OTC, by prescription in oral form, or as non-prescription nasal sprays and drops)

- ✓ Combinations of antihistamine (OTC and prescription) and decongestant products (available in oral form) are also used for multisymptomatic relief, as I discuss in the section "Two for the Nose: Combination Products"

- ✓ Nasal corticosteroid sprays (available only in prescription form)

- ✓ Mast cell stabilizer nasal sprays containing cromolyn (available OTC)

- ✓ Anticholinergic (drying) nasal sprays (available only in prescription form)

To get the most out of your treatment, take the time to know what each medication can do to relieve your symptoms. I explain the uses and benefits of each product in this chapter.

An informed patient is a healthier patient. If your doctor prescribes medication for your allergic rhinitis (or any ailment), don't hesitate to inquire about the product, why it's being prescribed, and any possible side effects. For further information on what you should know, see Chapter 14.

Blocking Your Histamines: Antihistamines

As the name indicates, antihistamines are medications (available in tablet, capsule, liquid, and nasal spray forms, or by injection) that counter the effects of *histamine* — a chemical substance released by the body as the result of injury or in response to an allergen. *First-generation* (sedating) OTC antihistamines have been in use since 1942 and are frequently the first medication option for allergic rhinitis sufferers. I discuss the important differences between OTC and most newer, *second-generation* (nonsedating or less sedating) antihistamines in the section "Newer antihistamines," later in this chapter.

Both first- and second-generation antihistamines block the effects of histamine and are most effective in controlling or alleviating symptoms of sneezing, runny nose, and itchy nose, eyes, and throat. However, these medications may not reduce nasal congestion. As a result, they're frequently combined with a decongestant to relieve symptoms of congestion. In addition, antihistamines produce various side effects, depending on the type of product (OTC or prescription), dosage levels, and course of medication.

As an asthma patient, don't be afraid to use antihistamines, depending on your specific condition and your doctor's advice. In the past, product information labels advised asthma patients not to use antihistamines because these medications theoretically dry out the airways. However, studies show that the improvement of nasal symptoms produced by antihistamines improves the lung functions of many people with asthma.

Histamine hints

As I explain in Chapter 1, *mast cells* (among the cells that line your nose and respiratory tract) produce and release a chemical substance called histamine. You may only become aware of histamine when your immune system releases massive amounts of this chemical into nasal tissue as a reaction to injury or in the presence of an allergen. After being released from the mast cells, histamine seeks out "receptor" sites located in the nasal lining tissues.

Think of these receptors sites as locks. Histamine inserts itself like a key into the receptor site and triggers the familiar hay fever symptoms of allergic rhinitis. Antihistamines attach to the receptors before histamine gets to them. Because receptors accept only one chemical at a time, if antihistamines block histamine, allergic symptoms won't be triggered.

A dose of prevention

Many people tend to use antihistamines only as rescue medications. However, these products usually work much better and give greater relief if taken preventively. Taking an antihistamine to relieve your symptoms is like closing the barn door after your horse has already bolted. You're not going to get that horse back (although by closing the door, you'll at least prevent any others from escaping).

Antihistamines usually work best when taken on a regular basis before allergen exposure occurs. For example:

✔ If you're allergic to ragweed pollen, start using your medication at the beginning of August — before ragweed pollens are released in the middle of the month — and continue using the medication until after ragweed season is through. Even if you're exposed to significant amounts of allergen, you'll usually experience far fewer symptoms by using this type of preventive approach.

✔ If you know that animal dander triggers your allergic rhinitis and you plan to visit someone who has pets, take your antihistamine two to five hours beforehand. Also, remember to continue with the antihistamine after you leave, until you have an opportunity to change your clothing because dander probably will be on your clothes.

First-generation OTC antihistamines

The most common variety of antihistamine medications is first-generation nonprescription products that are available in OTC form. Hundreds of these nonprescription antihistamine products line drugstore and supermarket shelves. Most of these products, however, are just different brand names for a few of the same active ingredients, such as:

✔ Brompheniramine maleate — the active ingredient in Dimetapp

✔ Chlorpheniramine maleate — the active ingredient in Chlor-Trimeton

✔ Clemastine fumarate — the active ingredient in Tavist-1

✔ Diphenhydramine hydrochloride — the active ingredient in Benadryl

Although first-generation OTC antihistamines can relieve allergic rhinitis symptoms, such as sneezing, runny nose, and itchy nose, eyes, and throat, they also produce side effects that can significantly interfere with your daily life. These OTC antihistamines can cross from the bloodstream into your brain, where they affect histamine receptors in the central nervous system, resulting in drowsiness — the most serious and potentially dangerous side effect.

Consider these factors when taking nonprescription antihistamines:

✔ Many states in the United States consider people who take first-generation OTC antihistamines to be under the influence of drugs. The Federal Aviation Administration (FAA) prohibits pilots from flying if they take OTC antihistamines within 24 hours of flight time. Similar restrictions on the use of first-generation OTC antihistamines apply to truck and bus drivers and operators in other transportation industries.

✔ Operating heavy machinery or engaging in activities that require alertness, coordination, dexterity, or quick reflexes while taking first-generation OTC antihistamines is dangerous.

✔ Avoid alcohol, sedatives, antidepressants, or other types of tranquilizers while taking first-generation OTC antihistamines.

✔ First-generation OTC antihistamines can also produce other side effects including the following:

  • Dizziness

  • Dryness of mouth and sinus passages

  • Gastrointestinal irritation or distress

  • Nasal stuffiness

  • Urine retention (which can aggravate existing prostate problems)

✔ Recent studies show that children with allergic rhinitis who take diphenhydramine (the active ingredient in Benadryl) for their symptoms score significantly lower on learning ability tests than children who receive equivalent doses of loratadine (the second-generation OTC antihistamine Claritin).

In my experience, many asthma patients don't tolerate the side effects of first-generation nonprescription antihistamines. As a result, they're less likely to take a long-term or even mid-term preventive course of a first-generation nonprescription antihistamine medication. Instead, patients may resort to these older OTC antihistamines as quick, short-term fixes after allergens trigger their allergic rhinitis symptoms. This approach often leads to a pattern of debilitating, recurring symptoms that can increase the chances that asthma patients' respiratory ailments will worsen and thus diminish their quality of life.

Newer antihistamines

Many people assume that OTC medications are somehow safer than prescription products. In the case of antihistamines, however, the reverse may be true. Due to significant advances in research since the development of first-generation antihistamines more than 50 years ago, several of the newer, second-generation antihistamines have fewer side effects. (However, the majority of the existing prescription antihistamines are still of the older, first-generation type, and just like all the first-generation OTC antihistamines, they can potentially cause drowsiness.) Some of the benefits of these newer second-generation medications include

✔ Not crossing the blood-brain barrier, which means that second-generation products are nonsedating, such as fexofenadine (Allegra), loratadine (Alavert and Claritin) — reclassified by the FDA as an OTC product in 2002 — and desloratadine (Clarinex), or cause only mild sedative effects, as in the case of cetirizine (Zyrtec).

✔ Side effects other than drowsiness, such as dry mouth, constipation, urine retention, or blurred vision, occur less frequently or are much less noticeable with second-generation antihistamines.

✔ Although second-generation antihistamines, whether prescription or OTC (such as loratadine — the active ingredient in Alavert and Claritin), can cost more than most first-generation nonprescription antihistamine products, the more recently developed products work longer and require only one or two doses per day to prevent or relieve allergic rhinitis symptoms.

✔ For the most part, second-generation products work as rapidly as the first-generation drugs. For example, desloratadine (Clarinex), loratadine (Claritin), and cetirizine (Zyrtec) usually start functioning within 30 minutes.

✔ Overall, patients who use second-generation antihistamines usually experience much less disruption or impairment in their daily lives.

Because of these factors, second-generation antihistamines (see Table 12-1) can greatly improve the treatment of allergic rhinitis. In my experience, asthma patients are far more likely to stick with second-generation antihistamines for the prescribed course, which often results in a more effective prevention of allergic rhinitis symptoms and a significant improvement of their respiratory symptoms and overall condition.

Table 12-1		Second-Generation Prescription (and OTC) Antihistamines		
Active Ingredient	*Formulation*	*Brand Name*	*Total Usual Daily Dose for Children under 12 Years (See Formulation Details)*	*Total Usual Daily Adult Dose*
Cetirizine	5 mg, 10 mg tablet (ages 12 years and older), syrup, 5 mg per teaspoon (2–5 years)	Zyrtec	Syrup, ½ teaspoon (2.5 mg) once per day for ages 2–5 years; 1–2 teaspoons (5–10 mg) once per day for ages 6–11 years	1 tablet once per day
Cetirizine (with 120 mg pseudoephedrine)	5 mg tablet (12 years and older)	Zyrtec-D	Not approved for children under 12 years of age	1 tablet twice per day
Desloratadine	5 mg tablet	Clarinex	Not approved for children under 12 years of age	1 tablet once per day (12 years and older)
Fexofenadine	30 mg tablet (6–11 years)	Allegra-Pediatric	1 tablet twice per day	Not applicable
Fexofenadine	60 mg capsule, 60 mg tablet (12 years and older)	Allegra	Not approved for children under 12 years of age	1 capsule twice per day
Fexofenadine	180 mg tablet (12 years and older)	Allegra-24 Hour	Not approved for children under 12 years of age	1 tablet once per day
Fexofenadine (with 120 mg pseudoephedrine)	60 mg tablet (12 years and older)	Allegra-D	Not approved for children under 12 years of age	1 tablet twice per day
Loratadine	10 mg tablet (6 years and older)	Claritin	1 tablet once per day (6 years and older)	1 tablet once per day

(continued)

Table 12-1 *(continued)*

Active Ingredient	Formulation	Brand Name	Total Usual Daily Dose for Children under 12 Years (See Formulation Details)	Total Usual Daily Adult Dose
Loratadine	10 mg tablet (rapidly disintegrating) (6 years and older)	Claritin RediTabs	1 tablet once per day (6 years and older)	1 tablet once per day
Loratadine	10 mg tablet (rapidly disintegrating) (6 years and older)	Alavert	1 tablet once per day (6 years and older)	1 tablet once per day
Loratadine (with 120 mg pseudo-ephedrine)	5 mg tablet (12 years and older)	Claritin-D 12 Hour	Not approved for children under 12 years of age	1 tablet twice per day
Loratadine (with 240 mg pseudo-ephedrine)	10 mg tablet (12 years and older)	Claritin-D 24 Hour	Not approved for children under 12 years of age	1 tablet once per day
Loratadine	Syrup, 5 mg per teaspoon (for ages 2–11 years)	Claritin Syrup	2 teaspoons (10 mg) once per day for ages 6–11 years; 1 teaspoon (5 mg) once per day for ages 2–5 years	2 teaspoons (10 mg) once per day
The following drugs are no longer available in the United States.				
Astemizole	10 mg tablet (12 years and older)	Hismanal	Not approved for children under 12 years of age	1 tablet once per day
Terfenadine	60 mg tablet (12 years and older)	Seldane	Not approved for children under 12 years of age	1 tablet twice per day
Terfenadine (with 120 mg pseudo-ephedrine)	60 mg tablet (12 years and older)	Seldane-D	Not approved for children under 12 years of age	1 tablet twice per day

mg = milligram

Seldane and Hismanal issues

When used in combination with certain systemic antifungals (such as keto-conazole), antibiotics (such as erythromycin), any medical condition that may affect liver function, and even if taken with grapefruit juice, Seldane and Hismanal (no longer available in the United States but still sold in Canada and other countries) can — in rare cases — produce abnormal and potentially fatal heart rhythms. Make sure that you inform your doctor about any and all medications you already take — including OTC products — when you receive a prescription for another drug.

Understanding the pros and cons of OTC Claritin and Alavert

The approval of loratadine (Alavert, Claritin) in 2002 as an OTC product may at first glance seem like great news for asthma and allergy sufferers. After all, you can buy medications formulated with loratadine right off the shelf at your local drug store, and those products now cost less than when you had to have your doctor prescribe them. However, since loratadine's OTC reclas-sification, many physicians are concerned about some insurers and managed-care providers' actions to no longer provide coverage of the cost of other second-generation prescription-only antihistamines.

The problem with that bottom-line approach is that patients and their condi-tions vary widely. In some cases, even though loratadine may be the least expensive second-generation antihistamine available, it may not be the most effective drug for preventing and relieving your allergy symptoms. For this reason, both the American College of Allergy, Asthma, and Immunology (ACAAI) and the American Academy of Allergy, Asthma, and Immunology (AAAAI), which are national organizations of allergists and immunologists dedicated to quality patient care through research, advocacy, and public edu-cation, issued a statement in November 2002 concerning limited insurance coverage for second-generation antihistamines.

That statement points out that these cost-cutting attempts will reduce access to treatment for millions of patients with asthma and allergies and will also have a negative effect on the health and safety of the general public. If your doctor determines that the most effective drug for your allergies is a second-generation prescription antihistamine (such as Allegra, Clarinex, or Zyrtec), you shouldn't have to worry whether or not your health plan will cover the cost of that medication. In essence, the ACAAI and AAAAI are trying to make sure that you and your physician will make the decisions about your health in the exam room, rather than by number crunchers in HMO boardrooms. (For more on my concerns about the way managed-care plans can limit patients' access to the most effective treatments for their conditions, see Chapter 3.)

Dosing a.m. to p.m.

As part of their cost-cutting efforts, some managed-care organizations experiment with a dosing schedule that consists of prescribing a nonsedating second-generation antihistamine during the day and a less expensive, sedating OTC antihistamine at night. Although the concept may seem logical in theory, the reality can actually cause many problems. Because antihistamines continue to act in the body for a long time, the sedative side effects of the first-generation product may persist during the day. Studies show that using a first-generation product at night leads to sedation, performance impairment, and decreased alertness the next day.

Antihistamines and children

Treating children with any type of illness can be quite a challenge, and allergic rhinitis is certainly no exception. Besides the difficulty of getting children to actually take medications, parents also need to be concerned about side effects. In this regard, some of the second-generation antihistamines, such as the following, can be especially useful when treating children with allergic rhinitis:

- ✔ **Loratadine (Claritin):** Your doctor can prescribe this medication in a once-a-day kid-friendly syrup or rapidly disintegrating tablet form (Alavert, Claritin RediTabs) for children as young as 6 years.

- ✔ **Cetirizine (Zyrtec):** Your doctor can prescribe this medicine for children as young as 2 years in a once-a-day syrup form.

Antihistamine nasal sprays

On the front lines of allergic rhinitis treatment, a recent addition to the antihistamine arsenal in the United States is *azelastine hydrochloride*. The FDA approved azelastine for use as a nasal spray under the product name Astelin. Remember these basic facts about this nasal spray:

- ✔ Azelastine hydrochloride is highly effective for the treatment of seasonal allergic rhinitis symptoms, such as sneezing, runny nose, and itchy nose, eyes, and throat.

- ✔ In contrast to most oral antihistamines, studies show that azelastine often helps reduce nasal congestion (stuffy nose), which may make it particularly useful in dealing with the congestion that often accompanies allergic rhinitis due to late-phase reactions (see Chapter 6).

✔ You can use azelastine nasal spray in combination therapy with nasal corticosteroid sprays or oral antihistamines in cases that require greater prevention or relief. (See "Using Nasal Corticosteroids," later in this chapter, for more information on these sprays.)

✔ The recommended dosage for azelastine is two sprays in each nostril twice a day for patients older than 12 years and one spray in each nostril twice a day for children ages 5 to 11 years.

✔ The spray usually starts to take effect within three hours.

✔ The FDA approved azelastine hydrochloride for the treatment of *vasomotor rhinitis* (nonallergic rhinitis; see Chapter 7) for ages 12 years and older. The recommended dosage is two sprays in each nostril twice a day.

✔ Side effects may include a bitter taste and drowsiness in cases of prolonged use.

Decongesting Your Nose

People commonly use decongestants to relieve their stuffy noses. You can find decongestants in two forms: systemic decongestants in tablet, capsule, or liquid forms, and decongestants in the form of nasal sprays or nose drops. Unlike antihistamines, no second-generation decongestants have yet been developed.

Oral decongestants

Nonprescription oral decongestants are among the most widely used OTC products in the world, and you can find them in various tablet, capsule, and liquid forms. These medications work by shrinking blood vessels, thus reducing the amount of fluid that leaks into tissues lining the nose, thereby decreasing nasal congestion. The most commonly used decongestants are pseudoephedrine and phenylephrine.

Pseudoephedrine is the most frequently used active ingredient in OTC oral decongestants, such as Sudafed, and in antihistamine-decongestant combinations such as Actifed and Dimetapp. This drug is the "D" (standing for decongestant) in the commonly used second-generation products known as Allegra-D, Claritin-D, and Zyrtec-D.

Remember the following information before using this type of decongestant:

✔ Systemic decongestants are often combined with other drugs, such as antihistamines, *antipyretics* (fever reducers), *analgesics* (pain relievers), *antitussives* (cough suppressants), or expectorants to provide multi-symptom relief for headaches, fever, cough, sleeplessness, and other symptoms of the common cold, flu, allergic rhinitis, and other ailments.

✔ Oral forms of systemic decongestants can cause side effects, such as sleeplessness, nervous agitation, loss of appetite, dryness of mouth and sinuses, difficulty urinating, high blood pressure, and heart palpitations if used consistently over a long period of time.

If you have a medical condition, such as arrhythmia, coronary heart disease, hypertension, hyperthyroidism, glaucoma, diabetes, enlarged prostate, or urinary dysfunction, don't take any product containing a decongestant (even OTC) without first checking with your doctor.

✔ Because of the stimulant effect of oral decongestants, use them cautiously with children. (Believe it or not, most of the parents in my practice aren't interested in unduly stimulating their kids.)

Nasal decongestants

Nonprescription decongestant nasal sprays and nose drops can provide quick and effective short-term relief of nasal congestion. However, only use them occasionally, and not for more than three to five days in a row, because long-term or consistent use can result in adverse effects such as *nasal rebound* (see the nearby sidebar of the same name).

Never use decongestant nasal sprays and drops with children under the age of 6 without a doctor's supervision. If you use them properly, OTC decongestants generally produce few side effects other than occasional sneezing and dry nasal passages. The most common OTC decongestant drugs and brand-name medications include

✔ Naphazoline, found in Privine

✔ Oxymetazoline, found in Afrin, Allerest, Dristan Long Lasting, and Sinex Long Lasting

✔ Phenylephrine, found in Neo-Synephrine, Sinex, and Little Noses (one-eighth percent formula for infants and children)

✔ Xylometazoline, found in Otrivin

The dosage levels and usage frequency of these medications vary depending on each product's formulation and method of application. As always, carefully read all product instructions and warnings before using any medication.

Nasal rebound

No, nasal rebound isn't a new basketball technique. This condition, more formally known as *rhinitis medicamentosa,* results from prolonged overuse of OTC decongestant nasal sprays and drops. Overusing such medications can irritate and inflame the mucous membranes in your nose more than before you used the spray, leading to more serious nasal congestion.

Unfortunately, some people increase their use of the product as their congestion worsens, leading to a vicious cycle in which more use produces more congestion. When this happens, higher doses don't clear the congestion — they only make it worse. To break this vicious cycle, stop using your OTC decongestant. Your doctor may also need to prescribe a short course of oral and/or nasal corticosteroids to clear your nasal congestion and allow you to tolerate the discontinuation of the OTC decongestant.

Remember, the warning on the label that directs you not to use the nasal decongestant spray or drops longer than three to five days really means three to five days and no more. If your stuffy nose persists beyond this point, consider using an oral decongestant.

The long-lasting products require no more than two doses a day to remain effective, but other short-acting products may work for only one to four hours. Therefore, you may need to apply short-acting products several times a day, as long as you don't exceed safe dosage levels and don't use the product continuously without checking first with your physician.

Two for the Nose: Combination Products

Antihistamines and decongestants can often be more effective in treating the full range of allergic rhinitis symptoms if you combine them in one preparation. You can find numerous oral OTC combination products in tablet, capsule, and liquid forms on store shelves.

An antihistamine, such as chlorpheniramine or brompheniramine, is often combined with a decongestant, such as pseudoephedrine. These products are also frequently combined with other active ingredients — pain relievers, cough suppressants, and fever relievers, for example — to provide relief for a variety of ailments, such as cold and flu symptoms.

The onset of action and dosage frequency vary with different products. Tablets and capsules generally come in two varieties:

✔ **Rapid release:** These medications start working quickly but usually lose effectiveness within four hours.

✔ **Sustained release:** As you may expect, these products work the opposite way; they act slower but last longer than rapid release medications — usually six to eight hours or longer.

Non-drowsy OTC formulas may contain pain relievers, fever reducers, cough suppressants, or other active ingredients for multisymptom relief but don't contain first-generation antihistamines, which cause drowsiness. Therefore, these formulas don't usually provide relief from the sneezing, runny nose, and itchy nose, eyes, and throat that are significant symptoms of allergic rhinitis.

The decongestant in combination products can still cause sleeplessness, nervous agitation, loss of appetite, dryness of mouth and sinuses, high blood pressure, and heart palpitations, especially in older patients. Likewise, the antihistamine in combination products can still cause drowsiness. For example, the antihistamine diphenhydramine (Benadryl) is the active ingredient in many popular sleep aids, such as Nytol. See the following section for more details.

Analyzing the upside and downside

Because of their sedative effects, OTC antihistamines are generally thought of as *downers*. Likewise, because decongestants act as stimulants, they're considered *uppers*. You may think that combining these two types of drugs in a single OTC product cancels out both the sedative and stimulant side effects. However, a person may experience both the upper and downer effects at the same time — the worst of both worlds, in other words — resulting in an agitated, jittery form of drowsiness.

If my patient's condition warrants a combination product, I usually prescribe a nonsedating antihistamine formulated with a decongestant, such as Allegra-D, or possibly a less sedating antihistamine formulated with a decongestant, such as Zyrtec-D. The decongestant (pseudoephedrine) in these products usually doesn't produce as great a stimulant effect as other decongestants, such as phenylpropanolamine, which the FDA recently removed from the market. As a result, the patient gets the benefits of both a nonsedating antihistamine and a less stimulating decongestant action, minimizing the adverse downer or upper side effects.

Most OTC liquid forms are short-acting, which means that they usually require up to four doses a day. However, you may prefer to use liquids, especially syrup forms that often contain flavorings (and sometimes sweeteners), to treat children as well as adults who have trouble swallowing tablets and capsules. Another option in these cases is to use prescription chewable formulations of these products, such as AH-Chew Chewable Tablets.

One size fits all may not suit your condition

Although combination antihistamine and decongestant products may work well when you need quick relief, the products are less viable for long-term use because you can't adjust the dosage levels of the individual active ingredients. Each dose, whether in tablet, capsule, or liquid form, delivers the same amount of antihistamine and decongestant (as well as other active ingredients) to your system whether you need relief from one symptom or the full range of ailments.

If you're considering switching combination products because the one you use doesn't seem effective, check the active ingredients on other medications to make sure that you don't buy the same antihistamine and decongestant combination under a different brand name.

Using Nasal Corticosteroids

The most effective medication currently available for controlling the four major symptoms of allergic rhinitis — sneezing, itching, runny nose, and nasal congestion — is *nasal corticosteroid spray.* Patients and the general public commonly refer to these corticosteroid products as *steroids* or *cortisone.* However, in this book, I use the proper term *corticosteroid* for these types of nasal sprays so as to avoid confusion.

The negative perception that some people have of steroids is mostly due to attempts by some athletes to build up muscle mass by abusing *anabolic steroids.* In fact, the types of steroids used in corticosteroid nasal sprays are a completely different type of drug than anabolic steroids (which are actually male hormones).

The spray is available by prescription only, and is administered by an *aqueous* (non-CFC propellant) mechanical pump. The following information can help you and your doctor decide whether nasal corticosteroids can work for you:

✔ Nasal corticosteroid sprays suppress the inflammation of nasal passages, thereby clearing your nose for easier breathing.

✔ Nasal corticosteroid sprays are most effective if you use them daily as preventive medications. For a guide to safe dosage levels, see Table 12-2.

Never exceed dosage levels with these products to minimize the possibility of the medication causing systemic side effects, such as those associated with oral corticosteroids.

✔ Nasal corticosteroid sprays provide gradual relief of allergic rhinitis symptoms. Initially, you may need to use the medication for several days before the spray suppresses the inflammation. Full effectiveness may require two to three weeks of daily application.

✔ Only use nasal corticosteroids if your nose is clear enough for the spray to penetrate. If your nose is seriously congested, you may need to use a nasal decongestant for only the first three to five days just prior to administering the nasal corticosteroid spray.

✔ In order to prevent injuring your *septum* (the bone that divides the nose into two nostrils), direct the spray away from the septum and slightly in the direction of your ears. You may even want to spray the product once in the air to judge the force of the spray before using it in your nose.

✔ Using an aqueous (AQ) formulation of a nasal corticosteroid, because of its gentler action on the nasal lining, can often minimize the typical adverse side effects of nasal corticosteroid sprays, such as nasal irritation, burning, drying, and nosebleeds.

Although some evidence indicates that nasal corticosteroid sprays are highly effective and safe for children, some doctors are concerned about the possible effects the sprays may temporarily have on the growth rate of children who use them. If your child uses a nasal corticosteroid spray, make sure that your child's physician knows about your concerns so he can accurately monitor your youngster's growth.

Table 12-2		Nasal Corticosteroid Sprays		
Active Ingredient	*Formulation*	*Brand Name*	*Total Usual Daily Dose for Children under 12 Years (See Formulation Details)*	*Total Usual Daily Adult Dose*
Beclomethasone	42 mcg per inhalation	Beconase AQ, Vancenase AQ	1–2 sprays each nostril twice per day (6–11 years)	1–2 sprays each nostril twice per day

Active Ingredient	Formulation	Brand Name	Total Usual Daily Dose for Children under 12 Years (See Formulation Details)	Total Usual Daily Adult Dose
Beclomethasone	84 mcg per inhalation	Vancenase AQ Double Strength	1–2 sprays each nostril once per day (6–11 years)	1–2 sprays each nostril once per day
Budesonide	32 mcg per inhalation	Rhinocort Aqua	1–4 sprays each per day (6–11 years)	1–2 sprays each nostril once per day
Flunisolide	25 mcg per inhalation	Nasarel, Nasalide	1 spray each nostril three times per day or 2 sprays each nostril twice per day (6–11 years)	2 sprays each nostril twice per day
Fluticasone	50 mcg per inhalation	Flonase	1 spray each nostril once per day; may be increased to 2 sprays each nostril once per day (4–11 years)	2 sprays each nostril once per day or 1 spray each nostril twice per day; may be decreased to maintenance dose of 1 spray each nostril once per day
Mometasone	50 mcg per inhalation	Nasonex	1 spray each nostril once per day; may be increased to 2 sprays each nostril once per day (3–11 years)	2 sprays each nostril once per day
Triamcinolone	55 mcg per inhalation	Nasacort AQ	2 sprays each nostril once per day (6–11 years)	2 sprays each nostril once per day

mcg = microgram

Steroids to avoid

Although nasal corticosteroid sprays are highly effective and generally safe for both adults and children when administered under a physician's care, using other forms of steroids is less advisable and potentially unsafe. The following steroids are potentially harmful to you:

✔ Oral corticosteroids: I advise using quick bursts of short-acting oral steroids (such as prednisone or methylprednisolone) only in cases of severe nasal rebound or nasal polyps, where a decongestant nasal spray

can't penetrate sufficiently to decongest your nose. In such cases, you may require a short course of oral corticosteroids to sufficiently clear your congestion so you can use a nasal corticosteroid spray.

✔ Intranasal injections: Cortisone shots into the nose aren't appropriate treatment for allergic rhinitis because of their potential for serious side effects, including vision disturbances and possibly even blindness.

Cromolyn Sodium

Cromolyn sodium, an anti-inflammatory OTC nasal spray, may be highly effective in controlling symptoms of allergic rhinitis when you use it properly. (You can find this medicine under the brand name Nasalcrom.) Cromolyn sodium stabilizes mast cells, thereby preventing the release of histamine and other chemical mediators that can cause nasal inflammation.

To help determine whether cromolyn sodium nasal spray might work for you, check out these facts about its recommended use and effectiveness:

✔ Cromolyn sodium is most effective if you start using it two to four weeks before exposure to allergens. In cases of occupational allergic rhinitis or of limited exposure to allergens, using the spray immediately prior to an isolated, single, allergen exposure (before mowing the lawn or visiting a home with pet), if your nasal passages aren't already congested, may also provide some relief.

✔ If allergic rhinitis symptoms are already present, you may need a short course of a combination antihistamine-decongestant for the first few days that you use cromolyn sodium.

✔ Because cromolyn sodium has an excellent safety profile and produces no significant side effects, doctors may often prescribe it for children and pregnant women.

✔ You can purchase cromolyn sodium in a metered spray form. The recommended dosage for adults and children older than 6 is one spray in each nostril, three to six times per day at regular intervals. Only administer cromolyn sodium to children between 2 and 6 years of age under the supervision of a doctor.

Reducing Mucus with Anticholinergic Sprays

Ipratropium bromide is the active ingredient in the anticholinergic products (drying agents) that sell under the brand name Atrovent Nasal Spray. As the name of this drug class indicates, anticholinergics counter cholinergic activity by blocking *acetylcholine* — a neurotransmitter that stimulates mucus production — from attaching to chemical receptors in the nose. Therefore, these sprays reduce the amount of mucus in your nose.

Some basic facts about anticholinergic sprays include

- ✔ Ipratropium bromide effectively reduces runny nose, as seen in conditions such as *vasomotor* (nonallergic) rhinitis (see the nearby "Skier's nose" sidebar) or the common cold.

- ✔ Ipratropium bromide has little effect on other allergic rhinitis symptoms, such as stuffy nose, sneezing, or itchy nose.

- ✔ Your doctor can prescribe Atrovent Nasal Spray in two strengths — 0.03 percent for relief of runny nose associated with allergic and nonallergic rhinitis in adults and children older than 6, and 0.06 percent for relief of runny nose associated with the common cold in adults and children older than 12.

- ✔ Spray two sprays per nostril two to three times per day (0.03 percent) or three or four times per day (0.06 percent) at regular intervals for the recommended dosage.

Skier's nose

Ever notice how often skiers blow their noses? When I was training at National Jewish Hospital in Denver, I managed to get to the ski slopes occasionally. When I did, I noticed many boxes of tissues at the bottom of the ski lifts. As I discovered, the tissue boxes were there because of what people call *skier's nose,* which is triggered by cold air and is symptomatic of vasomotor rhinitis (see Chapter 7).

I've since found that Atrovent Nasal Spray works well to prevent skier's nose as well as jogger's nose, if you use it before being exposed to cold air, and also for treatment after symptoms appear. However, doctors also use anticholinergic eye drops similar to ipratropium bromide (the active ingredient) to dilate patients' eyes, so make sure that you keep the spray away from your eyes or you won't see that mogul coming right at you.

Treating Rhinitis with Leukotriene Modifiers

Leukotrienes play a significant role in asthma attacks. These chemicals, found in the mast cells that line the airways of the lungs and nose, enhance mucus production, constrict the bronchial passages, and promote further inflammation of the respiratory lining by attracting additional inflammatory cells into the airways.

Leukotriene modifiers, such as montelukast (Singulair) and zafirlukast (Accolate), approved for the treatment of asthma (see Chapter 15) are relatively newer drugs that competitively block leukotriene activity at the receptor site, thus decreasing the amount of mucus generated by exposure to allergens.

Studies have shown that leukotriene modifiers may effectively treat patients whose allergic rhinitis symptoms don't respond solely to antihistamines. If you're in that category, ask your doctor whether leukotriene modifiers may work for you. One of these drugs, Singulair, which the FDA recently approved for treatment of allergic rhinitis, also shows promise in treating symptoms of allergic conjunctivitis.

Keeping an Eye out for Allergic Conjunctivitis

Allergic conjunctivitis often coexists with allergic rhinitis. In fact, most of the same allergens involved in allergic rhinitis can trigger allergic conjunctivitis. Characteristic symptoms of this ailment include redness of the eyes and the underside of the eyelids, and swollen, itchy, and watery eyes.

Because the mechanisms of allergic rhinitis and allergic conjunctivitis are similar, conjunctivitis is often treated with some of the same types of drugs used to control rhinitis in solutions specifically formulated for safe use in the eye. Treatment can include

✔ **Prescription antihistamines:** Two newer second-generation prescription antihistamines, *levocabastine* (Livostin) and *emedastine* (Emadine), appear to be more effective than OTC antihistamines for the treatment of allergic conjunctivitis. Normal recommended dosage for both of these products is one drop per eye up to four times a day for up to two weeks.

✔ **OTC decongestants:** Products include Clear Eyes, Clear Eyes ACR, Visine A.C., Visine L.R., Visine Moisturizing, and Visine Original.

✔ **Combinations of OTC antihistamines and decongestants:** Product names include Naphcon-A, Vasocon-A, Ocuhist, Prefrin, and VasoClear.

✔ **Mast cell stabilizers:** This group of medications inhibits mast cells from releasing chemical mediators of inflammation, thus potentially preventing allergic symptoms from developing. These types of eye drop products include

- **Cromolyn sodium (Crolom, Opticrom):** As I mention earlier in the chapter, cromolyn sodium works best if you use it preventively, prior to allergen exposure. Likewise, administer it on a regular basis, four times a day. For infrequent allergen exposure (when visiting someone with pets, for example), use cromolyn sodium immediately before you visit. This product has also demonstrated some effectiveness in treating forms of *vernal conjunctivitis* (a chronic eye condition that can cause severe burning and intense itching and marked sensitivity to bright light).

- **Nedocromil sodium (Alocril):** This medication, already available in a metered-dose inhaler (MDI) formulation for the treatment of asthma (Tilade), has recently been approved in the United States as an ophthalmic solution. Your doctor can prescribe it for itching eyes associated with allergic conjunctivitis. He also can prescribe it for children as young as 3. This product provides effective relief of both the early and late-phase allergic response (see Chapter 6). The normal dosage for Alocril is one to two drops in each eye twice per day.

- **Lodoxamide (Alomide):** This drug isn't approved for use specifically for allergic conjunctivitis, but it has shown some effectiveness in clinical trials as a treatment for vernal conjunctivitis. Normal dosage is one to two drops per eye, four times per day, for up to three months.

✔ **Nonsteroidal anti-inflammatory drugs (NSAIDs):** Ketorolac (Acular) is a type of NSAID that can relieve the itching of seasonal allergic conjunctivitis. Normal dosage is one drop per eye, four times per day.

✔ **Combination antihistamine and mast cell stabilizer:** The most recent additions to allergic conjunctivitis eye products are olapatadine (Patanol), ketotifen (Zaditor), azelastine (Optivar), and epinastine (Elestat), which are available by prescription in the United States. The normal recommended dosage for Patanol is one drop in each affected eye twice per day, at an interval of six to eight hours. For Zaditor, the recommended dosage is one drop in each eye twice daily, every eight to twelve hours. The recommended dosage for Optivar and also for Elestat is one drop in each eye twice a day.

Doctors prescribe corticosteroid eye drops for severe cases of allergic conjunctivitis that are unresponsive to the medications I describe in the preceding section. However, monitor the use of corticosteroid eye drops closely because using these products improperly can lead to very serious adverse side effects. Don't ever use corticosteroid eye drops in cases where you suspect you have a viral infection of the eyes, such as herpes, because using these products may result in prolonging the course of and increasing the severity of the viral infection. In addition, prolonged use of these corticosteroid eye drops may result in glaucoma, vision disturbances, and cataract formations. Consider consulting a qualified ophthalmologist before routinely using corticosteroid eye products.

Patients with allergic conjunctivitis should use eye drops during peak pollination seasons in addition to their other prescribed medication for allergic rhinitis to minimize eye discomfort. Try not to rub your eyes. Even though they may itch, rubbing them usually only makes matters worse. Instead, gently rinsing your eyes with clean water or a soothing OTC sterile irrigating solution can often wash away pollen and help relieve your symptoms.

If you experience severe allergic conjunctivitis, your doctor may prescribe an oral antihistamine, eye drops, and/or a combination of two different eye drop products for maximum relief of your symptoms.

Chapter 13

Treating Your Ear, Nose, and Throat Symptoms

In This Chapter

▶ Knowing the complications of untreated or poorly managed allergies

▶ Diagnosing sinus and ear infections

▶ Clearing the nosy road to your ears and sinuses

*B*ecause many people refer to allergic rhinitis as *hay fever,* they often think that this allergic condition is just a nuisance rather than a serious disease. However, allergic rhinitis isn't a simple problem. Allergic rhinitis is an ailment that often requires serious attention and management, not only because the symptoms can worsen your asthma and severely affect your quality of life, but also because ineffective treatment can lead to serious complications, such as *sinusitis* (an inflammation of the sinuses) and *otitis media* (an inflammation of the middle ear).

Other conditions, such as *tonsillitis* (an inflammation of the tonsils), adenoid disease, and chronic cough can also be worsened by *postnasal drip* (nasal discharge that trickles down the back of your throat). This characteristic symptom of allergic rhinitis, which usually increases in severity when the ailment is poorly managed, can result in the spread of bacteria-laden mucus that irritates and/or infects the throat's lining.

In addition, ineffectively treated allergic rhinitis and resulting postnasal drip can also adversely affect asthma patients with gastroesophageal reflux disease (GERD). This digestive disorder, which is the third most common cause of chronic cough in North America, is a trigger of asthma symptoms in a large number of asthmatics, especially in cases of nonallergic, adult-onset asthma. (See Chapter 5 for a more extensive discussion on GERD.)

This chapter explains the causes and symptoms of sinusitis and otitis media, and the appropriate methods of preventing and treating these ailments.

Complicating Your Allergies and Asthma: Sinusitis

If you've ever had cold or nasal symptoms that didn't seem to go away, you may have actually been suffering from a form of sinusitis. This often painful condition develops as a result of swollen nasal and sinus passages that frequently result from allergic rhinitis. Many asthma patients often confuse sinusitis symptoms with the symptoms of a cold, flu, or allergy.

Sinusitis is one of the most common health problems in the United States. Current estimates are that sinusitis affects 35 million people each year. Because of the congestion and discomfort that sinusitis causes, it's one of the most common reasons for doctor visits in the United States.

Consult a doctor as soon as you suspect you may have sinusitis. Complications, such as aggravation of asthma, recurrent bronchitis, otitis media, and nasal polyps, can occur if you manage your sinusitis poorly. Chronic sinus infections can result in swollen adenoids that may require surgery to remove. On a more positive note, studies show that asthma patients who effectively manage their sinusitis can significantly improve their respiratory symptoms.

Recognizing common causes

In a significant number of sinusitis cases, allergic rhinitis precedes the start of a sinus infection. Research shows that more than half of all children in the United States who receive treatment for sinusitis also have allergic rhinitis.

Vasomotor rhinitis, a nonallergic form of rhinitis that results from sudden temperature changes or exposure to tobacco smoke, pollutants, and other irritants (see Chapter 7), can also contribute to sinusitis. Swimmers, divers, fliers (passengers, as well as flight crews), and other people with this form of rhinitis who frequently experience pressure and weather changes may be particularly prone to developing sinusitis if they don't effectively manage their rhinitis symptoms.

Other factors (you may have one or more of these) that can also increase your chances of developing sinusitis include

- **Upper respiratory viral infections:** Viruses, such as those associated with the common cold, are the most frequent causes of sinusitis.
- **Bacteria:** The same family of germs that can cause acute otitis media (*Streptococcus pneumonia, Haemophilus influenza, Moraxella catarrhalis*) can cause acute bacterial sinusitis. Unlike viral infections, this type of sinusitis responds to antibiotic therapy.

✔ **Fungal:** This type of sinusitis infection can develop in otherwise healthy patients who have been on long-term antibiotic treatment or have been taking oral corticosteroids on a chronic basis. *Aspergillus* is the most common fungus that causes these types of cases and is also frequently implicated in cases of *allergic fungal sinusitis.* Characteristic signs and symptoms of this recurring fungal infection, which can often affect individuals with allergic rhinitis and/or asthma, are sinus infections and *nasal polyps* (growths in the nose).

✔ **Nasal rebound:** Overuse of OTC nasal decongestants can also predispose you to sinusitis. (See Chapter 12 for more information.)

✔ **Anatomical obstructions:** Nasal polyps, other growths, enlarged adenoids (particularly in children), and a deviated nasal septum (the great divide between the nostrils — see Chapter 7 for more details) can increase your chances of developing sinusitis.

✔ **Other diseases:** Patients with cystic fibrosis, in which abnormally thick mucus is produced and the function of the *cilia* (tiny hair-like projections of certain types of cells that sweep debris-laden mucus through the airways) is impaired, frequently suffer from sinus infections. In addition, AIDS and other immune-deficiency diseases often weaken the body's defenses to the point where bacteria and viruses can cause many types of infections, including sinusitis. These patients with compromised immune systems may be particularly vulnerable to various forms of fungal sinus infections.

Sinus science

Allergists refer to the sinuses that surround your nose — called *paranasal sinuses* — when they discuss sinusitis. *Para* is Greek for around or near; *nasal,* of course, refers to the nose; and *sinus* is Latin for a hollow place. Your sinuses are hollow cavities in the bones that surround your nasal cavity (see Figure 13-1), hence sinusitis, which means inflammation (itis) of the sinuses.

The three types of paranasal sinuses come in pairs (one on each side of the nose) and are named for the bones that house them. They include

✔ **Maxillary sinuses:** The largest of the sinuses, these sinuses are located in your cheekbones.

✔ **Frontal sinuses:** These sinuses reside in your forehead above your eyes.

✔ **Ethmoid sinuses:** These sinuses are immediately behind your eyes and nose.

The other sinus affected by sinusitis is the *sphenoid* sinus, located behind your nose near the base of your brain.

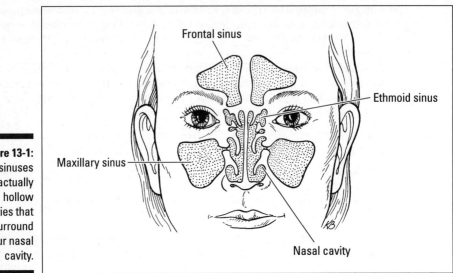

Figure 13-1:
Your sinuses
are actually
hollow
cavities that
surround
your nasal
cavity.

Frontal sinus

Ethmoid sinus

Maxillary sinus

Nasal cavity

Sinus infections most often affect the maxillary, frontal, and ethmoid sinuses. The most common complication affects the orbit around the eye, causing *cellulitis* and possibly forming an *abscess* (a localized collection of pus surrounded by inflamed tissue). Patients with this type of infection may look as though they've been severely punched in the eye. Because the sphenoid sinus is near the brain, an infection in this area, although rare, is usually associated with infections in all the other sinuses (*pansinusitis*) and can have very serious consequences if infected fluids spread to the central nervous system. Untreated sinusitis has the potential to lead to life-threatening conditions, such as *meningitis* (an infection of the membranes that envelop the brain and spinal cord) and brain abscesses.

Your maxillary sinuses are present at birth, along with immature ethmoid sinuses, which begin to fully develop when you're between 3 and 7 years old. Therefore, contrary to previous medical opinion, children under 5 can experience sinus infections that require appropriate therapy. If your young child has allergic rhinitis, effectively treating his or her condition is vital in reducing the risk of developing sinusitis.

Practical sinus

Sinuses are a vital part of your body's defense against the airborne bacteria, viruses, irritants, and allergens that you constantly inhale. Under normal circumstances, the mucus in your sinuses traps most of these intruders. Cilia sweep the particle-laden mucus through connecting *ostia* (sinus drainage openings) into your nasal passages, which then drains into your throat. From your throat, the mucus moves into your stomach, where your digestive system can neutralize and eventually eliminate the offending substances.

In addition to helping clear your upper respiratory tract of particle-laden mucus, your sinuses serve other important roles. For example, your sinuses act as:

- ✔ Air pockets that lighten your skull — otherwise, your head would be too heavy for your neck. Calling someone an airhead is actually an anatomically correct statement.

- ✔ Resonance chambers that provide space for your voice to resonate.

- ✔ Climate adjusters, warming and humidifying the air that you inhale.

- ✔ Insulators, which also warm the base of your brain, located directly behind your nose.

- ✔ Shock absorbers, protecting the inside of your skull from injury.

Allergic rhinitis irritates the nasal and sinus lining, causing the linings to swell, which narrows the sinus drainage openings into the nasal cavity. At the same time, your immune system's allergic response to allergic rhinitis increases mucus production. This combination of increased mucus flow and a swollen sinus lining overwhelms the cilia's abilities to sweep out the mucus, which then becomes infected.

Think of a swiftly flowing stream. If the stream dams up, the water usually stagnates and turns into a breeding ground for all sorts of organisms. The same process applies to your sinuses, which is why it's crucial to avoid letting them turn into swamps.

How long has this been goin' on?

Although no universal definition exists for the various presentations of sinusitis, most doctors base their sinusitis classifications on the duration and types of symptoms involved. Therefore, doctors often use the following terms to classify cases of sinusitis:

- ✔ **Acute sinusitis:** Symptoms of acute sinusitis persist for up to three to four weeks, although some doctors may diagnose symptoms that continue for up to eight weeks as acute. Typical symptoms of acute sinusitis include

  - • Upper respiratory infection.

  - • Runny nose with infected mucus that often appears as cloudy, thick, yellowish, or greenish nasal discharge.

- Cloudy, yellowish, or greenish postnasal drip (often of such a quantity that you may need to swallow frequently).

- Facial pain or pressure around cheeks, eyes, and lower nose (mainly in adults, less commonly in children), especially while bending over or moving vigorously (for example, during exercise).

- Nasal congestion, headache, fever, and cough.

- A reduction or loss of the sense of smell, pain in upper teeth or the upper jawbone, and bad breath.

- In some children, nausea and vomiting due to gagging on infected mucus. Some children have persistent nocturnal cough and *halitosis* (bad breath).

✔ **Chronic sinusitis:** When your condition lasts longer than four weeks, doctors usually consider you a chronic sufferer. In many cases, chronic sinusitis can last for months with combinations of the same symptoms as acute sinusitis, although you may not have a fever. For this reason, many people with chronic sinusitis think that they suffer from frequent or constant colds.

✔ **Recurrent sinusitis:** Doctors usually define recurrent sinusitis as three or more episodes of acute sinusitis per year. The recurring episodes may occur as a result of different causes. If you have recurrent sinusitis, your doctor may refer you to an allergist to determine whether allergies are the underlying cause of your condition. (See Chapter 11 for more details on allergy testing.)

Diagnosing sinusitis

Often, your doctor can diagnose sinusitis based on your symptoms and medical history. Your doctor may ask questions like the following:

✔ When did you first notice the symptoms?

✔ What hurts? Where do you feel the pain?

✔ Does your family have a history of allergies and sinus problems?

✔ What have you done to treat your symptoms? What sorts of medications have you taken, and what has been their effect?

Your doctor also conducts a physical exam of your nose and sinuses in order to confirm diagnosis. This exam may include

✔ Taking your temperature to check for fever and listening to your chest to see whether the infection has spread to your lungs.

✔ Lightly tapping your forehead and cheekbones to check for sensitivity in your frontal and maxillary sinuses.

✔ Looking for infected mucus in your nose and the back of your throat. This exam may require insertion of a flexible fiber-optic device, known as an *endoscope* or a fiber-optic rhinoscope, so your doctor can clearly view potentially infected areas.

Your doctor may use sophisticated imaging techniques to confirm the diagnosis of sinusitis. *Computed tomography* (CT) is currently the gold standard and, in many cases, is replacing the use of less-accurate sinus X-rays. A CT scan, also known as a *CAT scan,* is a diagnostic test that combines the use of X-rays with state-of-the-art computer technology. This test uses a series of X-ray beams from many different angles to create cross-sectional images of your body — in this case, of your head and sinuses. With computer assistance, these images are assembled into a three-dimensional picture that can display organs, bones, and tissues in great detail.

Determining the best course of treatment

To effectively treat your sinusitis, you need to effectively manage your allergic rhinitis. In many cases, appropriately treating your allergic rhinitis also improves your sinusitis. As I explain in Chapter 10, avoidance and allergy-proofing are crucial tools you can use to effectively treat your allergies. Chapter 12 provides you with an in-depth explanation of allergy medications that you may find appropriate for your condition.

In addition to addressing your allergic rhinitis, doctors can also prescribe a variety of treatments for sinusitis, ranging from medication to irrigation to surgery.

Antibiotics

Antibiotics are the most common medications that doctors prescribe to clear up the bacterial (not viral) infection in your sinuses. When taking antibiotics, keep the following in mind:

✔ Because the blood flow to your sinuses is poor, you may need to take your prescribed antibiotics for a while before you notice a beneficial effect. However, most cases of acute sinusitis respond to antibiotic treatment within two weeks.

✔ In cases of chronic sinusitis, don't be surprised if your doctor prescribes a six- to eight-week course of antibiotic therapy with combined use of intranasal steroids (see Chapter 12) to eliminate your bacterial infection.

✔ In some cases of acute or chronic sinusitis, you may notice a sudden improvement in your symptoms soon after you start a course of antibiotics, and you may consider stopping the medication at that point. However, take the complete course of antibiotics to ensure that all the bacteria have been completely eliminated.

Other medications

In addition to prescribing antibiotics to clear up the bacterial infection in your sinuses, your doctor may also prescribe medications to treat symptoms of allergic rhinitis, which I describe extensively in Chapter 12.

Irrigation

Your doctor may advise you to use a nasal douche cup, nasal spray bottle, nasal bulb syringe, Water Pik with nasal attachment, or some other type of nasal wash device to irrigate your nostrils with warm saline solution. You can use these devices at home to relieve pressure and congestion in your nasal passages. Ask your doctor for specific instructions on how to use nasal wash devices.

Get steamed

Your doctor may also advise a simple home remedy to help clear your sinuses and relieve discomfort. This remedy consists of inhaling steam to liquefy and soften crusty mucus while moisturizing your inflamed passages.

Use the following method for inhaling steam:

1. **Boil water in a kettle on the stove.**

2. **Carefully pour the boiling water in a pan or basin on a low table.**

3. **Sit at the table and drape a towel over your head, leaning over the pan or basin to form a kind of human tent with your head as the pole.**

4. **Hold your face a few inches above the steaming water and breathe the steam through your nose for approximately ten minutes.**

Two steam treatments a day may provide relief. However, you still need to deal with the underlying cause of the sinus infection, so I don't advise relying solely on this home remedy as the only therapy for your infectious sinusitis.

Sinus surgery

If other treatment methods don't provide effective relief, you may need surgery, especially if physical obstructions, such as a deviated septum or nasal polyps, contribute to your condition. However, if allergic rhinitis is the underlying cause of your sinusitis, surgery alone won't resolve your sinus problems. You must continue managing your allergic rhinitis to avoid further complications. By the same token, treating your allergies alone won't reverse the damage that sinusitis may have already caused.

If your doctor thinks that surgery is advisable, she will refer you to an ear, nose, and throat specialist, or ENT, otherwise known as an *otolaryngologist* (remember that word for your next Scrabble game — you could score big). Before you consider surgery, make sure your doctor thoroughly reviews your medical history and evaluates your clinical condition.

Never hesitate to ask your surgeon for further information concerning your planned surgical procedure, such as how long the procedure takes, where and when it will be performed, any possible complications that may occur, and how soon you can get back to work or school.

The good news about surgery for your sinuses is that the two most common procedures are minimally invasive. An ENT specialist can perform them on an outpatient basis with local anesthesia, although he may use general anesthesia in certain cases. The two procedures most often used are

✔ **Antral puncture and irrigation:** This procedure opens up your sinuses so they can drain and irrigate properly, but is used less often now since the advent of fiber-optic surgery.

✔ **Functional endoscopic sinus surgery:** This procedure is more complex than antral puncture and irrigation. Functional endoscopic sinus surgery often involves enlarging the ethmoid and maxillary sinus openings into the nasal cavity and removing and cleaning the infected sinus membranes, resulting in improved drainage. This procedure re-establishes the ventilation of your ethmoid, maxillary, and frontal sinuses. Otolaryngologists perform this type of surgery with high-tech computer-assisted instruments and navigation devices to ensure pinpoint accuracy.

An ounce of prevention . . .

If you have allergic rhinitis, consider taking the following preventive measures to keep your sinuses clear if you come down with an upper respiratory infection (such as the common cold) or experience an allergy attack:

✔ **Take the appropriate medications.** See Chapter 12 for a complete listing.

✔ **Drink plenty of water.** Water keeps your mucus thin and fluid so your sinuses can drain more easily.

✔ **Be nice to your nose.** Blow it gently, preferably one nostril at a time.

✔ **Avoid flying.** If you have to travel by air while you have a cold or an allergy attack, use a topical nasal decongestant spray prior to takeoff. The spray prevents the sudden pressure changes from blocking your sinuses and ears.

✔ **Avoid swimming.** You probably won't feel like going to the beach or the pool if you have a cold or allergy attack, and your sinuses won't enjoy the pressure changes that swimming and diving involve (scuba diving wouldn't be a good idea either).

Otitis Media

Otitis media is an inflammation of the middle ear, as well as a condition in which fluid accumulates in your ear. This condition is in contrast to *otitis externa,* which affects the external auditory canal, known commonly as *swimmer's ear.* Based on the definitions I provide of sinusitis and rhinitis (see Chapter 7), you can probably already guess what *otitis* means: an inflammation (*itis*) of the ear (*otikos* in Greek). *Media* means middle, by the way. Infectious organisms, such as bacteria and viruses, often affect the middle ear. Otitis media can often develop as a result of allergic rhinitis and from complications of sinusitis.

Middle ear infections and fluid in the ear are especially common in young children and infants. In fact, otitis media is the most common reason in the United States for pediatric visits, with doctors treating at least 10 million children annually for ear infections. Otitis media can have serious consequences for youngsters, in particular by adversely affecting a child's development and learning ability due to potential hearing loss.

The most common forms of otitis media are

- ✔ **Acute otitis media (AOM):** This condition involves inflammation and infection of the middle ear and Eustachian tube. The peak incidence is between 6 months and 1 year of age, decreasing with age and with fewer episodes after 7 years of age.

- ✔ **Otitis media with effusion (OME):** Doctors also refer to this condition as serous otitis media — fluid in the middle ear. This condition, which occurs commonly in children ages 2 to 7 years, can lead to hearing loss if not treated properly.

Revealing common causes

In a significant number of cases, allergic rhinitis precedes an ear infection. A long-term study of 2,000 children found that 50 percent of the patients with chronic and recurrent ear infections who were 3 years of age and older had allergic rhinitis.

Other conditions that can increase your chances of developing ear infections include

- ✔ Sinusitis. The same factors that can lead to sinus infections, such as exposure to allergens, tobacco smoke, pollutants, and other irritants, can also contribute to ear infections.

- ✔ Enlarged adenoids.

✔ Unrepaired cleft palate.

✔ Nasal polyps.

✔ Pacifier use by babies.

✔ Defective or immature immune system.

✔ Benign or malignant tumors.

✔ Teething. Some physicians believe that teething in young children can also contribute to ear infections, but no one has established a direct connection.

Many of the conditions in the previous list affect infants and young children. Always ask your physician to check your child's ear for infection and fluid in the middle ear anytime he or she is ill.

Getting an earful

The visible part of your ear — that funny-looking protrusion on the side of your head — is only the tip of the iceberg. Most of your ears' functions take place inside your skull in chambers, tubes, and passages that register and conduct sound and also provide your sense of balance.

Figure 13-2 shows the parts that make up the ear:

✔ **Outer ear:** Also known as the *pinna,* this structure is what many people think of as the ear. The primary function of this skin-covered flap of elastic cartilage is to funnel sound into the middle ear and to keep your eyeglasses on the side of your head.

✔ **Middle ear:** This air-filled chamber is bordered by the *tympanic membrane* (commonly known as the *eardrum*) and small bones that enable your eardrum to function. Through its connection (the *Eustachian tube*) to the *nasopharynx* (back of the nose), your middle ear also equalizes the air pressure on both sides of your eardrum.

✔ **Inner ear:** Your inner ear contains sensory receptors that provide your hearing and balance. The hearing receptors are enclosed in the *cochlea,* a fluid-filled chamber, while the balance receptors are in the semi-circular canals (refer to Figure 13-2).

✔ **Eustachian tube (ET):** Your Eustachian tube is an extension of the middle ear that connects to the nasopharynx. The ET, which is often the origin of ear infections, serves three important functions:

- The ET provides ventilation for your middle ear.

- The ET helps equalize air pressure inside your ear, buffering the eardrum from the force of external air, and helps dissipate the energy of sound waves from your inner ear into your throat.

- Because your ET is closed most of the time, it serves as an important barrier to viruses, bacteria, irritants, and allergens that enter your middle ear. Similar to the function of your sinuses, cilia in the middle ear sweep debris-laden mucus from your middle ear through the ET into the back of your nasal cavity. The cilia prepare the mucus for drainage into your throat and eventually into your stomach.

The ET briefly opens to allow the cilia to sweep mucus away when you swallow, yawn, sniff, or strain. In many children, however, the ET doesn't fully develop until age 6, causing the ET to ineffectively ventilate, clear, or protect the middle ear. Therefore, large numbers of young children get middle ear infections.

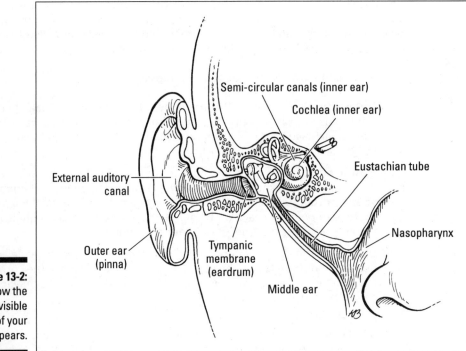

Figure 13-2:
See how the less visible part of your ear appears.

Acute otitis media (AOM)

Many people suffer *acute otitis media* — an inflammation and infection of the middle ear and Eustachian tube — in early childhood. The main symptoms include

- ✔ Earache — sometimes with intense, stabbing pains — and fever. Occasionally, vomiting and diarrhea accompany this symptom.

- ✔ Possible hearing loss and occasional dizziness and ringing in the affected ear.

- ✔ With infants, high fever, irritability, and a tendency to pull on the affected ear.

- ✔ In some cases, discharge of infected fluid from the middle ear (if your eardrum has been perforated).

An AOM infection generally develops as a result of an allergic, bacterial, or viral ailment that inflames your nose, sinuses, middle ear, and Eustachian tube. Your ET may swell shut, trapping infected fluid, which then presses on your eardrum, causing the pain you associate with an earache. If you don't rectify this situation, infected fluids can eventually reach the membranes that cover your brain, leading to meningitis and even possibly death.

Because sinusitis and otitis media often coexist, doctors usually treat these conditions with the same medications. Treatment of AOM usually includes a course of antibiotics (available by prescription only) to rid your middle ear of infection. The antibiotic drugs that doctors commonly prescribe include

- ✔ Amoxicillin (Amoxil) or amoxicillin/potassium clavulanate (Augmentin)

- ✔ Clarithromycin (Biaxin) or azithromycin (Zithromax)

- ✔ Trimethoprim-sulfamethoxazole (Bactrim or Septra)

- ✔ A third-generation cephalosporin antibiotic, such as cefuroxime (Ceftin), cefpodoxime (Vantin), cefprozil (Cefzil), and cefixime (Suprax)

If you're allergic to penicillin, make sure your doctor knows. Some people who have penicillin allergies may also have adverse reactions to cephalosporin medications.

Otitis media with effusion (OME)

When you have otitis media with effusion (OME, also known as *serous otitis media*), your middle ear traps infected or sterile fluid. The most common symptoms of OME are

- ✔ Plugged-up ears (similar to the discomfort that you may experience when descending in an airplane)
- ✔ Some hearing loss

Children with OME may not show obvious symptoms. However, if your child acts inattentive (other than the obvious times when children don't seem to hear you asking them to clean their room), doesn't seem to hear well (for example, he or she always wants the television volume turned up loud), and/or talks loudly, make sure your doctor examines your child's ears. Undetected or poorly treated OME can result in hearing loss, poor language development, learning disorders, and eventual behavioral problems.

OME treatments can also include nonprescription oral decongestants and nasal decongestant sprays, as well as topical nasal corticosteroid sprays. (For more information on these types of medicines, see Chapter 12.)

For children with chronic OME that lasts more than six to eight weeks, your pediatrician may refer your child to an ENT specialist for surgery. The most common OME treatment procedures are

- ✔ **Adenoidectomy:** If your child's Eustachian tube is chronically blocked and your child is more than 3 years old, your doctor may recommend removing your child's adenoids. (Removing the tonsils is no longer an effective or appropriate procedure for treatment of ear problems.)

- ✔ **Myringotomy:** The ENT surgeon makes a small incision in the eardrum that permits drainage of the trapped fluid. This procedure is helpful both for diagnostic purposes (to identify infecting organisms) and to relieve the severe pain, pressure, and fever associated with an acute middle ear infection.

- ✔ **Tympanostomy:** This procedure includes surgically inserting small plastic tubes (known as *pressure equalization* or *PE tubes*) in the eardrum to equalize air pressure in the ear and to allow drainage of fluid from the middle ear and Eustachian tube down to the nasopharynx. ENT surgeons usually perform tympanostomies with a general anesthetic, and occasionally with local anesthetic (for older children or adults), as an outpatient procedure. In most cases, doctors recommend that PE tubes remain in place for 6 to 18 months or until they fall out. Children often don't notice the tubes after they've been in place for a while. Generally, children with tubes shouldn't go swimming. However, in some cases, an ENT surgeon may fit your child with earplugs, making water activities a possibility.

Diagnosing ear infections

The first step in diagnosing suspected ear infections usually involves examining your middle ear. Your doctor usually uses an *otoscope* (a metal instrument you've probably seen before) to look for an obvious sign of infection. AOM often appears as a swollen, red, inflamed bulging of the tympanic membrane (eardrum) with poor or no movement. OME can appear as a pink or white opaque, withdrawn tympanic membrane with poor or no movement.

Other diagnostic procedures for both AOM and OME may include

- ✔ **Audiometry:** This procedure evaluates the effect of chronic middle ear effusions on a person's hearing. Audiometry is especially important for children because hearing loss can cause delayed speech and language development.

- ✔ **Tympanometry:** This procedure measures the eardrum's response at various pressure levels and helps to diagnose middle ear effusions and Eustachian tube dysfunction.

Taking preventive measures

As with sinusitis, one of the most important steps you can take to prevent ear infections, if you also have allergic rhinitis, is to effectively treat your allergies, which includes using the avoidance measures that I describe in Chapter 10 and also the appropriate medications, if necessary, to manage allergic rhinitis symptoms, as I explain in Chapter 12.

You also need to take the preventive measures that I describe in the "Complicating Your Allergies and Asthma: Sinusitis" section of this chapter to keep your sinuses clear if you have an allergy attack or a cold or other upper respiratory infection.

Part IV

Controlling Asthma with Medications

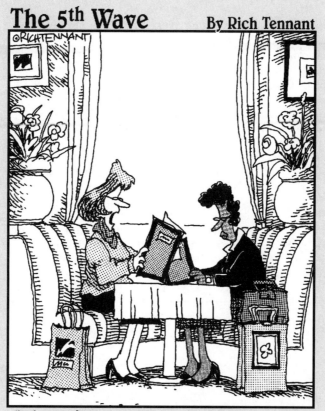

"When I feel an asthma attack coming on I try to relax, take 2 puffs of my rescue inhaler, and then follow up with a facial, a massage, and a 3 hour lunch."

In this part . . .

In this part, I get into the nitty-gritty of asthma therapy with four chapters devoted to the medications that physicians prescribe for effective short-term and long-term treatment of asthma symptoms.

In Chapter 14, I present an overview of the different categories of asthma medications, and I also offer detailed information on the proper use and maintenance of inhaled medication delivery devices, including inhalers and nebulizers. Chapter 15 provides an in-depth account of long-term asthma medications, while Chapter 16 does the same for short-term drugs. Both chapters include extensive information on when and how doctors prescribe these products, general dosage guidelines, and potential adverse side effects that may occur in some cases. I also highlight recently approved new medications that are just now hitting the market.

Chapter 17 looks to the future as I survey the most exciting and innovative advances occurring in asthma research today. Some of this research has the potential for enabling physicians to soon go beyond managing respiratory symptoms and actually treat the root cause of asthma.

Chapter 14

Knowing Asthma Medications

· ·

· ·

*T*reatment with medications, which doctors refer to as *pharmacotherapy,* is a crucial component of your asthma management plan (see Chapter 2). As with the other aspects of your asthma management plan — self-monitoring (most commonly by using a peak-flow meter, as I explain in Chapter 4); keeping track of your symptoms (usually with a symptom diary; see Chapter 4); avoiding possible asthma triggers (see Chapter 5); and educating yourself about your disease (this entire book) — adhering to your doctor's instructions for taking prescribed medications is vital in effectively treating your condition.

Given the choice, most people would rather not take medications on a regular basis. After all, you have places to go, people to meet, things to do. Remembering to inhale, swallow, or receive an injection of a prescribed medication at the right time in the proper manner can every now and then seem like a nuisance.

Physicians who care for people with asthma are very aware that patients prefer not to take medications on a regular basis. However, asthma is more than the coughing, wheezing, or other symptoms that you may occasionally experience. If you have persistent asthma — like the majority of asthmatics in the United States — some degree of airway inflammation and *hyperreactivity* (increased sensitivity) is always present, even when you aren't noticing any obvious respiratory symptoms and therefore feel fine. Controlling that inflammation is the key to keeping your condition from getting out of hand.

As I explain in this chapter, for the vast majority of asthma patients, treatment with at least some form of controller (long-term) and/or rescue (short-term) medication is almost always an essential component of reducing the severity and frequency of your symptoms, and in some cases even eliminating them and improving your overall quality of life.

BERGER BIT

Understanding the medicine that you take

An informed patient is a healthier person. In fact, making sure that you understand all aspects of your treatment is your responsibility as a patient. Don't hesitate to inquire about medications your doctor prescribes for your asthma (or any ailment, for that matter). I advise knowing the following information about your prescription before you leave your doctor's office and begin using a medication:

✓ The name of the medication, the prescribed dose, how often you should take it, and over what period of time you must use it. Your doctor may provide an instruction card with this information. This card can greatly assist you in communicating with other doctors about the medications you're taking, and it may prove vital in an emergency situation. Likewise, ensuring that the product's name is clearly written is important, because the drug and brand names of many medications sound alike.

✓ The way the drug works, any potential adverse side effects that may result, and what you should do if any of these side effects occur.

✓ What you should do if you accidentally miss a dose or take an extra dose of the medication.

✓ Any cautions about potential interactions between your prescription and other medications you already take or may take, including over-the-counter (OTC) antihistamines, decongestants, pain relievers, vitamins, or nutritional supplements.

✓ Any effects your prescription may have on various aspects of your life, such as your job, school, exercise or sports, other activities, sleeping patterns, and diet.

✓ If the medication is for your child, make sure that you know how your child's dosage may differ from an adult's.

✓ If you're pregnant or nursing a child, make sure that you inform your doctor about these situations.

✓ Be sure your doctor knows about any adverse reactions you've had to any drugs in the past, including both prescription and OTC preparations.

Use only those products that are clearly identified to treat the symptoms you experience. Carefully read the product instructions and only take the medication according to your doctor's directions.

Occasionally, doctors need to prescribe medications *off label* (beyond the manufacturer's official recommendations) in order to achieve maximum improvement in a particular patient's condition. A patient's health and well-being is a doctor's primary commitment, and sometimes treatments need to be individualized, such as using high-dose inhaled corticosteroids in cases of severe persistent asthma.

In addition to the printed information that doctors may provide concerning the drugs they prescribe, you can also request materials from the National Council on Patient Information and Education, 4915 Saint Elmo Ave., Suite 505, Bethesda, MD 20814-6082; tel: 301-656-8565, fax: 301-656-4464; e-mail: ncpie@ncpie.info; Web site: www.talkaboutrx.org.

Taking Your Medicine: Why It's Essential

Asthma is a chronic condition requiring chronic treatment. Therefore, treat your asthma the way people with high blood pressure or heart disease or diabetes treat their ailments: by taking medications preventively, on a regular basis. Most asthmatics get into trouble with their disease from too little rather than too much treatment. As I explain in Chapter 2, patients who take their medications as directed can prevent the majority of emergency room visits and hospitalizations that asthma causes.

Your physician's goal is to determine the most appropriate medications to help you control your symptoms and achieve your best possible lung function without adverse side effects. Therefore, routinely take the drugs that your doctor prescribes, because they're essential to managing your condition and because they can help significantly improve your quality of life. Without using the medications that your doctor prescribes, you're likely to have a much more difficult time controlling your asthma.

Looking at asthma's changing dynamics

Because asthma is a chronic disease, the vast majority of asthmatics need to take appropriate long-acting, preventive ("controller") medications throughout their lifetime in order to control the underlying airway inflammation that characterizes this disease.

However, asthma is also a dynamic condition. As a result, the combination — and dosages — of medications that your doctor prescribes for you may vary over time. For this reason, consistently consulting your physician about your medication regimen is vital — regardless of whether or not you're experiencing noticeable respiratory symptoms, instead of deciding on your own whether or not to take a particular medication.

In some cases, your physician may need to step up your medication to obtain better control of your symptoms, while in other instances, your doctor may recommend stepping down your level of medication if you've been able to consistently achieve good control of your symptoms. (See Chapter 4 for details on the stepwise approach to asthma management.)

Tracking your asthma condition

In addition, because the frequency and character of your symptoms are liable to change throughout your lifetime, your doctor needs to assess your condition on a regular basis, through lung-function tests (usually with spirometry), as well as by evaluating your peak expiratory flow rate, or PEFR (see Chapter 4).

This enables your physician to determine whether your current treatment plan is optimal for your current condition, or if it requires adjustment.

Your asthma condition and severity level may also require adjustment due to factors such as:

✔ Seasonal changes, especially those that involve sudden variations in climate and weather, as well as increases or decreases in pollen and mold counts.

✔ Moving to a new building, neighborhood, city, and/or region, which can result in exposure to different types and levels of allergens and irritants.

✔ Occupational changes, which may also expose you to different types and levels of allergens and irritants.

✔ Change in exercise and activity patterns.

✔ Change in medical condition, especially if it requires the use of a medication not previously used that has the potential to cause an adverse drug interaction.

Consult with your physician about any other prescription or OTC medications you may be already taking or may think of taking for other medical conditions, even for relief of minor aches and pains. In some cases, adverse drug interactions can occur between these products and your prescribed asthma medications.

Regular medical visits also enable your doctor to evaluate your inhaler/ nebulizer technique (see "Delivering Your Dose: Inhalers and Nebulizers," later in this chapter). Your doctor will want to make sure that you are able to derive the maximum benefit from the medication administered by your delivery device.

Effective asthma pharmacotherapy can help you achieve the following goals in managing your condition:

✔ Preventing and controlling your asthma symptoms

✔ Reducing the frequency and severity of your asthma episodes

✔ Reversing your airway obstruction and maintaining improved lung function

In this chapter, I explain and discuss the types of medications that doctors prescribe and recommend to treat asthma, and I also show the proper ways of using different delivery systems designed to administer many of these products.

You can find more detailed information on the specific active ingredients and brand names of individual asthma drugs in the two chapters that follow this one. In Chapter 15, I get in-depth with long-term (controller) drugs, while Chapter 16 focuses on quick-relief (rescue) products.

Getting the Long and Short of Asthma Medications

Asthma pharmacotherapy involves two basic classes of medications. These medications are

- **Long-term control medications:** Doctors prescribe these products as part of a regular, preventive regimen (most often with daily doses) to achieve and control the underlying airway inflammation that characterizes asthma. For this reason, many of the products in this class are sometimes referred to as *anti-inflammatory drugs* or *controlling drugs*.

- **Quick-relief medications:** At times, you may need these products — often called *rescue drugs* or *relieving drugs* — to provide prompt relief of severe and sudden airway constriction and airflow obstruction that can occur when your asthma symptoms unexpectedly worsen.

Your doctor may prescribe products from both classes of medications as part of your long-term asthma management program. The specific combination that your doctor prescribes depends on your asthma's severity and other factors, such as:

- **Your age.** Doses and products for infants, toddlers, children under 12, and the elderly often vary from those doses and products that doctors prescribe for children over 12 and adults. See Chapter 18 for more information about asthma and children and Chapter 20 for details about asthma and the elderly.

- **Your medical history and physical condition.** For example, your doctor may adjust dosages and/or products if you're pregnant or nursing (as I explain in greater detail in Chapter 19).

- **Any other ailments that may affect you, as well as other medications you may take to treat those conditions.** Letting your doctor know about any and all medications you may be using (including OTC ones for minor aches and pains, as well as vitamin supplements and herbal remedies) is essential in order to avoid potential adverse interactions between those products and the asthma medications your doctor may prescribe.

- **Any sensitivities you may have to particular drugs or to certain ingredients in the formulations of particular medications.** Some patients may experience tremors or jitteriness when using an older bronchodilator, such as albuterol (Proventil, Ventolin). However, these patients may experience fewer adverse side effects from a newer, improved broncholdilating formulation, such as levalbuterol (Xopenex) and will therefore be more likely to adhere to their asthma medication regimen.

Toning your lungs, not your muscles

The attempts by some athletes to build up muscle mass by abusing anabolic steroids (related to *testosterone*) have led many people to harbor negative perceptions about all steroids. Understanding that corticosteroids rarely, if ever, cause the adverse side effects often associated with inappropriate use of anabolic steroids is vital.

In fact, the corticosteroids in the inhaled and oral corticosteroid products often prescribed for asthma patients are a completely different type of drug than anabolic steroids, which are actually synthetic male hormones. The confusion is largely due to the common use of the term *steroid,* which really is a general term for any of the hormones with related chemical structures produced by specific glands in the body. These hormones include testosterone from the *testes,* estrogen from the *ovaries,* and corticosteroids (related to *cortisone*) from the *cortex* (outer layer) of the *adrenal gland* (glands above the kidneys).

Most medical professionals, including myself, consider *corticosteroid* the proper term — rather than *steroid* — for the types of inhaled and oral products that I describe in this chapter.

Controlling asthma with long-term medications

If used in an appropriate, consistent manner, long-term control medications can reduce existing airway inflammation and may also help prevent further inflammation. However, your doctor should make sure you understand that these types of drugs aren't advisable for rescue relief of a severe asthma episode. For this reason, your asthma management plan should also include a prescribed quick-relief medication (most often a quick-relief bronchodilator, as I explain in "Relieving asthma episodes with quick-relief products," later in this chapter).

Long-term control medications include the following categories of drugs:

- ✔ Anti-inflammatory drugs, such as inhaled corticosteroids (beclomethasone, budesonide, ciclesonide, flunisolide, fluticasone, mometasone, triamcinolone), oral corticosteroids (methylprednisolone, prednisolone, prednisone), and inhaled mast cell stabilizers (cromolyn and nedocromil). These drugs are available in metered-dose inhaler (MDI), dry-powder inhaler (DPI), or compressor-driven nebulizer (CDN) formulations (see "Delivering Your Dose: Inhalers and Nebulizers," later in this chapter).

- ✔ Long-acting bronchodilators, such as inhaled salmeterol, formoterol, and oral forms of albuterol. Although most long-acting bronchodilators require at least 10 to 30 minutes to begin providing relief and four to six hours to reach full effect, a newer DPI formulation of formoterol (Foradil), approved by the FDA in 2001, starts working in most patients within one to three minutes.

✔ A combination of the inhaled corticosteroid fluticasone with the long-acting bronchodilator salmeterol, approved by the FDA in 2000. This product, available under the brand name Advair Diskus, treats both airway constriction and inflammation and is one of the most commonly prescribed asthma medications in the United States.

✔ Sustained release methylxanthine bronchodilators, such as oral theophylline.

✔ Leukotriene modifiers, such as oral montelukast, zafirlukast, and zileuton, available as tablets. If your physician decides that this category of drugs is suitable for your condition, you may benefit from the ease and convenience of taking tablets, which may help you more effectively adhere to the pharmacotherapy aspect of your asthma management plan. (The FDA has also approved montelukast in pediatric formulations as chewable tablets and oral granules for young children and babies.)

✔ Anti-IgE antibodies, which represent an exciting new development in asthma treatment, as I explain in Chapter 17. Omalizumab/rhuMAb-E25 (Xolair), which physicians administer by injection, is the first drug in this class to be approved by the FDA. (See Chapter 6 for a detailed discussion of IgE antibodies and the immune system.)

Relieving asthma episodes with quick-relief products

The primary function of quick-relief drugs, also known as *rescue medications*, is to promptly reverse acute airflow obstruction and relieve constricted airways during an asthma episode. Your doctor may also prescribe a quick-relief product, such as an inhaled beta$_2$-adrenergic bronchodilator, prior to exercise to prevent symptoms of exercise-induced asthma, or EIA.

Quick-relief medications include

✔ **Short-acting beta$_2$-adrenergic bronchodilators.** These adrenaline-like drugs work by rapidly relaxing the smooth muscles in your airways, causing your airways to open, usually within five minutes of inhaling the medication. Inhaled or aerosol forms of these drugs provide the most effective, prompt relief of acute bronchospasms, and many doctors consider beta$_2$-adrenergic bronchodilators the medication of choice for treating asthma symptoms that suddenly worsen and for preventing EIA.

Drugs in this class include albuterol (Proventil, Ventolin), bitolterol (Tornalate), metaproterenol (Alupent), pirbuterol (Maxair), and terbutaline (Brethaire, Brethine, Bricanyl). A recently approved new version (single isomer) of albuterol known as *levalbuterol* (Xopenex), a short-acting beta$_2$-adrenergic bronchodilator, is available in nebulizer (CDN) formulations for patients 6 and older.

✔ **Anticholinergics, which may provide added relief when combined with inhaled short-acting beta$_2$-adrenergic bronchodilators.** These drugs block *acetylcholine* (a neurotransmitter that stimulates mucus production) and therefore help reduce mucus in your airways. These drugs also relax the smooth muscle around the lungs' large and medium airways.

Ipratropium bromide (Atrovent) is the most widely used anticholinergic in the United States and is usually prescribed in combination with short-acting beta$_2$-adrenergic bronchodilators to dilate your airways.

✔ **Oral corticosteroids, also referred to as systemic corticosteroids.** Doctors prescribe these for use in asthma attacks in addition to their use as long-acting medications. During moderate-to-severe asthma episodes, your doctor may use oral corticosteroids to rapidly gain control over worsening symptoms. In such cases, oral corticosteroids can help your other quick-relief medications work more effectively, resulting in a more rapid reversal or reduction of airway inflammation, speeding recovery, and reducing the rate of relapse.

✔ Because prolonged use of oral corticosteroids can lead to adverse systemic side effects, doctors typically prescribe these drugs only as a last resort, and discontinue them (by gradual tapering) as soon as symptoms are under control.

Taking asthma medications prior to surgery

Anesthesia administered during surgery may depress lung functions, so make sure your surgeon is aware of your asthma and the medications you take to control it. (Your surgeon should evaluate both your lung functions and medication use prior to surgery.)

Your doctor may prescribe a short course of oral corticosteroids to improve your lung function starting just prior to surgery. If you've taken oral corticosteroids within the six months prior to surgery, your doctor may also prescribe intravenous hydrocortisone on a set schedule during surgery, with a rapid taper of the dose within 24 hours after your procedure.

Delivering Your Dose: Inhalers and Nebulizers

Understanding how to use inhalers and nebulizers is an important aspect of effectively treating your asthma. If your medication doesn't go where it's supposed to go, you don't benefit from it. One of the unique aspects of treating a respiratory condition is that the proper use of an inhaler is just as important as the medication itself in the inhaler: The objective is to get the medication to the area of your lungs where it can work most effectively.

The major advantages of delivering drugs directly into your lungs with inhaled delivery systems include the following:

- You can more effectively administer higher concentrations of medication into your airways.

- You can reduce the risk of systemic side effects that may occur when you use oral forms of these medications.

- You receive relief from inhaled drugs faster than with oral products.

Protecting your airways and the ozone at the same time

You're probably familiar with the issue of replacing ozone-depleting chlorofluorocarbons (CFCs) with less damaging propellants in refrigerators, air-conditioning systems, and aerosol sprays, particularly in hair, deodorant, and fragrance products. This issue especially affects people with asthma because many metered-dose inhaler (MDI) formulations use CFCs as propellants. A temporary medical exemption allows pharmaceutical companies to continue using CFCs. This exemption is presently scheduled for phase-out by 2005, but it may be extended.

As a result, pharmaceutical companies continue to develop more environmentally friendly propellants for MDI products. Hydrofluoroalkane (HFA), a new nonchlorinated propellant, recently won FDA approval for use in inhaled medications. Proventil HFA, Ventolin HFA (albuterol), and QVAR-HFA (beclomethasone) are the first ozone-friendly products on the market with this propellant, which delivers medication to the lungs more effectively than the CFC propellants developed in the 1950s.

In most cases, because of a lower velocity propellant spray and smaller particle size, a non-CFC propelled product allows more of the medication to get into the smaller, more peripheral airways of your lungs.

Using a metered-dose inhaler

An MDI consists of a canister of pressurized medication that fits into a plastic actuator sleeve and connects to a mouthpiece. An MDI propels medication at more than 60 miles per hour (a lot faster than my first car!), and that medication needs to make a sharp turn to effectively get into the airways of your lungs. Therefore, most of the medication sprayed from the MDI never even reaches your lungs. For example, the spray can coat your mouth, the end of your tongue, or the back of your throat. In the best-case scenario, your small airways receive only 10 to 20 percent of the inhaled drug.

Millions of people with asthma breathe easier thanks to inhalers, but properly using these devices is crucial to their success. Many people experience difficulty controlling their asthma because they use their inhalers incorrectly.

Taking your metered dose correctly

When prescribing your inhaled medication, your physician should instruct you on how to properly use an MDI. Likewise, she should review your inhaler technique at subsequent office visits. The following are some important instructions that apply to using most MDI products.

1. **Remove the cap and hold the encased inhaler upright.**

2. **Shake the inhaler.**

3. **Tilt your head back slightly and breathe out slowly.**

4. **Depending on your physician's specific instructions, open your mouth with your head 1 to 2 inches away from the inhaler or position the inhaler in your mouth.**

5. **Press down on the inhaler to release medication as you start inhaling or within the first second of inhaling; continue inhaling as you press down on your inhaler.**

   Breathe in slowly through your mouth, not your nose, for three to five seconds. Press your inhaler only once while you're inhaling (one breath for each puff). Make sure you breathe evenly and deeply.

6. **Hold your breath for ten seconds to allow the medicine to reach deep into your lungs.**

7. **Repeat puffs as your prescription dictates.**

   Waiting one minute between puffs may permit the second puff to reach into the airways of your lungs better.

Getting the right dose from your MDI

Two important factors that can affect the dosage you receive from your MDI include the following:

- ✔ **Loss of prime:** People who use inhalers often keep several around the house or office so that backup medication is always handy. Keeping too many back-up inhalers around can lead to infrequent inhaler activation and *loss of prime*. Loss of prime occurs when the inhaler's propellant evaporates or escapes from the metering chamber after days or weeks of nonuse. If you haven't used an inhaler recently, waste a puff of medication (often less than a full dose) into the air before inhaling your first dose to ensure that you receive the full potency of your medication.

- ✔ **Tail-off:** In a misguided attempt to economize, many inhaler users try to squeeze every last drop of medication from their MDIs. However, research indicates that this practice may actually contribute to the documented rise in asthma deaths and poor quality of life for some people with asthma because of a phenomenon known as *tail-off*. As an MDI reaches its empty stage, dose reliability becomes increasingly unpredictable. Therefore, don't use your MDI beyond the labeled number of doses, even if you think that some medication remains.

Using new, improved MDIs versus generic brands

Many patients have found that the recently developed Maxair Autohaler, which is formulated to deliver pirbuterol (a short-acting beta₂-adrenergic bronchodilator), is a simpler, user-friendly way of delivering medication to the airways compared to many other MDIs. That's mainly because the Autohaler is the only breath-activated MDI approved by the FDA, and requires less coordination to use. The Autohaler also doesn't require the use of a holding chamber, or spacer (see the section "Using holding chambers," in this chapter).

Given the more sophisticated design and effectiveness of the Autohaler and of various dry-powder inhalers as well as the recently approved Advair Diskus (which I discuss later in this section), you may wonder why generic MDIs continue to be prescribed.

The reason for that is simple: dollars and cents. As I explain more extensively in Chapter 3, a bottom-line attitude has taken over the healthcare industry, and too often, in the name of cost containment, physicians prescribe low-cost generics rather than brand-name products. Many asthma patients may not be receiving the treatment they really require because too often their physicians prescribe generic medications rather than costlier brand-name products, such as the Autohaler, which feature more advanced drug formulations and easier-to-use inhalation systems.

Using holding chambers

Doctors recommend *holding chambers* (also known as spacers) for younger children, as well as people who can't use an MDI correctly. A holding chamber is a hollow device that extends the space between the opening of the inhaler and your mouth. The holding chamber traps and suspends particles of medication as the inhaler releases them, allowing you to inhale your dose over a span of one to six breaths, depending on the particular device you use.

Use a holding chamber when taking inhaled corticosteroids with an MDI to minimize the possibility of developing an oral yeast infection and to improve delivery of the medication to your lungs.

Holding chambers come in various shapes and sizes. Several of these devices (such as AeroChamber and E-Z Spacer) have both a mouthpiece for adults, as shown in Figure 14-1, and a mask for infants and small children, as shown in Figure 14-2.

Using a dry-powder inhaler

DPIs, as their name implies, dispense medication in a dry-powder formulation. DPIs come in different shapes and sizes and can deliver bronchodilators as well as anti-inflammatory medications. In recent years, the FDA has approved DPI formulations of the four following long-acting drugs:

- ✔ Budesonide, an inhaled corticosteroid, distributed in the United States as Pulmicort Turbuhaler

- ✔ Fluticasone, also an inhaled corticosteroid, available as Flovent Rotadisk to be used with the Diskhaler device

- ✔ Salmeterol, a long-acting bronchodilator, marketed as Serevent Diskus

- ✔ Fluticasone and salmeterol in combination, marketed as Advair Diskus

DPIs are easy to use and very effective, if you operate them properly. The medication particles in the dry powder are so small that they can easily reach the tiniest airways. Keep in mind that, unlike most MDIs with a few types of DPIs, you may not taste or feel the medication when using the device. If you've administered the medication properly, however, you will receive its benefit.

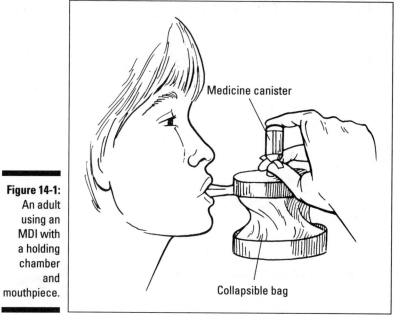

Figure 14-1: An adult using an MDI with a holding chamber and mouthpiece.

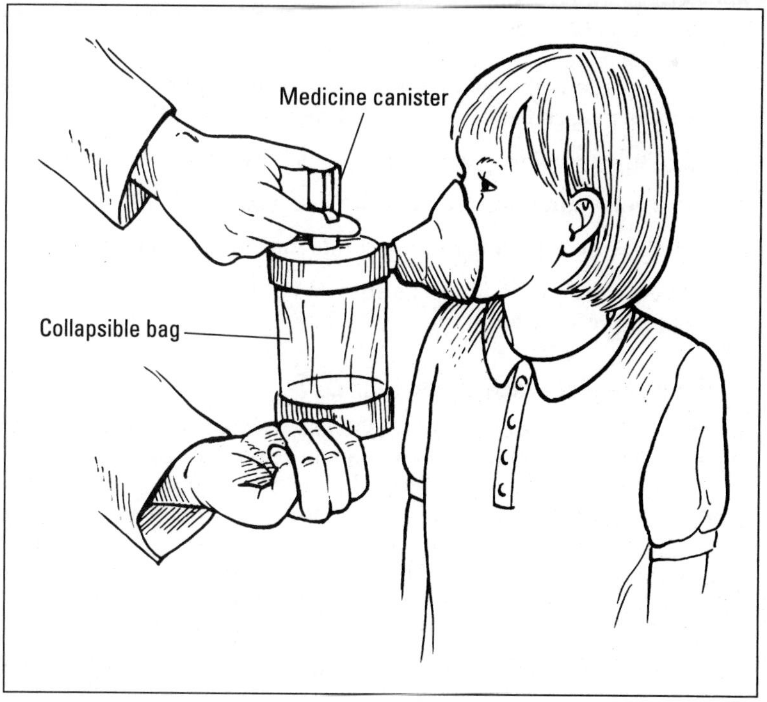

Medicine canister

Collapsible bag

Figure 14-2: A child using an MDI with a holding chamber and mask.

Medicine canister

Collapsible bag

Some of the specific benefits of using a DPI include the following:

- ✔ Children as young as 4 can use these devices.

- ✔ For many people who have poor MDI technique or who have difficulty coordinating the steps required for properly inhaling medication from an MDI, a DPI is often an excellent alternative, especially for children.

- ✔ One inhalation from a DPI often provides the same dosage as two puffs of a comparable medication from an MDI.

- ✔ Because some DPIs have dose counters, you can easily tell when your inhaler is almost empty.

- ✔ Cold temperatures don't reduce the effectiveness of DPIs.

- ✔ DPIs don't use chlorofluorocarbons (CFCs), so they don't damage the planet's ozone layer.

DPI instructions

Although DPIs don't require using a holding chamber, you still need to use your DPI in a specific way. Because every DPI works a little differently, make sure you know how to use the one your doctor prescribes. As with an MDI (see "Using a metered-dose inhaler"), your physician should instruct you on how to properly use your DPI and should review your inhaler technique at subsequent office visits. The following are important, general instructions on the proper use of most DPIs:

1. **Follow the manufacturer's instructions to prime your DPI and then load a prescribed dose of the dry-powder medication.**

2. **Breathe out slowly and completely (usually for three to five seconds).**

3. **Put your mouth on the mouthpiece and inhale deeply and forcefully.**

4. **Hold your breath for ten seconds and then exhale slowly.**

5. **Repeat the procedure as outlined by your physician until you've taken the correct number of doses.**

Getting the right dose from your DPI

In addition to the steps in the previous section, keep the following points in mind in order to obtain the most benefit from your DPI:

- ✔ **Your DPI is breath-activated.** That means you can control the rate at which you inhale the dry powder. However, you do need to inhale with sufficient force (minimal flow rate) in order to assure delivery of the medication to the smallest airways of your lungs. In order to be truly effective, using a DPI requires closing your mouth tightly around the inhaler's mouthpiece and inhaling steadily, deeply, and forcefully.

✔ **Make sure the dry powder in your DPI stays dry to avoid caking or clumping, which can affect the dose's reliability.** For DPIs with caps, make sure you always replace the cap after using the product. Don't ever wash a DPI that still contains medication.

✔ **In contrast with the operation of an MDI, you don't need to shake your DPI just before using it in order to assure delivery of the proper dose.** In fact, shaking some DPIs can result in losing dry powder.

Using a multidose-powder inhaler

Advair, a recently approved combination of fluticasone (an inhaled cortico-steroid) with salmeterol (a long-acting beta$_2$-adrenergic bronchodilator), is formulated in a new type of delivery device known as a Diskus. As with other DPIs, the Diskus is breath-activated, and for the majority of patients, it's easier to use than most MDIs.

The FDA approved this product, the first of its kind, to treat both the underlying inflammation that characterizes asthma and the airway constriction that often results from episodes of respiratory symptoms. Evidence suggests that using Advair Diskus usually reduces airway inflammation within one or two weeks (sometimes longer in certain cases), while the medication's bronchodilation effects are usually felt within 30 to 60 minutes. However, remember that Advair Diskus isn't a replacement for a quick-relief drug that your doctor prescribes for you to use if your respiratory symptoms worsen.

Important advantages of Advair Diskus include the following:

✔ Each dose of Advair is effective for up to 12 hours. The normal dosage is one inhalation twice per day (for patients 12 years and older): once in the morning and once at night. This medication schedule is often more practical for patients than most MDI medications. As a result, patients using Advair Diskus are liable to be more successful in adhering to an asthma management plan.

✔ Using the Diskus requires far less coordination than most MDIs.

✔ The built-in Diskus dose counter lets you keep track of every dose.

Operating your Diskus

If your physician prescribes Advair Diskus for you, make sure she explains the proper use of it.

The following are important, general instructions when using the Diskus:

1. **While holding the device in one hand, place the thumb of your other hand on the device's thumb grip and push away until the mouthpiece appears and snaps into position.**

2. **Hold the Diskus in a level, horizontal position with the mouthpiece facing you and slide the lever away from you as far as it goes until it clicks.**

   The "click" means the Diskus is ready for use.

3. **Exhale, while holding the Diskus level but away from your mouth (never exhale into the Diskus mouthpiece).**

4. **Place the mouthpiece to your lips, breathe in quickly and deeply through the Diskus (don't breathe in through your nose).**

5. **Remove the Diskus from your mouth and hold your breath for about ten seconds or as long you find comfortable; exhale slowly through your mouth.**

6. **Close the Diskus when you have completed taking a dose.**

   To do so, place your thumb once again on the thumb grip and slide it back toward you as far as it goes. The Diskus clicks shut, and the lever returns to its original position. The device is ready for your next dose, which you should take in approximately 12 hours (unless your doctor has advised you differently).

7. **After taking your Diskus dose, rinse your mouth with water without swallowing.**

Getting the right dose from your Diskus

Beyond the general Advair Diskus instructions I list in the previous section, keep the following points in mind to get the most out of this medication:

✔ Don't advance the lever more than once when preparing your dose. Also, don't play with the lever.

✔ Avoid tilting the Diskus when using it. Only use it in a level, horizontal position.

✔ Never try to take the Diskus apart.

✔ Always keep the Diskus dry. Never wash any part of the device, including the mouthpiece.

Using nebulizers

A *nebulizer* is an air compressor connected to a generator. Nebulizers deliver medication as a mist that is easy to inhale, which often brings rapid symptom relief. These medication-delivery systems, sometimes known as *breathing machines,* are especially useful when a child is too young or too sick to use other devices. In addition to standard, home plug-in models, you can purchase portable nebulizers with battery packs or cigarette lighter adapters to use in a vehicle.

Although at times a bit more expensive in terms of the initial purchase price, the newer jet nebulizers are preferable to older units. The slight cost difference between these newer nebulizers and their precursor evaporates after patients begin using the more modern machines and realize how much more effectively they deliver medication throughout the airways.

Doctors typically recommend jet nebulizers as the delivery device for administering Pulmicort Respules, a commonly prescribed CDN formulation of the inhaled corticosteroid drug budesonide.

Doctors may prescribe nebulizer therapy for adults to reduce or eliminate hospital or emergency room visits, especially for severe persistent asthma sufferers. Many nebulizer users find that the device allows them more effective relief than metered-dose inhalers. Therefore, if you're experiencing sudden-onset, severe asthma attacks on a frequent basis, you may benefit greatly from having a nebulizer prescribed for home use.

Remember these general guidelines when using a nebulizer with a mouthpiece:

- Place your mouth over the mouthpiece and breathe in and out.

- Make sure that you breathe through your mouth and not your nose.

  You or your child can use a facemask that covers the mouth and nose with the nebulizer. Some nebulizer manufacturers also offer colorful, kid-friendly pediatric masks. These masks usually feature animal shapes and can help in making the process of using a nebulizer more attractive — even fun in some cases — for young children.

- Have an extra nebulizer mask on hand when using the device, especially if you're administering the medication to a young child. (If you have a young child, you can probably imagine any number of reasons why that extra mask might come in handy).

- When using a nebulizer on your child, don't "blow by" or mist the medication in your child's face. A nebulizer requires a closed system to provide effective treatment (I explain this aspect in greater detail in Chapter 18).

- Use all the medication in your nebulizer. (Doing so normally takes 7 to 15 minutes, depending on the type of nebulizer you're using.)

Cleaning your medication delivery system

Rinse your MDI, holding chamber, and nebulizer daily and wash these devices weekly with a mild detergent to keep them clean and free of medication build-up. Don't use harsh chemicals in washing your delivery devices, and make sure to follow the manufacturer's instructions for maintenance and care. Also, don't forget any MDIs that have been sitting in a drawer, backpack, briefcase, or handbag for a long time.

Remember to always keep the cap on your inhaler when you're not using it. If the cap accidentally becomes dislodged, make sure you that you properly clean your inhaler before using it again.

Chapter 15

Looking at Asthma Controller Drugs

In This Chapter

▶ Controlling your asthma with long-term drugs

▶ Understanding why anti-inflammatory products are often vital for asthma patients

▶ Combining certain types of drugs for optimal long-term asthma control

*A*sthma is more than coughing, wheezing, shortness of breath, chest tightness, and other respiratory symptoms that may come and go. If you have persistent asthma, as is the case for a majority of asthmatics, some airway inflammation and *hyperreactivity* ("twitchiness") will almost always be present through your lifetime, even during periods when you aren't experiencing obvious symptoms.

As a result, an essential aspect of treating asthma is the regular and preventive use of long-term control medications, also known as *anti-inflammatory drugs* or *controlling drugs*, which your physician prescribes to control your airway inflammation. Along with these products, your doctor should also prescribe quick-relief medications (often called *rescue drugs* or *relieving drugs*) — such as short-acting bronchodilators — to be used appropriately on an as-needed basis during an asthma episode, and/or prior to allergen exposure or exercise. (See Chapter 16 for more on rescue drugs.)

Your doctor usually prescribes medications from at least one or more of the following classes of drugs as part of your long-term asthma management plan:

✔ Anti-inflammatories, which include inhaled corticosteroids, oral corticosteroids, and mast cell stabilizers

✔ Long-acting bronchodilators

✔ Sustained release methylxanthines

✔ Leukotriene modifiers

✔ IgE blocker, a recently developed anti-IgE therapy that physicians administer by injection

I discuss each of these categories of long-term asthma medications extensively throughout this chapter and also provide general dosage information for specific drugs.

Controlling Airway Inflammation with Corticosteroids

Corticosteroids provide the most potent and consistently effective long-term control of moderate to severe symptoms of asthma. With their anti-inflammatory action, these drugs can

- Decrease swelling in your airways
- Make your airways less hyperresponsive ("twitchy") to asthma triggers
- Reduce mucus production in your airways

Corticosteroids may also prevent irreversible damage (known as *remodeling* — replacing healthy tissue with scar tissue) to the airway (see Chapter 2).

Inhaled corticosteroids

Doctors generally consider inhaled corticosteroids the *primary controller* or *maintenance therapy* for patients with moderate and severe persistent asthma, because of the drugs' anti-inflammatory properties. Doctors use these drugs because the inhaled forms directly deliver the medication to the airways with minimal side effects (see Table 15-1). Consistent and appropriate (as determined by your doctor) use of inhaled corticosteroids can also reduce the need for oral (or *systemic*) corticosteroids, which may cause serious adverse side effects when used long-term.

Inhaled corticosteroids usually start reducing airway inflammation after a week of regular administration, reaching their full effect within four weeks. However, although these drugs can work well as preventives, if you develop severe symptoms — from a sudden high exposure to potent asthma triggers, for example — you need to use a quick-relief medication (usually a bronchodilator that your doctor prescribes) as part of your asthma management plan.

Table 15-1 **Inhaled Corticosteroid Medications**

Active Ingredient	Formulation	Brand Name	Total Usual Daily Child Dose (Under 12)	Total Usual Daily Adult Dose
Beclomethasone	MDI (HFA P&B): 40 mcg or 80 mcg	QVAR-HFA	(Ages 5–11) 40 mcg: 2 puffs twice per day 80 mcg: 2 puffs twice per day	40 mcg: Low dose: 1 puff twice per day 80 mcg: Low dose: 1 puff twice per day Med. dose: 2 puffs twice per day High dose: 4 puffs twice per day
Budesonide	Turbuhaler (DPI): 200 mcg/dose Respules (CDN): 0.25 mg, 0.5 mg per 2 mL unit dose	Pulmicort Turbuhaler, Pulmicort Respules	DPI: Low dose: 1 inhalation Med. dose: 1 to 2 inhalations High dose: More than 2 inhalations CDN (12 months–8 years): Initial dose: 0.5 mg, starting as single dose or 0.25 twice per day, not to exceed 1 mg; High dose (for patients on oral corticosteroids who need to convert to inhaled corticosteroids): Total of 2 mg per day	DPI: Low dose: 1 to 2 inhalations Med. dose: 2 to 3 inhalations High dose: More than 3 inhalations CDN: Low dose: 0.5 mg twice per day Med. dose: 1 mg twice per day High dose: 2 mg twice per day
Budesonide with formoterol	MDI (HFA): 80/4.5 mcg (pediatric formulation) 160/4.5 mcg (ages 12 and above)	Symbicort*	(Ages 6–11) Two inhalations of the 80/4.5 mcg formulation twice per day	One to 2 inhalations of the 160/4.5 mcg formulation twice per day

(continued)

Table 15-1 (continued)

Active Ingredient	Formulation	Brand Name	Total Usual Daily Child Dose (Under 12)	Total Usual Daily Adult Dose
Ciclesonide*	MDI (HFA): 40 mcg (pediatric formulation) 80 mcg/puff 160 mcg/puff	Alvesco*	(Ages 6–11) 40 mcg: 2 puffs once per day	Low dose: 2 puffs once per day of 80 mcg High dose: 2 puffs once per day of 160 mcg
Flunisolide	MDI: 250 mcg/puff	Aerobid, Aerobid-M	MDI (Aerobid, Aerobid-M):	MDI: Low dose: 2 to 4 puffs
Flunisolide HFA*	MDI (HFA): 85 mcg/puff	Aerospan (HFA)*	Low dose: 2 to 3 puffs Med. dose: 4 to 5 puffs High dose: More than 5 puffs MDI (HFA): 1 to 2 puffs twice per day	Med. dose: 4 to 8 puffs High dose: More than 8 puffs MDI (HFA): 2 to 4 puffs twice per day
Fluticasone	MDI: 44, 110, 220 mcg/puff Flovent Diskus (DPI): 50, 100, 250 mcg/dose Flovent Rotadisk (DPI): 50, 100, 250 mcg/dose	Flovent	MDI: Low dose: 2 to 4 puffs of 44 mcg Med. dose: 4 to 10 puffs of 44 mcg or 2 to 4 puffs of 110 mcg High dose: More than 4 puffs of 110 mcg or more than 2 puffs of 220 mcg	MDI: Low dose: 2 to 6 puffs of 44 mcg or 2 puffs of 110 mcg Med. dose: 2 to 6 puffs of 110 mcg High dose: More than 6 puffs of 110 mcg or more than 3 puffs of 220 mcg

Table 15-1 (continued)

Active Ingredient	Formulation	Brand Name	Total Usual Daily Child Dose (Under 12)	Total Usual Daily Adult Dose
			DPI: Low dose: 2 to 4 inhalations of 50 mcg Med. dose: 2 to 4 inhalations of 100 mcg High dose: More than 4 inhalations of 100 mcg or more than 2 inhalations of 250 mcg	DPI: Low dose: 2 to 6 inhalations of 50 mcg Med. dose: 3 to 6 inhalations of 100 mcg High dose: More than 6 inhalations of 100 mcg or more than 2 inhalations of 250 mcg
Fluticasone with salmeterol	Diskus (DPI) in 3 formulations: 100, 250, or 500 mcg of fluticasone with 50 mcg of salmeterol	Advair Diskus	Not yet approved for children under 12	One inhalation twice per day
Mometasone	Twisthaler (DPI): 200 mcg/dose	Asmanex*	Recommended dose is 1 inhalation per day	Recommended dose is 1 to 2 inhalations per day
Triamcinolone	MDI: 100 mcg/puff	Azmacort	Low dose: 4 to 8 puffs Med. dose: 8 to 12 puffs High dose: More than 12 puffs	Low dose: 4 to 10 puffs Med. dose: 10 to 20 puffs High dose: More than 20 puffs

*Awaiting approval in the United States (under development as an MDI HFA formulation). Doctors usually divide the daily dosage into two doses. In some cases, you may take your daily dosage in one dose, depending on your doctor's advice. Note: mg = milligram; mcg = microgram; CDN: compressor-driven nebulizer; MDI: metered-dose inhaler; DPI: dry-powder inhaler; HFA (hydrofluoroalkane); P & B: press and breathe.

Knowing your inhaled corticosteroid devices and formulations

Doctors can prescribe inhaled corticosteroids in metered-dose inhaler (MDI), dry-powder inhaler (DPI), or compressor-driven nebulizer (CDN) formulations (see Chapter 14).

Because the pressurized canisters of some MDI medications are packaged in plastic sleeves of the same color, knowing which strength your doctor specifically prescribes for you is especially important.

Monitoring children who take inhaled corticosteroids

Although all available evidence indicates that inhaled corticosteroids are highly effective and safe for children, some concern exists about the possible temporary effects on the growth rate in children who use these products.

If your child's asthma doctor prescribes inhaled corticosteroids, make sure that he accurately monitors your child's growth.

Taking inhaled corticosteroids more effectively

In order to avoid the rare occurrence of an oral yeast infection or hoarseness (due to yeast infection in the throat) from using inhaled corticosteroids, make sure that you thoroughly rinse your mouth with water, or even a mouthwash, without swallowing, after using any of these products.

Use a holding chamber, sometimes known as a spacer (see Chapter 14 for more information), with an MDI formulation of inhaled corticosteroids to improve delivery of the medication to the airways and further reduce the risk of developing an oral yeast infection or hoarseness of the throat.

Oral corticosteroids

In severe asthma cases, early use of oral corticosteroids can prevent relapses and reduce the need for hospitalization. They're also essential for treating patients who don't respond quickly to bronchodilators (see Table 15-2). In addition, doctors may use oral corticosteroids to gain prompt control of asthma when starting long-term therapy.

If overused, these drugs can cause systemic adverse side effects, including fluid retention, altered blood sugar levels, weight gain, peptic ulcers, mood alteration, high blood pressure, reduced bone density, and impaired immune functioning. For this reason, oral corticosteroids are often the last medications that doctors add to your pharmacotherapy and the first ones they remove — after they determine that your symptoms are under control.

If you suffer from severe, persistent asthma, your doctor may prescribe a course of alternate-day, single morning oral corticosteroid therapy to control symptoms while reducing the risk of adverse side effects.

Table 15-2 **Oral Corticosteroid Medications**

Active Ingredient	Formulation	Brand Name	Total Usual Daily Child Dose (Under 12)*	Total Usual Daily Adult Dose*
Methylprednisolone	2, 4, 8, 16, 32 mg tablets	Medrol	0.25 to 2 mg per kg of the child's weight in a single daily dose or single dose every other day as needed for control of symptoms. Doctors may also prescribe a short course "burst" of 1 to 2 mg per kg of the child's weight per day, for a maximum of 60 mg per day, for 3 to 10 days.	7.5 to 60 mg in a single daily dose or single dose every other day as needed for control of symptoms. Doctors may also prescribe a short course "burst" of 40 to 60 mg per day as a single dose or 2 divided doses for 3 to 10 days.
Prednisone	15 mg/5 mL solution	Orapred		
Prednisolone	5 mg tablets	Prednisolone		
Prednisolone	5 mg/5 mL solution 15 mg/5 mL solution	Prelone		
Prednisolone	1 mg/mL solution	Pediapred		
Prednisone	1, 2.5, 5, 10, 20, 25 mg tablets	Deltasone, Prednisone		

*Dosages apply to all listed products.
Note: 1 kg (kilogram) = 2.2 pounds; mg = milligram; mL = milliliter.

Preventing Respiratory Symptoms with Mast Cell Stabilizers

Mast cells are important players in the inflammatory process (see Chapter 6 for more information about mast cells). These cells exist in large numbers in your lungs and nose. When triggered (usually by allergens), mast cells release several substances, including histamine and leukotrienes, which cause inflammation and also lead to airway constriction and increased mucus production.

Mast cell stabilizers (see Table 15-3) used in long-term treatment of asthma, such as inhaled cromolyn and nedocromil, inhibit the release of mast cell mediators, thus preventing or reducing inflammation. (See Chapter 5 for an explanation of airway inflammation.) However, to properly prevent asthma symptoms, both cromolyn and nedocromil need to reach deep into your lungs.

Table 15-3		Mast Cell Stabilizer Medications		
Active Ingredient	**Formulation**	**Brand Name**	**Total Usual Daily Child Dose (Under 12)**	**Total Usual Daily Adult Dose**
Cromolyn	MDI: 1 mg per puff; CDN: 20 mg per *ampule* (vial of solution)	Intal	MDI: 1 to 2 puffs four times per day or as needed prior to exercise or allergen exposure (ages 5–11) CDN: 1 ampule four times per day or as needed prior to exercise or allergen exposure (ages 2–11)	MDI: 2 to 4 puffs four times per day or as needed CDN: 1 ampule four times per day or as needed prior to exercise or allergen exposure
Nedocromil	MDI: 1.75 mg per puff	Tilade	One to 2 puffs four times per day or as needed prior to exercise or allergen exposure (ages 6–11)	Two to 4 puffs four times per day or as needed prior to exercise or allergen exposure

Note: mg = milligram; CDN: compressor-driven nebulizer; MDI: metered-dose inhaler.

Cromolyn

Cromolyn can be effective in certain patients, either alone or with a bronchodilator, in preventing the symptoms of persistent mild-to-moderate asthma. Doctors sometimes recommend cromolyn in a nasal formulation (Nasalcrom), which is available as an over-the-counter (OTC) product, to prevent allergic rhinitis symptoms (see Chapter 12).

Your doctor may also prescribe cromolyn medications for asthma treatments in CDN or MDI forms.

Prescribing cromolyn for young children and pregnant women

Because cromolyn has an excellent safety profile and produces no significant side effects, doctors sometimes use it in CDN form to treat young children (see Chapter 18). For similar reasons, doctors also prescribe MDI formulations of cromolyn to control pregnant women's respiratory symptoms (see Chapter 19).

Cromolyn especially helps to suppress symptoms triggered by unavoidable exposures to asthma triggers, such as animal dander, pollen, and viral respiratory infections. Your doctor may prescribe this drug during pollen season, winter months, or if you experience routine exposures to pets.

Taking cromolyn prior to pollen exposure and exercise

To prevent pollen-induced symptoms, start taking inhaled cromolyn at least one week before pollen season begins. Taking inhaled cromolyn 30 minutes before exposure to animal dander — during (preferably) brief visits with people who have pets, for example — can often reduce the risk of developing asthma symptoms.

Cromolyn can prevent or reduce exercise-induced asthma (EIA) symptoms if you take it 15 to 30 minutes before exercising. (I discuss exercise-related respiratory symptoms in Chapter 9.)

Nedocromil

Although different from cromolyn, nedocromil can also provide similar long-term anti-inflammatory benefits. As with cromolyn, nedocromil maintains an excellent safety profile. The main differences between the two drugs include the following:

✔ At regular dosage levels, nedocromil may be more effective than cromolyn, because it can start preventing airway inflammation in three days. (Refer to Table 15-3 for dosage information.)

✔ At recommended doses, doctors find nedocromil a more effective tool than cromolyn for preventing symptoms of EIA in some patients.

✔ Only patients older than 6 who suffer mild persistent asthma should use nedocromil.

✔ Nedocromil is only available as an MDI formulation.

Some patients find the taste of nedocromil unpleasant. To reduce the aftertaste, your doctor may recommend using a holding chamber (see Chapter 14) or sipping water before or after inhaling nedocromil.

Prepping for mast cell stabilizers with other drugs

If your airways are already inflamed or constricted, you may need a one-week course of oral corticosteroids (or 30 days of inhaled corticosteroids) to sufficiently reduce the existing airway inflammation. Doing so helps to ensure that the inhaled cromolyn or nedocromil work effectively as preventive medications.

Your doctor may also prescribe a bronchodilator to reduce airway constriction prior to inhaling cromolyn or nedocromil for the first month that you take these drugs.

Knowing when mast cell stabilizers may not be enough

Although appropriate long-term, routine use of cromolyn and nedocromil can reduce the intensity of your asthma symptoms, neither drug is helpful in managing an asthma episode if one occurs. If you suffer an asthma attack, you may need to use a short-term rescue bronchodilator, as your asthma management plan specifies. However, even during an asthma episode, your doctor may advise you to continue using cromolyn or nedocromil to maintain the drug's preventive effect, in addition to any other prescribed treatment.

Dilating Your Airways with Long-Acting Bronchodilators

REMEMBER

Doctors prescribe long-acting beta$_2$-adrenergic bronchodilators for long-term prevention of asthma symptoms, usually with anti-inflammatory medications such as inhaled corticosteroids and/or occasionally mast cell stabilizers (cromolyn or nedocromil). In addition to relaxing your airway's smooth muscles, long-acting beta$_2$-adrenergic bronchodilators can also increase the anti-inflammatory effect of inhaled corticosteroids if you use them on a consistent, long-term basis.

Because long-acting bronchodilators can dilate the airways for up to 12 hours per dose, doctors often prescribe these products to control nighttime asthma symptoms. Serevent, a long-acting bronchodilator in DPI (Serevent Diskus) and MDI formulations (see Table 15-4), works well to prevent episodes of nighttime asthma and EIA, if taken 30 minutes before exercising, and also enhances the effect of inhaled corticosteroids when used together. Serevent Diskus is approved for use in patients as young as 4 years old. Both the MDI and the Diskus device contain the same medication. However, one inhalation of the Diskus is equal to two puffs of the MDI.

Table 15-4	Long-Acting Beta$_2$-Adrenergic Bronchodilators			
Active Ingredient	*Formulation*	*Brand Name*	*Total Usual Daily Child Dose (Under 12)*	*Total Usual Daily Adult Dose*
Albuterol (sustained release tablet)	4 or 8 mg extended-release tablets	Volmax, Proventil Repetab	0.3 to 0.6 mg per kg of child's weight, not to exceed 8 mg total per day (ages 6–11)	1 tablet (4 or 8 mg) twice per day, not to exceed 32 mg total per day
Formoterol	Aerolizer (DPI)	Foradil	One 12 mcg capsule by inhalation twice per day (ages 6–11)	One 12 mcg capsule by inhalation twice per day

(continued)

Table 15-4 (continued)

Active Ingredient	Formulation	Brand Name	Total Usual Daily Child Dose (Under 12)	Total Usual Daily Adult Dose
Salmeterol	Diskus (DPI): 50 mcg/ inhalation	Serevent	DPI: 1 inhalation twice per day (ages 4–11)	DPI: 1 inhalation twice per day
	MDI: 21 mcg/puff		MDI: Not yet approved for children under 12	MDI: 2 puffs twice per day

Note: 1 kg (kilogram) = 2.2 pounds; mcg = microgram; DPI: dry-powder inhaler; MDI: metered-dose inhaler.

Combining two drugs: Advair

The introduction of Advair (refer to Table 15-1), a combination of an inhaled corticosteroid (fluticasone) and a long-acting beta$_2$-adrenergic bronchodilator (salmeterol), represents a *complementary* (an enhanced anti-inflammatory effect compared to either therapy alone) blend of medications.

According to recent studies of patients with persistent asthma who had previously been treated with inhaled corticosteroids, Advair (initially available in a Diskus DPI device) improved lung functions by 25 percent on average as compared to 15 percent with fluticasone (Flovent) alone and 5 percent with salmeterol (Serevent) alone.

Researchers have found that taking one dose of Advair is superior to taking two separate doses of fluticasone and salmeterol at the same time. Advair truly represents a significantly more convenient and effective form of combination asthma therapy that treats airway constriction and inflammation, which probably explains why Advair has become one of the most commonly prescribed asthma medications in the United States.

Understanding timing: Why long-acting products may not always be enough

Effectively using these long-acting products may also reduce your need for quick-relief bronchodilators. However, long-acting bronchodilators, such as salmeterol (Serevent), take longer to kick in (ranging from 10 to 30 minutes and reaching peak effectiveness in four to six hours) and don't work as well as rescue medications if asthma episodes develop.

Currently, the only long-acting bronchodilator with a rapid onset of action in the United States is formoterol (Foradil), which the FDA approved in 2001. Available in a DPI formulation, this drug starts working in most patients within one to three minutes.

If you experience an asthma attack, continue using the quick-relief medication your doctor prescribes. If you have a heart condition, make sure your doctor knows this before prescribing long-acting beta$_2$-adrenergic bronchodilators. In some cases, these products can cause an elevated heartbeat.

Enhancing anti-inflammatory effectiveness

Never consider long-acting beta$_2$-adrenergic bronchodilators a substitute for an anti-inflammatory medication, such as inhaled corticosteroid. Long-acting bronchodilators should never be used by themselves but only as an addition to anti-inflammatory treatment. Using long-acting bronchodilators with inhaled corticosteroids enables you to reduce your inhaled corticosteroid dose, while maintaining equal or better control of your asthma. Studies provide strong evidence that adding a long-acting bronchodilator to your pharmacotherapy enhances the effectiveness of your existing inhaled corticosteroid medication.

Relieving Nighttime Asthma with Theophylline

The principal *methylxanthine* (chemical class related to the caffeine family) drug that doctors prescribe for asthma treatment is *oral theophylline*. Doctors most often use theophylline in conjunction with inhaled corticosteroids. Your doctor may prescribe theophylline to reduce the frequency and severity of your persistent asthma symptoms and possibly to decrease the amount of inhaled corticosteroids you may need to take. Because of the drug's long-acting effects, which can last from 8 to 24 hours, doctors often use theophylline to control nighttime asthma symptoms, particularly for patients with mild to moderate persistent asthma.

Since the development of more effective products, such as inhaled corticosteroids and safer inhaled bronchodilators (which achieve more consistent results and produce fewer adverse side effects), doctors don't prescribe theophylline as much as in the past (see Table 15-5).

Table 15-5		Methylxanthine Medications		
Active Ingredient	**Formulation**	**Brand Name**	**Total Usual Daily Child Dose (Under 12)***	**Total Usual Daily Adult Dose***
Theophylline	400, 600 mg tablets	Uni-Dur Uniphyl	Starting dose of 10 mg per kg of child's weight per day	Starting dose of 10 mg per kg of patient's weight per day
Theophylline	100, 200, 300, 450 mg tablets	Theo-Dur	Younger than 1 year: Maximum 5 mg per kg of child's weight per day	Usual max: 800 mg per day
Theophylline	100, 200, 300, 400 mg capsules	Theo-24	Older than 1 year: Maximum 16 mg per kg of child's weight per day	
Theophylline	50, 75, 100, 125, 200, 300 mg capsules/ tablets	Slo-bid Gyrocaps Theolair		

*Dosages apply to all methylxanthine products.
Note: 1 kg (kilogram) = 2.2 pounds; mg = milligram

Watching out for theophylline's undesirable side effects

Although doctors consider theophylline safe, the drug can cause a variety of undesirable side effects, such as nausea, vomiting, stomach cramps, diarrhea, and tremors. Poor school performance has occasionally been linked to children who were taking theophylline for their asthma. If you're taking a theophylline medication (usually in the form of tablets or capsules) and experience any of these types of side effects, immediately report those symptoms to your doctor.

Various factors, such as viral infections, alcohol, heart failure, and taking other medications, can impede your liver's ability to eliminate theophylline from your system. This impediment can result in higher than desirable levels of the drug in your body, leading to the side effects that I mention in the preceding paragraph, or more serious adverse side effects, such as increased irritability, insomnia, or behavioral problems — symptoms similar to what you experience after drinking too much coffee. In rare cases, excessive theophylline levels in your blood can create toxic central nervous system effects, potentially causing a coma, convulsions, or even death. Therefore, your physician should closely monitor your dosage and any change in your clinical condition.

Bad combinations: Adverse interactions with theophylline

Conversely, factors such as smoking, an overactive thyroid, a high-protein diet (featuring red meat), and certain medications, including Phenobarbital, rifampicin (Rifampin), and phenytoin (Dilantin), can increase your liver's rate of metabolizing and processing theophylline, thus often requiring an increase in dosage of the drug.

Make your doctor aware of any other medications that you take for asthma, as well as for any other ailments, if she considers prescribing theophylline. Your physician may use a standard blood test to determine whether the level of theophylline in your body is optimal.

If you suffer an asthma attack, don't take theophylline as a rescue medication. Instead, use an appropriate quick-relief bronchodilator, as prescribed by your doctor, to relieve your acute symptoms.

Reducing Respiratory Symptoms with Leukotriene Modifiers

Leukotrienes are chemicals that constrict the bronchial tubes, cause mucus secretion, and produce other adverse effects characteristic of asthma. Leukotriene modifiers are a class of drugs that prevent the activity of leukotrienes (montelukast, zafirlukast) or block their synthesis (zileuton). Regular use of these drugs can, in some asthma patients, substantially reduce respiratory symptoms.

Leukotriene modifiers can begin to work within an hour. However, these drugs often require a few days to a week of regular use to reach their full effect. Some asthmatics who have taken leukotriene modifiers over an extended period of time have reduced the amount of long-term inhaled corticosteroids or other inhaled medications needed to control their asthma symptoms.

In the United States, leukotriene modifiers are available by prescription in tablet form for the long-term management of asthma (see Table 15-6), and include the following products: montelukast (Singulair), zafirlukast (Accolate), and zileuton (Zyflo). The FDA also approved montelukast for allergic rhinitis (see Chapter 12), and this drug shows promise as well in treating allergic conjunctivitis.

Table 15-6		Leukotriene Modifiers		
Active Ingredient	*Formulation*	*Brand Name*	*Total Usual Daily Child Dose (Under 12)*	*Total Usual Daily Adult Dose*
Montelukast	10 mg tablet (ages 15 and older); 5 mg chewable tablet (ages 6–14); 4 mg chewable tablet (ages 2–5); 4 mg oral granules (ages 12–23 months)	Singulair	One 5 mg chewable tablet (ages 6–14) per day (in the evening) One 4 mg chewable tablet (ages 2–5) per day (in the evening) One packet of 4 mg oral granules (ages 12–23 months) per day (in the evening) Can be administered directly into the baby's mouth or mixed with soft food (applesauce, carrots, rice, or ice cream are recommended)	One 10 mg tablet per day (in the evening)
Zafirlukast	20 mg tablet (12 and older); 10 mg tablet (ages 6–11)	Accolate	One 10 mg tablet twice per day (ages 7–11)	One 20 mg tablet twice per day
Zileuton	300 mg, 600 mg tablet	Zyflo	Not approved for children under 12	2,400 mg daily: Two 300 mg tablets or one 600 mg tablet four times per day

Note: 1 kg (kilogram) = 2.2 pounds; mg = milligram

In addition, the FDA has recently approved a pediatric, oral granule formulation of montelukast (Singulair) for ages 12 to 23 months. You administer the medication directly into the baby's mouth or by mixing it with the baby's soft food. According to the product insert, the recommended foods are apple-sauce, carrots, rice, or — talk about making the medicine go down nice and easy — ice cream.

Compared with other categories of asthma drugs, some patients find leukotriene modifiers more user-friendly, because they're formulated as tablets and oral granules. As a result, you may find taking these medications on a regular basis more convenient than other products. That should in turn mean that you'll be more likely to successfully adhere to your asthma management program.

Understanding the importance of leukotrienes in asthma

Leukotrienes are potent biochemical substances that play a significant role in asthma attacks. These chemical mediators of inflammation are stored in special immune system cells (known as *mast cells*). They're released on exposure to allergy and asthma triggers and precipitating factors. (See Chapter 5 for details on the various factors that can trigger your respiratory symptoms.)

After they're released, leukotrienes induce inflammation, increase mucus secretions, attract and activate inflammatory cells in your airway, and promote the production of IgE antibodies, thus playing an active role in both allergic reactions and asthma episodes. (I discuss leukotrienes and other chemical mediators of inflammation more extensively in Chapter 6.)

Watching out for adverse side effects

Leukotriene modifiers can sometimes reduce respiratory reactions in patients with sensitivities to aspirin and nonsteroidal anti-inflammatory drugs (NSAIDs). If you suffer from these types of sensitivities, however, continue avoiding aspirin and NSAIDs while taking leukotriene modifiers, because reactions still may occur.

Although studies have shown that the newer prescription NSAIDs, known as COX-2 inhibitors, including celecoxib (Celebrex) and rofecoxib (Vioxx), appear not to trigger the same types of reactions in susceptible individuals as the older NSAIDs, the patient inserts for these newer medications still warn about the possibility of adverse reactions. So, I'm echoing that warning as well. Avoidance (see Chapter 5) is still the best approach when dealing with any type of drug sensitivity.

Looking at leukotriene modifiers, adverse interactions, and your liver

Because certain leukotriene modifiers can inhibit particular liver activities, make sure your doctor is aware of any other medications that you take. For example, in some cases, your liver may have trouble processing certain antibiotics and anti-seizure medications if you take leukotriene modifiers. If you take zileuton, make sure your doctor monitors your liver. Because of its potential effects on your liver, zileuton may also interfere with theophylline, warfarin (Coumadin), an anti-blood clotting medication used to reduce the risk of strokes, or beta-blockers (used for treating high blood pressure or migraine headaches), such as propranolol (Inderal).

Phenobarbital or Rifampin can increase your liver metabolism, thus breaking down certain other medications, such as montelukast, more rapidly if you take them concurrently. For this reason, your doctor should closely monitor your respiratory symptoms.

Alerting yourself to special issues with zafirlukast

Co-administration of the leukotriene modifier zafirlukast (Accolate) with other medications can affect the blood levels of zafirlukast. When used in combination with theophylline, zafirlukast blood levels may decrease by as much as one-third, while with aspirin, zafirlukast blood levels can increase by close to 50 percent.

Lower blood levels of zafirlukast may result in less than optimal control of your respiratory symptoms; elevated levels can produce side effects such as headache, or in some cases, nausea. Therefore, always make sure that your doctor knows about all medications you're taking, even OTC drugs, for any and all ailments.

Leukotriene modifiers aren't rescue medications. If you suffer an asthma attack, use a quick-relief bronchodilator as your asthma management plan specifies. However, continue taking your prescribed leukotriene modifiers during your asthma episode, because the drug often enhances the effectiveness of quick-relief medications.

Introducing the Newest Therapy on the Block: IgE Blocker

One of the most promising and novel approaches to asthma treatment is anti-IgE therapy, which the FDA approved in June 2003. The first drug in this class, omalizumab/rhuMAb-E25 (Xolair), is a *recombinant human monoclonal antibody* (rhuMab), which is an anti-IgE antibody.

This medication holds great promise for patients with moderate-to-severe allergic asthma because the treatment is specifically designed to block IgE from initiating the allergic response that typically triggers respiratory symptoms in the vast majority of asthmatics. (See Chapter 17 for further details.) Omalizumab/rhuMAb-E25 is designed to be administered once every two to four weeks by injection, with the exact dosage tailored to each patient's body weight and baseline level of circulating IgE.

Clinical trials have shown that appropriate use of this more targeted form of treatment resulted in less frequent respiratory symptoms among patients with moderate to severe allergic asthma. In studies of patients with allergy-related asthma who were treated with omalizumab/rhuMAb-E25, more than half of the participants not only experienced fewer asthma episodes, they also were able to stop using their inhaled corticosteroid medication.

As with the other medications I discuss in this chapter, remember that even if you're receiving anti-IgE therapy, you may still need to use any other asthma medications prescribed by your physician to control your respiratory symptoms.

Chapter 16

Treating Asthma Episodes

- -

In This Chapter

▶ Relieving asthma symptoms with short-term medications

▶ Considering anticholinergic therapy

▶ Controlling worsening respiratory symptoms with oral corticosteroids

- -

*Y*ou can use quick-relief drugs, also known as *rescue medications,* for the rapid treatment of acute airway obstruction and constriction that can occur during an asthma attack. Your doctor usually prescribes these medications along with long-term medications (see Chapter 15) as part of an overall asthma management plan.

Quick-relief medications serve two main purposes:

- ✔ **Short-term relief.** To prevent a worsening of respiratory symptoms prior to exposure to asthma triggers, and/or before engaging in exercise or other strenuous activities that could trigger symptoms of exercise-induced asthma (EIA), as specified by your physician.

- ✔ **Rescue.** In cases where an asthma condition suddenly worsens — perhaps due to unanticipated exposure to allergens, irritants, or precipitating factors — quick-relief medications are essential for reversing rapidly deteriorating respiratory symptoms.

The following are the three types of medications that doctors commonly prescribe for short-term relief and rescue treatment of asthma:

- ✔ Short-acting beta$_2$-adrenergic bronchodilators

- ✔ Anticholinergics, which may provide added relief when combined with inhaled short-acting beta$_2$-adrenergic bronchodilators

- ✔ Oral corticosteroids, also referred to as systemic corticosteroids, which doctors prescribe in closely supervised courses to reestablish control of a patient's asthma in cases of sudden, severe worsening of respiratory symptoms

I discuss these three categories of short-term asthma medications in detail throughout this chapter and also list general dosage information for specific drugs in each class.

Relieving Symptoms with Short-Acting Bronchodilators

The primary class of medications that physicians prescribe for rescue treatment of asthma is inhaled or aerosol formulations of short-acting beta$_2$-adrenergic (beta$_2$-agonist) bronchodilators. These adrenaline-like drugs work by rapidly relaxing the smooth muscles in your airways, causing your airways to open, usually within five minutes of inhaling the medication.

In comparison to beta$_2$-adrenergic pills and syrups, physicians consider inhaled or aerosol forms of bronchodilators the therapy of choice for treating asthma symptoms that suddenly worsen, and for preventing EIA. When administered in their inhaled or aerosol formulations, beta$_2$-adrenergic bronchodilators work faster, produce fewer side effects, and provide the most effective, prompt relief of acute respiratory symptoms.

To prevent EIA, your doctor may recommend that you inhale a dose of your prescribed short-acting beta$_2$-adrenergic bronchodilator 15 to 30 minutes before you begin to exert yourself. (See Chapter 9 for a more extensive discussion of EIA.)

The principal short-acting beta$_2$-adrenergic bronchodilators prescribed in the United States include the following:

- Albuterol (Proventil, Ventolin)
- Bitolterol (Tornalate)
- Metaproterenol (Alupent)
- Pirbuterol (Maxair)
- Terbutaline (Brethaire, Brethine, Bricanyl)
- Levalbuterol (Xopenex), a new, improved version of albuterol, available in compressor-driven nebulizer (CDN) formulations for patients 6 and older

Table 16-1 provides detailed dosage information for individual short-acting beta$_2$-adrenergic bronchodilators.

Table 16-1		Short-acting Beta₂-Adrenergic Bronchodilators			

Active Ingredient	Formulation	Brand Name	Total Usual Daily Child Dose (Under 12)	Total Usual Daily Adult Dose
Albuterol	MDI: 90 mcg/puff, 200 puffs/canister Rotacaps (DPI; via Ventolin Rotahaler); 200 mcg / Rotacaps CDN solution with calibrated dropper: 5 mg/mL (0.5%) CDN unit dose bottle (nebule) 2.5 mg/3mL (0.083%); Tablets: 2, 4 mg; Syrup: 2 mg per 5 mL	Proventil, Proventil HFA, Ventolin, Ventolin HFA, Ventolin Rotacaps (available in MDI, CDN, tablet, and syrup)	MDI: Two puffs 4 times per day or as needed prior to exercise DPI: One capsule every 4 to 6 hours or as needed prior to exercise CDN solution: 0.05 mg per kg of child's weight in 2 to 3 cc of saline solution every 4 to 6 hours; CDN unit dose (2–11 years, more than 15 kg weight): 2.5 mg (one unit dose/nebule) 3 to 4 times per day; Tablets: (ages 6–11) Starting dose: One 2 mg tablet 4 times per day, maximum of 24 mg per day; Syrup: 1 teaspoon every 6 hours	MDI: Two puffs 4 times per day or as needed prior to exercise DPI: One capsule every 4 to 6 hours or as needed prior to exercise CDN: 1.25 to 5 mg in 2 to 3 cc of saline solution every 4 to 8 hours; CDN unit dose: 2.5 mg (one unit dose/nebule) 3 to 4 times per day; Tablets: Starting dose, one 2 mg or 4 mg tablet 3 to 4 times per day, maximum of 32 mg per day; Syrup: 1 to 2 teaspoons every 6 hours

(continued)

Table 16-1 (continued)

Active Ingredient	Formulation	Brand Name	Total Usual Daily Child Dose (Under 12)	Total Usual Daily Adult Dose
Albuterol	CDN: 0.63 mg/ 3mL (vial); 1.25 mg/ 3mL (vial)	AccuNeb	CDN: (ages 2–12) low dose 0.63 mg/ vial every 3 to 4 times per day; high dose 1.25 mg/ vial 3 to 4 times per day	Indicated for children 2–12
Bitolterol	MDI: 370 mcg/ puff 300 puffs/ canister CDN: 2mg/mL (0.2% solution: Usual dose 1.25 mL = 2.5 mg; Increased dose 1.75 mL = 3.5 mg; Decreased dose 0.75 mL = 1.5 mg (each mL contains 2 mg of bitolterol)	Tornalate	MDI: Not approved for children under 12 CDN: Not approved for children under 12	MDI: Two puffs every 8 hours, not to exceed 2 puffs every 4 hours or as needed prior to exercise CDN: 0.5 to 3.5 mg (0.25–1mL) in 2 mL of saline solution every 4 to 8 hours
Levalbuterol	CDN: (ages 6–11) 0.31 mg/3 mL nebule; (children over 12 and adults) 0.63 mg/ 3 mL nebule, 1.25 mg/ 3 mL nebule	Xopenex	CDN: (ages 6–11) 0.31 mg per nebule every 6 to 8 hours	Low dose: 0.63 mg per nebule every 6 to 8 hours; High dose: 1.25 mg per nebule every 6 to 8 hours if symptoms are acute or unresponsive to low dose

Active Ingredient	Formulation	Brand Name	Total Usual Daily Child Dose (Under 12)	Total Usual Daily Adult Dose
Metaproterenol	MDI: 0.65 mL/ puff, 200 puffs/ canister CDN: 0.4%, 0.6% vials; Tablet: 10 mg, 20 mg; Syrup: 10 mg per tsp	Alupent	CDN: Not approved for children under 12; Tablet (ages 6–9): 10 mg every 6 hours; (ages 9 and above) 20 mg every 6 hours; Syrup: (ages 6–9) 1 teaspoon every 6 hours; (ages 9 and above) 2 teaspoons every 6 hours	MDI: 1 to 2 puffs every 2 to 4 hours or as needed, 1 to 2 puffs 5 minutes before exercise CDN: Low dose: 0.4% vial every 4 hours as needed; High dose: 0.6% vial every 4 hours as needed; Tablet: 20 mg every 6 hours; Syrup: 2 teaspoons every 6 hours
Pirbuterol	MDI: 200 mcg/ puff 400 puffs/ canister Autohaler (breath-activated MDI): 200 mcg/puff 400 puffs/canister	Maxair	Not approved for children under 12	Two puffs 4 times per day or as needed prior to exercise; Don't exceed 12 puffs per day
Terbutaline	MDI: 90 mcg/ puff 300 puffs/ canister; Tablets: 2.5, 5 mg	Brethaire, Brethine, Bricanyl	MDI: Two puffs 4 times per day or as needed prior to exercise; Tablets: (ages 12–15) One 2.5 mg tablet 3 times per day, maximum of 7.5 mg	MDI: Two puffs 4 times per day or as needed prior to exercise; Tablets: One 5 mg tablet 3 times per day, maximum of 15 mg

Note: 1 kg (kilogram) = 2.2 pounds; mcg = microgram; mg = milligram; mL = milliliter; CDN: compressor-driven nebulizer; DPI: dry-powder inhaler; HFA: hydrofluoroalkane; MDI: metered-dose inhaler.

Using short-acting bronchodilators effectively

If you correctly use your prescribed long-term asthma medications pre-scribed by your physician, along with effectively avoiding allergens, irritants, and other potential triggers, you can control your asthma most of the time. However, given the unpredictable nature of most people's lives, you may experience instances where your respiratory condition suddenly worsens, most often due to unexpected and unavoidable exposure to certain asthma triggers. (See Chapter 5 for details of asthma triggers.)

When these situations occur, make sure you discuss with your doctor what type of short-acting bronchodilator might work for you, based on your spe-cific asthma condition, for the prompt relief of an asthma episode.

In my experience, the vast majority of patients who successfully adhere to their asthma management plan, especially by sticking to their regimen of long-acting asthma controller medications, are the ones who usually wind up using short-acting bronchodilators the least.

But, in those rare instances when these patients do need to resort to using their short-acting bronchodilator, they'll most often be able to quickly regain control of their condition before it seriously worsens.

Getting more bronchodilation per breath

In order to maximize the quick-relief action of short-acting beta$_2$-adrenergic bronchodilators, use these medications with the appropriate delivery devices. Holding chambers (spacers) and nebulizers work especially well, ensuring that your lungs receive short-acting bronchodilator medications. (See Chapter 14 for more information.)

If your short-acting bronchodilator isn't providing rapid relief of symptoms, determine if any of the following factors may be causing the problem:

- **You're not using the product properly.** Make sure that your doctor shows you the proper technique for using your inhaler and reviews your technique during office visits.

- **Your canister may be empty.** To check whether you need a new canis-ter, remove the container from the actuator sleeve and put it in water (a sink works well for this test). If the canister starts floating to the top, it's likely close to empty.

- **The mouthpiece (where you inhale) may be dirty or blocked.** Keep your inhaler clean. (Chapter 14 provides details about cleaning your mouthpiece.)

Choosing better bronchodilators

Don't use over-the-counter (OTC) inhaled bronchodilators such as AsthmaHaler, Bronkaid Mist, Primatene Mist, or similar products. In many cases, these OTC products provide much shorter relief than prescription inhaled short-acting beta₂-adrenergic bronchodilators, and they often contain *epinephrine* (adrenaline) or similar drugs.

Although epinephrine is used in emergency treatment and in self-injection kits, such as EpiPen or Twinject, for cases of severe asthma attacks and *anaphylaxis* (a potentially life-threatening reaction that affects many organs simultaneously), routine use of the drug can cause serious adverse side effects, including shakiness, an increase in blood pressure, or a rapid or irregular heartbeat. Because of this danger, avoid using OTC bronchodilators if you have a heart condition.

Avoiding potential adverse side effects of short-acting bronchodilators

The principal side effects of short-acting beta₂-adrenergic therapy, although relatively mild — especially when used in inhalation forms (in contrast with oral or injectable formulations) — can be tremors, increased heart rate, and palpitations. These side effects occur as a result of the drug's direct stimulation of the heart and skeletal muscles, and they often go hand in hand with the drug's *bronchodilator action* (airway dilation), especially at high and/or frequent dosages.

In most cases, patients experience few, if any, of the potentially unpleasant side effects of short-acting bronchodilators by using these medications only for the quick relief of worsening respiratory symptoms. As effective as quick-relief bronchodilators can be for rescue purposes — especially a recently approved product such as levalbuterol (see the "Introducing new and improved bronchodilation" section, later in the chapter) — only use short-acting bronchodilators as needed, rather than on a routine basis, especially if you have persistent asthma

Instead of using rescue products on a day-to-day basis to manage your respiratory symptoms, make sure that you're consistently taking long-term medications your physician prescribes (as part of your overall asthma management plan) to maintain control over your asthma condition. (See Chapter 15 for detailed information on long-term products.)

Bucking bronchodilator dependence: Avoiding overuse of your quick-relief product

If you find that you're taking more than eight puffs per day or using more than one canister (usually 200 puffs) of a short-acting bronchodilator per month, your asthma isn't adequately controlled. In that case, see your doctor so that he can properly adjust your asthma management plan.

Ensuring that your asthma management plan is as effective as possible may mean that you need to take long-term anti-inflammatory medication, such as inhaled corticosteroids, on a regular basis to control your asthma (see Chapter 15).

Contact your doctor immediately if you're using your short-acting beta$_2$-adrenergic bronchodilator more often than once every one to two hours. Overusing this type of rescue medication at that rate (more frequently than once every one to two hours) is a sign that your asthma symptoms are worsening.

In my 25 years of practice, I've never seen the overuse of inhaled short-acting beta$_2$-adrenergic bronchodilators correct worsening asthma symptoms. In fact, overusing your short-acting bronchodilator almost always worsens your condition because frequently using this medication doesn't address the real source of the problem — the underlying airway inflammation.

Taking many medicines can make matters worse

Using short-acting bronchodilators while also taking beta-blockers, such as Inderal, Lopressor, and Corgard (frequently prescribed for migraine headaches, high blood pressure, glaucoma, angina, or hyperthyroidism), may cancel out the benefits of both medications. If you need both medications, your doctor may recommend alternatives to beta-blockers or may prescribe ipratropium bromide as an alternative quick-relief medication for your asthma symptoms (see "Reversing Airflow Obstruction with Anticholinergics," later in this chapter). This potentially adverse interaction between products is a particularly good example of why you need to make sure that all your physicians know the medications that you're taking for all your medical conditions (see Chapter 3).

Introducing new and improved bronchodilation

Recently, with improved chemical technology, researchers have developed a new version of albuterol known as *levalbuterol* (Xopenex). This third-generation short-acting beta$_2$-adrenergic bronchodilator provides the same level of bronchodilation at one-fourth the dose of albuterol. As a result, the dose-dependent side effects typical of older short-acting bronchodilators, such as tremors, increased heart rate, and palpitations, are substantially reduced and even eliminated for many patients.

Levalbuterol has been particularly useful when given by CDN to especially sensitive groups, such as the elderly and children. Because the FDA hasn't yet approved levalbuterol for use in children under 6, physicians administer this drug *off-label* to that age group. Because albuterol (the parent compound of levalbuterol) has been safely used without any significant adverse effects for more than 25 years to treat infants and young children, physicians often feel comfortable prescribing levalbuterol (Xopenex) for children under age 6.

Quick fix versus long-term asthma management

Controlling asthma means treating the underlying inflammation of your airways. Don't substitute the quick fix of an inhaled short-acting beta$_2$-adrenergic bronchodilator for consistent, routine use of the appropriate long-term asthma medications that your doctor prescribes.

Think of your asthma as a smoldering campfire in your lungs. If you pay attention to the embers only *after* they flare up, containing the flames becomes a serious problem. The goal of your asthma management plan is to get your asthma under control to the extent that you only rarely use bronchodilators on an as-needed basis — usually to reduce the risk of symptoms when exposed to unavoidable asthma triggers or precipitating factors, especially exercise.

Also, beware of relying on inhaled short-acting bronchodilators, because the quick relief these products provide can also give you the false impression that your asthma is just a set of symptoms, rather than a serious, underlying medical problem. Imagine having a high fever and only taking a pain reliever to reduce your discomfort. You may temporarily feel better, but if the underlying cause of your high temperature is a severe inflammation, such as appendicitis, treating only the symptoms can lead to a very serious situation — in this case a ruptured appendix — because you may not realize the gravity of your condition, thus delaying necessary treatment.

Likewise, if zapping your wheezing with an inhaled short-acting beta$_2$-adrenergic bronchodilator is the only way you deal with your persistent asthma, you may feel fine for a short while. However, if you use your peak-flow meter (see Chapter 4) to check your peak expiratory flow rate (PEFR), or if your doctor performs a spirometry procedure (see Chapter 2), you quickly realize that your airflow is significantly decreased and your lung functions are below normal. When based solely on how they're feeling, the majority of asthma patients tend to underestimate the magnitude of their airway obstruction. Often, it isn't until they can objectively measure their airflow, typically by using a peak-flow meter, that they really become aware of their deteriorating condition.

Reversing Airflow Obstruction with Anticholinergics

Anticholinergic drugs block *acetylcholine* (a neurotransmitter that stimulates mucus production) and therefore help reduce mucus in your airways. These drugs also relax the smooth muscle around the large and medium airways of the lungs. Inhaled anticholinergics often work especially well when doctors combine their use with short-acting beta$_2$-adrenergic bronchodilators to open your airways.

Keep in mind that anticholinergics on their own have little effect on asthma symptoms triggered by exposure to allergens. These products also don't prevent symptoms of EIA.

Anticholinergic medications are usually most effective for patients who have partially reversible airflow obstruction or who are prone to producing greater amounts of mucus. Doctors frequently prescribe these products for patients with chronic bronchitis and emphysema, collectively referred to as *chronic obstructive pulmonary disease* (COPD).

The principal anticholinergic used in the United States is ipratropium bromide, a quick-relief drug that doctors often prescribe in conjunction with a short-acting beta$_2$-adrenergic bronchodilator for dilating the airways. Ipratropium bromide can provide greater bronchodilation when combined with a bronchodilator such as albuterol into a single inhaled product (Combivent). Table 16-2 lists general dosage information for anticholinergic medications.

Ipratropium bromide has an excellent safety profile and few potential adverse side effects. Those side effects can include dry mouth, airway secretions, and, in rare cases, wheezing. Don't accidentally spray this product in your eyes, because it can temporarily blur your vision.

Table 16-2	Anticholinergic Medications			
Active Ingredient	*Formulation*	*Brand Name*	*Total Usual Daily Child Dose (Under 12)*	*Total Usual Daily Adult Dose*
Ipratropium	MDI: 18 mcg/ puff 200 puffs/ canister	Atrovent	Not approved for children under 12	MDI: Two to 3 puffs every 6 hours, not to exceed 12 puffs per day
	Nebulizer (CDN): 0.5 mg/ 2.5 mL (vial)			CDN: One vial every 6 to 8 hours

Active Ingredient	Formulation	Brand Name	Total Usual Daily Child Dose (Under 12)	Total Usual Daily Adult Dose
Ipratropium + albuterol	MDI: 370 mcg/puff 300 puffs/canister	Combivent	Not approved for children under 12	Two puffs 4 times a day
Ipratropium + albuterol	Nebulizer (CDN): 0.5 mg (ipratropium), 2.5 mg/3.0 mL (vial)	DuoNeb	Not approved for children under 12	CDN: One vial 4 times a day

Note: mcg = microgram; mL = milliliter; CDN: compressor-driven nebulizer; MDI: metered-dose inhaler.

Because the use of anticholinergics may complicate prostate problems, physicians need to assess the condition of elderly male asthmatic patients prior to prescribing any medication that contains ipratropium bromide.

Looking at Short-Term, Rescue Use of Oral Corticosteroids

In addition to their use as long-acting medications, oral corticosteroids (see Chapter 15) can also play a quick-relief role in your asthma management. During moderate-to-severe asthma episodes, your doctor may use oral corticosteroids to rapidly gain control over worsening symptoms. In such cases, oral corticosteroids can help your other quick-relief medications work more effectively, resulting in a more rapid reversal or reduction of airway inflammation, speeding recovery, and reducing the rate of relapse.

A short course of oral corticosteroids generally lasts three to ten days, depending on the severity of your symptoms and your response to treatment. Don't suddenly stop taking oral corticosteroids without checking with your physician first.

If you use oral corticosteroids longer than two weeks, doctors frequently taper off the dosage to minimize side effects, instead of stopping the drug abruptly. This slow tapering allows most patients to regain their ability to produce their own natural corticosteroids from the *cortex* (outer layer) of their adrenal gland.

Prolonged use of oral corticosteroids can lead to adverse *systemic* (affecting multiple organs of your body) side effects, including fluid retention, altered blood sugar levels, weight gain, peptic ulcers, mood alteration, high blood pressure, reduced bone density, and impaired immune functioning. For this reason, doctors often prescribe these drugs only as a last resort, and discontinue (by gradual tapering) them as soon as symptoms are under control.

Chapter 17

Future Trends in Asthma Therapy

In This Chapter

▶ Looking ahead to improvements in managing asthma

▶ Understanding the importance of continuing asthma research

▶ Volunteering for clinical trials

During recent decades, the incidence of asthma has unfortunately risen. That's the bad news. But the good news is that continuing advances in medical science are providing doctors with increasingly more effective therapies to treat asthma patients and improve their quality of life. The even better news is that asthma therapy is only going to improve.

Based on the extensive experience I've gained during the last two decades while conducting clinical trials of new asthma drugs, I foresee more effective and innovative products on the horizon. In fact, the pharmaceutical industry, with significant specialty physician guidance and support, continues to develop new approaches to treating asthma.

The newer products will address the underlying airway inflammation that characterizes asthma even more successfully than has been possible until now. As a result, you can expect medications that more effectively treat the root cause of asthma, which would bring doctors and their patients a step closer to the goal of having patients achieve normal lung functions and complete control of symptoms with less need for taking medications on a regular basis.

So get out those sunglasses. As you see over the course of this chapter, the future of asthma therapy's so bright, you may need to wear shades.

Getting Better All the Time

No matter how good a product is, it can almost always be improved. In that spirit, researchers are continuing to develop more effective formulations and delivery devices for existing asthma medications. In this section, I explain the most notable developments in this area of asthma therapy.

Improving inhaled corticosteroids

The development of inhaled corticosteroids in the 1970s heralded a new age in asthma therapy. For the first time, anti-inflammatory drugs were available that could reduce swelling and mucus production in the airway, decrease airway *hyperreactivity* ("twitchiness") in response to asthma triggers, and in some cases even prevent *airway remodeling* (in which healthy, functioning tissue is replaced with non-functional scar tissue due to chronic airway inflammation).

In recent years, as pharmaceutical researchers have continued improving inhaled corticosteroids, most physicians have come to consider these products the therapy of choice for treating patients with moderate to severe asthma symptoms.

The newest generation of these drugs, which are currently in development or due for FDA approval as this book hits the stores, may provide even more effective therapy by directly targeting the lungs with greater accuracy while also reducing typical adverse side effects associated with inhaled corticosteroids. I'm particularly impressed with ciclesonide (Alvesco) and mometasone (Asmanex). These two drugs have shown great promise in clinical trials, especially in treating children with asthma.

Combining for complementary effect

Another promising trend in recent asthma pharmacology has been the development of products that combine an inhaled corticosteroid with a long-acting bronchodilator in order to achieve a complementary effect. Advair Diskus, which the FDA approved in 2000 and is now one of the most prescribed asthma drugs in the United States, combines fluticasone, an inhaled corticosteroid, and salmeterol, a long-acting bronchodilator.

This focus on complementary therapy is continuing and shows great promise with Symbicort, which the FDA should soon approve. This product combines budesonide, an inhaled corticosteroid, with formoterol, which is the only rapid-onset, long-acting bronchodilator available in the United States. In the near future, expect to see more products that combine formoterol, or other long-acting bronchodilators that are still in development, with some of the newer inhaled corticosteroids.

Special delivery: More effective devices

To really make a difference in effectively managing asthma, as well as other respiratory conditions, the inhaled medications that patients take — whether they're newly developed drugs or improved formulations of older products — need to reach as deep into the airways as possible. As a result, much of asthma medication development also focuses on improving delivery devices, especially inhalers.

Metered-dose inhalers (MDIs) have been standard delivery devices for asthma medications since the advent of beta$_2$-adrenergic bronchodilators and inhaled corticosteroids. However, many of these devices require a certain level of coordination for effective use (often requiring the patient to also use a holding chamber or spacer for optimal results) and at best only deliver 10 to 20 percent of the spray to the airways where it's really needed. Additionally, many MDI medications are formulated with ozone-depleting chlorofluorocarbons (CFCs) as propellants.

To overcome the shortcomings of older MDIs, newer inhaled asthma products, both recently approved ones and those still in clinical trials, offer the following improvements:

- **Environmentally friendly propellants.** The FDA approved Hydrofluoroalkane (HFA), a new non-CFC propellant for use in formulations of albuterol (Proventil HFA, Ventolin HFA) and beclomethasone (QVAR-HFA). Not only are these newer HFA-propelled products better for the ozone layer, but they also deliver medications to the lungs more effectively than the older CFC-based MDIs. You can soon expect to see more formulations of inhaled asthma drugs using HFA, or other soon-to-be approved non-CFC propellants.

- **User-friendlier MDIs.** The recently developed Maxair Autohaler is a prime example of this trend. The Autohaler, which is indicated for short-term relief of suddenly worsening respiratory symptoms, is a breath-activated MDI that delivers the short-acting beta$_2$-adrenergic bronchodilator pirbuterol without the need for a holding chamber and also requires less coordination to use compared to many other MDIs. Look for more delivery devices along these lines in the near future, especially for use with short-term or rescue medications.

✔ **Dry-powder inhalers (DPIs).** Rather than dispensing their product as an aerosolized spray, as do MDIs, these newer types of inhalers deliver asthma drugs in special dry-powder formulations. DPIs are also designed for easy use, and if operated properly, are very effective at delivering medication to the tiniest airways. The FDA has thus far approved DPI formulations of four inhaled products:

- Budesonide, an inhaled corticosteroid (Pulmicort Turbuhaler)

- Fluticasone, also an inhaled corticosteroid (Flovent Rotadisk, used with the Diskhaler device)

- Salmeterol, a long-acting bronchodilator (Serevent Diskus)

- Fluticasone and salmeterol in combination (Advair Diskus)

More DPI formulations are also in the pipeline, so breathe easy. Your doctor will continue to have a wider choice of simpler and more effective ways for delivering medications deeper into your airways than ever before.

Under Your Tongue: Swallow Immunotherapy

European researchers have recently developed a potential alternative to allergy shots, known as sublingual-swallow immunotherapy. Doctors in a few European countries are currently using the therapy to reduce symptoms of pollen allergies, a common trigger of asthma (see Chapter 5 for details on asthma triggers). This treatment, known by the less than lovely acronym of SLIT, consists of patients holding up to 20 drops of allergen extract under the tongue for as along as two minutes before swallowing.

Although some studies indicate that SLIT can indeed help reduce symptoms associated with allergic reactions to certain pollens, this exact form of the therapy still needs more research. For one thing, holding the required number of drops under your tongue for a definite amount of time isn't always that easy to do.

Perhaps more importantly, SLIT has mainly been prescribed as a self-administered therapy, with patients taking the drops at home rather than in a medical setting where doctors and nurses can make sure that the extract is taken properly. As a result, doctors and nurses can't monitor the patients to make sure that they get proper and immediate medical attention if the extract triggers a rare, serious adverse side effect (see Chapter 11).

However, I am intrigued by further advances in this concept of immunotherapy, especially the development of a disintegrating tablet form of SLIT, which gradually dissolves under the patient's tongue. Although this approach to SLIT is still at the trial stage in Europe, it could possibly simplify administration of immunotherapy and ensure that patients on their own would consistently adhere to the proper dosage and method of taking the extract.

Based on what my European colleagues have told me, and the studies I've seen, a disintegrating tablet form of SLIT could turn out to be the next potential breakthrough in immunotherapy in the United States, especially if the treatment can be developed to also provide effective treatment for a much wider range of allergens.

Blocking IgE: A Biotech Breakthrough

One way of effectively managing asthma and improving the quality of life of asthmatics is to attempt to block or interrupt the immune system's response to allergen exposure. (See Chapter 6 for an in-depth discussion of the immune system and its key players, including IgE.) To that end, the first-ever anti-IgE medication, a *recombinant human monoclonal antibody*, or rhuMab, known as omalizumab/rhuMAb-E25 (Xolair), has recently been developed and was approved by the FDA in June 2003.

This novel and more targeted form of therapy for asthma (and other allergic conditions) is specifically designed to block IgE — which the vast majority of people with allergies tend to overproduce — from playing its key role in triggering symptoms of allergic reactions. This anti-IgE antibody is designed to be administered in your physician's office once every two to four weeks by injection, with the exact dosage tailored to each patient's body weight and baseline levels of circulating IgE, as measured by a simple laboratory blood test.

As I explain in greater detail in Chapter 6, when a person's immune system with allergies is exposed to an allergen to which he or she has been previously sensitized, IgE antibodies prompt mast cells and basophils (among others) to initiate a complex chain of events that culminates in the release of potent chemical mediators of inflammation, such as histamine and leukotrienes. The action of these chemicals is the main cause of symptoms such as coughing, sneezing, watery eyes, and shortness of breath.

Omalizumab/rhuMAb-E25 (Xolair) represents an exciting advance in asthma management. Studies show that patients with moderate to severe allergic asthma who used Xolair had less frequent respiratory symptoms overall, and more than half of participants not only experienced fewer asthma episodes, but they also were able to stop using their inhaled corticosteroid medication.

Anti-IgE therapy provides an innovative way of treating asthma and other allergic disorders at an earlier stage, rather than after the allergic reaction and resulting symptoms have occurred. Researchers are also working on other promising monoclonal antibody medications, such as anti-IL-5 and perhaps anti-IL-8 (see the following section for more information).

Exploring the Frontiers of Asthma Therapy

Some of the most exciting and promising ongoing medical research focuses on the actual blocking of the immune system response that leads to airway inflammation and resulting airway hyperreactivity — the underlying cause of asthma. Although we're still years away from seeing FDA-approved products, the concept of isolating and neutralizing allergic reactions at the cellular level seems particularly promising.

Inhibiting interleukins

Among the key regulators of immune system functions, *interleukins* are a class of compounds produced by *lymphocytes* (which constitute 20 to 30 percent of the white blood cells in most human beings), by *macrophages* (cells that protect against infection and noxious substances), and by *monocytes* (large white blood cells formed in the bone marrow, which turn into macrophages after they enter the blood).

In recent years, researchers have identified two interleukin compounds, known as IL-5 and IL-8, as key components of the inflammatory process. Check out the following sections to read about research into new therapies using these compounds.

Anti-interleukin-5

Studies indicate that IL-5 plays an important role in the production of specialized white blood cells known as eosinophils. Chemical mediators attract eosinophils to the site of inflammation where these white blood cells in turn stimulate a prolonged response, which contributes to the late-phase reactions that asthma patients often experience (see Chapter 6). Studies also show that many people with allergic asthma have higher than average numbers of eosinophils in their bone marrow and *bronchial mucosa* (the internal lining of the airway).

Patients in recent clinical trials who were treated with *mepolizumab,* a newly developed anti-IL-5 monoclonal antibody, showed a marked reduction in the number of mature eosinophils and *eosinophil progenitors* (cells that can become eosinophils) in bone marrow, and an important decrease in levels of bronchial mucosa.

These results suggest that anti-IL-5/mepolizumab therapy may someday be an effective way of preventing the immune system from unleashing chemical mediators of inflammation when exposed to allergens.

Anti-interleukin-8

This interleukin compound seems to play a crucial role in cases of severe persistent asthma and sudden-onset fatal asthma. Many patients who suffer from these more serious forms of the condition produce above-normal levels of IL-8 and also of *neutrophils* (large white blood cells that appear under a microscope to be neutral-colored, hence the name). By attracting neutrophils to the airway *epithelium* (the membranous tissue that covers most of our internal surfaces and organs), IL-8 appears to foster airway inflammation, leading possibly to airway remodeling.

Although research is ongoing into ways of inhibiting or preventing the action of IL-8, some studies have also shown that salmeterol, an already approved and widely prescribed long-acting beta$_2$-adrenergic bronchodilator (see Chapter 15), may be effective in reducing the activity of IL-8.

Toll-like receptors (TLRs)

These proteins, which acquired their unusual name because the German scientist who first discovered them yelled out "toll" (German for *great*), alert the immune system to the presence of infectious agents such as viruses and bacteria. Toll-like receptors (TLRs), which reside on the surface of certain immune system cells, can also recruit other cells to attack infectious agents.

According to some researchers, TLRs can be used to enhance your immune system's response against actually harmful diseases, thus boosting your overall well-being. Conversely, this could help reduce the immune system's tendency — in those people with a genetic susceptibility to develop hypersensitivities and produce antibodies to otherwise harmless allergens — to trigger allergic responses when exposed to allergens.

Gene therapy

The completion of the U.S. Human Genome Project in April 2003 means that scientists are now much closer to identifying the proteins that make up human life. They're perhaps on the brink of isolating and blocking the inherited genetic mutations and abnormalities that can lead some people to develop hypersensitive immune systems and resulting conditions, such as allergic asthma.

One recent study of the DNA of asthmatics has shown that the process that leads to inflammation, and thus to characteristic respiratory symptoms of asthma, is actually due to a mutated gene. When the makeup of proteins produced by this sort of gene is established, scientists may be able to develop therapies that block the action of those proteins and keep the inherited condition from actually having an adverse effect.

Gene therapy may even make it possible to develop a vaccine for infants or young children that would provide them with a lifetime's immunity from asthma.

Keeping Research Alive: Clinical Trials and You

Studies around the world continue to show that asthma is almost always a life-long condition. The condition's extent and character may vary over a patient's life, but after a person has the disease, it will likely never go completely away. Medical researchers in New Zealand have recently confirmed this finding. (New Zealand is one of the countries hardest hit by asthma and a center of expertise in treating the condition.)

Even with new and improved treatments, those few patients who may actually outgrow their asthma will continue to be exceptional cases until doctors can pinpoint and correct the exact immune system malfunction that leads some people to develop asthma.

In order to keep improving asthma therapy, continued research into what causes the disorder and how to treat it more effectively is essential. And, in order for this research to be successful, the participation of human subjects is crucial. The more patients volunteer for studies and clinical trials, the quicker doctors can bring new and more effective treatments to market.

I encourage asthma patients, based on their physicians' advice, to consider enrolling in clinical trials of therapies that are still in development. In my own work as a principal investigator on many asthma and allergy research projects, I know the challenges of organizing and conducting the studies that are required in order to bring new medications to market.

One of the main reasons that pharmaceutical companies spend an average of $700 to $800 million dollars bringing new drugs from laboratory to market is the need for extensive clinical trials, which can often take seven years to complete. And at the end of this arduous process, only a small fraction of drugs actually receive FDA approval.

The high cost and financial gamble of pharmaceutical research and development (R&D) is, in turn, one of the main reasons the prices of prescription medication in the United States are so high. Pharmaceutical companies need to make back their investment in all their R&D from a relatively small number of products that do finally make it to market.

If more asthma patients participated in clinical trials, the process of developing new and more effective drugs and delivery devices could be accelerated to the benefit of asthmatics everywhere and may also result in products that would be less costly.

Part V
Special Asthma Conditions

The 5th Wave   By Rich Tennant

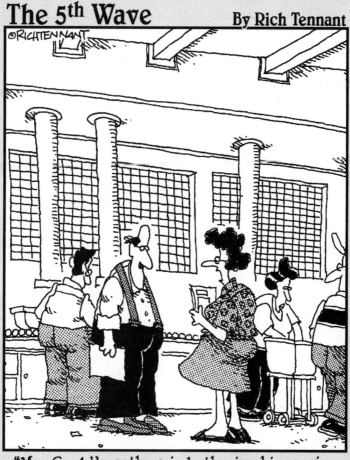

"Mr. Gould's asthma is bothering him again.
He says there's too much dust, mold and
nit—picking in the air."

In this part . . .

This part offers specifics about dealing with asthma successfully at different stages of life. In Chapter 18, I discuss asthma during childhood and the effective ways that parents can deal with a child's respiratory condition. Chapter 19 provides detailed information about continuing asthma treatment and managing your respiratory condition safely during pregnancy — when you're not just eating for two, you're also breathing for two. Chapter 20 covers special issues affecting elderly patients with asthma.

Chapter 18

Asthma during Childhood

*P*arents know that no one is more precious to them than their children. Therefore, parents want to treat any ailment that affects their youngsters as effectively as possible. If your child has asthma, the good news is that with a proper diagnosis, appropriate management, and a firm understanding of the disease, you can help your child effectively control his or her condition.

Unfortunately, some parents (and even some doctors) don't understand asthma well enough to recognize or diagnose the disease properly. Too often, this misunderstanding results in the misdiagnosis of children with asthma as instead having chronic bronchitis or recurring colds. In these cases, children may not receive the appropriate treatment and their symptoms may worsen, leading to severe asthma episodes that may require emergency measures to treat.

In fact, asthma — the most common chronic childhood disease in the United States — affects at least 5 million children. Current estimates are that only half of these youngsters receive accurate diagnosis and effective treatment.

However, these alarming asthma statistics don't need to continue. Treating your child's asthma early and aggressively, as well as practicing long-term preventive maintenance, can make the difference between a sickly youngster and a healthy, well-adjusted kid who rarely experiences the problematic symptoms.

Understanding Your Child's Asthma

Asthma is a chronic inflammatory disease of the airways that can make getting air in and especially out of the lungs difficult. Besides the serious health risks that asthma can pose for your child, properly managing the disease is vital for your youngster's overall growth: Anything that restricts proper breathing can impair his or her physical and mental development.

Asthma often begins in childhood and affects boys more commonly than girls. Most children who develop asthma experience their first symptoms of the disease before they reach their third birthday.

Look for the following signs and symptoms as possible asthma indicators in your child. (Keep in mind, however, that not every child with the disease experiences all these signs and symptoms.)

- ✔ Persistent coughing, wheezing, and recurring or lingering chest colds.

- ✔ An expanded or overinflated chest and hunched shoulders.

- ✔ Signs of coughing, wheezing, or extreme shortness of breath during or after exercise. These symptoms may signal the onset of exercise-induced asthma, or EIA (see "Participating in PE — exercise and asthma," later in this chapter).

- ✔ Snoring, especially in preschool children. According to recent studies, a strong association exists between snoring and asthma in children ages 2 to 5.

- ✔ Coughing at night, in the absence of other symptoms such as a cold.

Because you may find recognizing the preceding symptoms more difficult when observing infants and young children, watch for the following signs of possible asthma trouble:

- ✔ *Cyanosis,* due to severe airway obstruction blocking the normal flow of oxygen into the lungs, causes a very pale or blue skin color. This can occur in a very severe asthma attack and requires emergency treatment.

- ✔ Deep and rapid rib muscle movements, also known as *retractions,* which can occur when an infant or young child is having trouble breathing properly.

- ✔ Difficulty in nursing or eating.

- ✔ Lethargic activity and reduced responses, including not recognizing or responding to parents.

- ✔ Nasal flaring (rapidly moving nostrils), which can be a sign of severe asthma.

- ✔ Soft, shallow crying.

In addition to these signs, you also need to consider the presence of *atopy* (the genetic susceptibility for the immune system to produce antibodies to common allergens, which leads to allergy symptoms) as a key predisposing factor for your child developing asthma (see Chapters 2 and 6).

Atopic conditions, including food allergies (see Chapter 8), *allergic rhinitis* (hay fever — see Chapter 7), and *atopic dermatitis* (eczema — see Chapter 1), can indicate a potential predisposition for asthma, especially in infants and young children. In fact, more than three-quarters of all children who develop asthma also have allergies. In many cases, allergic reactions associated with the response to inhalant and ingested allergens can also cause flare-ups in a child with asthma.

Inheriting asthma

If you think that your child may have asthma, consider your family's medical history. Two-thirds of asthma patients have a close relative with the disease. Likewise, if you or your child's other parent has asthma, your child's chances of developing asthma are 25 percent; if *both* you and your child's other parent have asthma, your child's odds of developing asthma double to 50 percent.

However, asthma in your family doesn't guarantee that your child will develop asthma. Your child inherits the *tendency* to the disease, not the disease itself. If neither you nor your child's other parent has asthma, the odds of your child developing this disease are no greater than 15 percent.

Identifying children's asthma triggers

Although hereditary factors may increase your child's likelihood of developing asthma, environmental triggers and other precipitating factors usually bring on the symptoms. (See Chapter 5 for more detailed information on these triggers and precipitating factors.) Most physicians agree that viral respiratory infections are the most common triggers of asthma attacks in infants and young children.

The most serious air pollutant and irritant in terms of asthma is tobacco smoke. Parents absolutely should not smoke around a child, especially if the youngster has asthma. Even if your child is out (for example, at school), don't smoke in the home. The lingering odor of tobacco smoke can still trigger your child's asthma symptoms. According to numerous studies, exposure to maternal smoke is a major risk factor in the early onset of asthma in infancy. In fact, an infant whose mother smokes is almost twice as likely to develop asthma.

Controlling — not outgrowing — asthma

The idea that all children eventually "outgrow" asthma is a dangerous myth, and withholding treatment hoping that somehow your child's asthma will just go away is a misguided approach. As children grow, their lungs and airways become larger. If the amount of airway obstruction stays the same, the blockage may proportionally constitute a smaller part of the total airway diameter, thus resulting in fewer symptoms as an adult. In addition, many children do have fewer symptoms and a decrease in airway hyperreactivity as they grow older, but early and aggressive treatment of asthma significantly contributes to a better outcome.

Your child's sensitivities, however, may not entirely disappear, and the possibility exists that a lack of treatment could result in irreversible airway changes. Clear and compelling evidence shows that early diagnosis and treatment results in fewer asthma symptoms.

Your child's asthma symptoms may diminish or may no longer be apparent, but the increased airway sensitivity remains — just as your child's fingerprints stay the same even though his or her body grows and develops. Asthma isn't a disease that you can really cure; it's a condition that you must control.

Treating early to avoid problems later

In my practice, many adult patients are referred to me with severe asthma. In many cases, their conditions may not have deteriorated to such an extent if only their asthma had been properly treated during childhood. The first two years after asthma has been diagnosed generally are considered to be the time when aggressive medical treatment can dramatically improve the potential for maintaining normal lung functions in your child.

Unfortunately, some parents only focus on immediately treating serious asthma attacks instead of managing the child's condition on a consistent, everyday basis. This approach is misguided. Don't watch and wait to see how asthma affects your child. If your child has a persistent cough, shortness of breath, lingering colds, or other early signs of asthma (see the symptoms and signs I list in the first part of this section), make sure that a doctor checks your child's lung functions. This testing can help to determine whether asthma is, in fact, the cause of your child's symptoms.

Identifying Childhood-Onset Asthma

When dealing with a child, particularly one who is very young, what may seem an obvious and easily identifiable asthma diagnosis isn't always the case. Asthma is a complex condition with many possible combinations of symptoms that can vary widely from patient to patient. In fact, your child's symptoms can change over time.

The process of diagnosing your child's condition should include the following steps:

✔ A complete medical history

✔ A physical examination

✔ Lung-function tests

✔ Any other tests that your doctor considers necessary to determine the nature of your child's ailment

To diagnose your child's asthma, your doctor should establish the following key points:

✔ Your child experiences episodes of airway obstruction.

✔ The airway obstruction is at least partially reversible.

✔ Your child's symptoms result from asthma, not other potential conditions that I explain in the "All That Wheezes Isn't Asthma" section, later in this chapter.

Taking your child's medical history

A thorough and complete medical history is vital to diagnosing your child's condition. In addition to asking about the symptoms and signs of childhood asthma that I describe in "Understanding Your Child's Asthma," earlier in this chapter, your doctor may also inquire about the following:

✔ Any family history of allergies and/or asthma. (As I explain in the "Inheriting asthma" section of this chapter, genetics play a major role in asthma development.)

✔ Any exposures your child receives to common asthma triggers, such as inhalant allergens and irritants — especially tobacco smoke — or any other substances, as well as the precipitating factors that I describe in "Identifying children's asthma triggers," earlier in this chapter.

✔ Any times your child has been hospitalized for respiratory problems. Your doctor should also ask about any medications that your child takes, whether for respiratory symptoms or for other conditions.

Examining your child for signs of asthma

The focus of a physical exam for children with suspected asthma usually involves the following:

✔ Checking for signs of hunched shoulders, chest deformities, and pale skin.

✔ Examining your child's breathing passageways, from nose to chest. (See Chapter 2 for details of physical exams.)

✔ Looking for evidence of other atopic diseases, such as allergic rhinitis or atopic dermatitis, which may indicate a predisposition to asthma.

✔ Observing your child's breathing rate and rhythm. Your doctor listens with a stethoscope to the chest and back over areas of your child's lungs to check for the following signs and sounds of airway obstruction:

  • Wheezing or other sounds not usually associated with normal breathing

  • Unusually prolonged exhalations

  • Rapid, shallow respirations (panting) in more severe cases

Testing your child's lungs

After taking your child's medical history and performing a physical examination, your doctor may conduct lung-function tests if your child is older than 4 or 5 years old. These tests are vital in diagnosing asthma because they can tell whether airway obstruction has limited or affected your child's lung functions.

To diagnose asthma in children older than 4 or 5, doctors often use a procedure known as spirometry. *Spirometry* involves using a *spirometer* (pulmonary function machine) to measure your child's airflow, before and 15 minutes after he or she inhales a short-acting bronchodilator, to determine improvement in lung function. See Chapter 2 for more details on spirometry.

Spirometry tests are difficult, if not impossible, to perform on children under 4 years old. However, by age 6, most children are quite capable of performing accurate and reliable spirometry (if they *feel* like it!). To properly diagnose an infant or young child with asthma, your doctor may need to rely on your child's medical history and physical examination. In some cases, your doctor may prescribe a trial course of a nebulized beta$_2$-adrenergic bronchodilator and/or anti-inflammatory medications to evaluate your child's response.

All That Wheezes Isn't Asthma

Although the misdiagnosis of asthma (often as bronchitis) is a frequent problem in treating childhood respiratory conditions, in some cases, other ailments can cause symptoms that resemble asthma. These other ailments include

- ✔ Abnormal development of blood vessels, known as *vascular rings,* around the trachea (windpipe) and esophagus

- ✔ Congenital heart disease, often leading to congestive heart failure

- ✔ Cystic fibrosis

- ✔ Viral and/or bacterial bronchitis or pneumonia

- ✔ Viral bronchiolitis (RSV), a serious respiratory infection that can occur in the first two years of life

  RSV may resemble an acute asthma attack. This disease characteristically occurs during the winter months in children under 2 years of age. Studies have shown that more than half of children who experience infections of viral bronchiolitis and who have a family history of allergy go on to develop asthma.

- ✔ Vocal cord dysfunction (VCD)

Numerous cases also exist in which children suddenly start wheezing because a coin, food particle, or other foreign body has become lodged in their windpipe, respiratory tube, or esophagus. If you suspect that a foreign object is lodged somewhere in your child's respiratory system, seek medical help immediately.

Focusing on Special Issues Concerning Childhood Asthma

After your child's doctor has diagnosed your child's asthma, the doctor should develop an appropriate asthma management plan, in consultation with you and your child (if he or she is old enough to participate). Your child's plan should consist of specific avoidance, medication, monitoring, and assessment measures, and it should also provide steps that you and/or your child can take in case his or her asthma symptoms suddenly worsen.

The basic components of an appropriate and effective asthma management plan include

✔ **Reducing your child's level of exposure to asthma and allergy triggers.** I describe these triggers in "Identifying children's asthma triggers," earlier in this chapter. (For detailed tips and information on avoidance measures, trigger control, and allergy-proofing, see Chapter 5.)

✔ **Monitoring your child's peak-flow rates.** Your doctor should show you and your child (if your youngster is older than 4 years old) how to use a peak-flow meter. (See "Peak-flow meters and school-age children [ages 5 to 12]," later in this chapter.) Using this simple device at home and school to measure peak expiratory flow rates (PEFR) can help detect early deterioration of asthma, prompting you or your child to make the appropriate change in medications or, if needed, to seek medical attention.

Children and their parents very often don't perceive the early symptoms of worsening asthma without a peak-flow meter. As a result, you may not understand or notice when your child's asthma symptoms worsen, thus critically delaying the proper medical treatment. (For detailed instructions on using peak-flow meters, see Chapter 4.)

✔ **Assessing and monitoring your child's lung functions during regular office visits.** These tests and assessments, as well as the PEFR numbers that you (or your child) record in an asthma symptom diary (see Chapter 4), are vital to tracking how your child's condition develops and responds to prescribed treatment.

✔ **Using long-term preventive medications that control your child's underlying airway inflammation, congestion, constriction, and hyperresponsiveness.** (See Chapter 2 for details of how asthma affects the body.)

✔ **Implementing an asthma management plan for your child's school or daycare.** Prepare an emergency asthma management plan, which specifies short-term, fast-acting rescue medications for use only in the event that your child's condition suddenly deteriorates. This type of action plan should also clearly explain how to adjust your child's medications in response to particular signs, symptoms, and PEFR levels. Likewise, this action plan should tell you (or your child) when to call for medical help. (See "Handling Asthma at School and Daycare," later in this chapter, for more information.)

✔ **Educating yourself, your child, your child's teacher, and your family.** This education can involve information and resources that your doctor, clinic staff, and patient support groups provide or recommend, as well as relevant books, newsletters, videos, and other helpful materials. (See the appendix for information on these resources.)

Teaming up for the best treatment

Integrate any treatment your youngster may receive from an asthma specialist (an allergist or pulmonologist) and your child's asthma management plan with the general care that your pediatrician, family doctor, and/or primary care physician provides. A team approach by your child's physicians can eliminate the risk of different doctors prescribing treatments for various childhood ailments that may, in combination, produce adverse side effects.

Managing asthma in infants (newborns to 2 years old)

The most difficult part of treating an infant with asthma is that the child isn't old enough to tell you what's wrong. Unfortunately, no devices are currently available for practicing physicians to use in order to measure infants' lung functions. Special techniques do exist at a few major medical centers at this time, but scientists only use them for research purposes and not in clinical practice. Therefore, determining the extent and type of your baby's respiratory problems can present some unique challenges. In these cases, your doctor mainly relies on medical history (including family history), physical examination, and response to medical therapy.

Depending on your child's condition, your doctor may prescribe some of the following medications to control your baby's asthma:

✔ If your infant's asthma symptoms are mild or intermittent, his or her doctor may prescribe an inhaled, short-acting beta$_2$-adrenergic in a nebulizer or oral beta$_2$-adrenergic syrup to reduce airway obstruction. Your doctor also can prescribe a recently approved pediatric, oral granule formulation of montelukast (Singulair) for ages 12 to 23 months. Administer the medication directly into the baby's mouth or by mixing it with the baby's soft food. According to the product insert, the recommended foods are applesauce, carrots, rice, or ice cream.

✔ If your child suffers from more severe symptoms, your doctor may prescribe a daily, long-term preventive medication, such as cromolyn (Intal) via nebulizer or inhaler; nedocromil (Tilade) via inhaler; an inhaled corticosteroid (Flovent) via inhaler; or a nebulizer form of budesonide (Pulmicort Respules). Because of your child's young age, administering any of these medications with an inhaler requires using a holding chamber (spacer) and a mask. Occasionally, your child's doctor may also recommend theophylline in a syrup, tablet (crushed), or capsule (sprinkled) form. (See Chapters 14 and 15 for information on asthma medications and delivery devices.)

Physicians prescribe theophylline syrup or suggest emptying beaded contents of a theophylline capsule on food such as applesauce so that your baby can easily ingest the medication.

✔ In the event that your child suffers a severe asthma episode, your child's doctor may prescribe a short course of oral corticosteroids, available in syrup form (Orapred, Prelone, Pediapred) or as a tablet (prednisone).

Using a nebulizer with your infant or toddler

If your doctor prescribes nebulizer therapy for your infant or toddler, make sure that you, as well as any other person who may be taking care of your child (such as a nanny, babysitter, and/or daycare provider), understand how to use a nebulizer appropriately and effectively. Using this device may challenge an older child, but for an infant or toddler who may be struggling to breathe, using a nebulizer can prove especially difficult. Chapter 14 provides more detailed instructions and tips on using nebulizers properly and effectively.

When using a nebulizer with a very young child (your doctor should give you specific advice based on your child's condition), make stress reduction — for both you and your child — your first consideration. Try making the use of the nebulizer a more pleasant experience and maybe even a special daily occasion. Hold and cuddle your child first, and then slowly but firmly move the mask closer to your youngster's face.

If your child isn't experiencing sudden-onset severe respiratory symptoms, you can introduce the mask initially, before running the air compressor component of the machine. The air compressor can be noisy, and it may frighten your child at first. If your child suffers more severe symptoms, hold the mask fairly close to his or her face and then slowly move it closer until the mask is properly in place.

Listening to your children

Because children under 2 years old aren't able to use a peak-flow meter, you may consider using a stethoscope to listen to your child's lungs. Some parents find that using a stethoscope can help them detect an asthma attack in their infant or young child at an earlier stage and may enable them to more accurately report their youngster's asthma symptoms to their child's physician.

Consult your child's physician to see whether using a stethoscope can help you. Likewise, ask your doctor for instructions on using the device properly. Keep in mind that a stethoscope detects breathing problems only if your child's lung function drops by about 25 percent.

Delivering nebulizer doses properly

Keep in mind that a "blow by" (holding the nebulizer several inches from your child's face and merely misting the medication) doesn't help your child because the medication doesn't effectively enter his or her airways, which is where your child needs the medicine. In order to properly deliver your child's medications, the nebulizer must work as a closed system, with the mask fitting snugly on your child's face, covering both the nose and mouth.

As with many other situations that involve very young children, you can use music, appropriate toys, a special cartoon video, or other types of entertainment as a helpful distraction for your little one. If all else fails, remain firm and steady, and make sure that your child receives the necessary medicine. Even the smallest infants ultimately discover that nebulizer treatments make them feel better. Eventually, that realization makes the time you spend administering nebulizer therapy more effective, comfortable, and rewarding for both you and your child.

Treating toddlers (ages 2 to 5 years): Medication challenges

Few medications are available in the United States for children ages 2 to 5 years. The Food and Drug Administration (FDA) has recently approved the use of montelukast (Singulair), a leukotriene modifier (see Chapter 15), in a 4-milligram chewable tablet, for use in this age group. However, inhaled topical corticosteroids and long-acting inhaled beta$_2$-adrenergic (beta$_2$-agonist) bronchodilators (or nonsedating antihistamines for allergic rhinitis) aren't specifically formulated for children under 4 years. Therefore, nebulizer use can be extremely important during the toddler and early school-age years (see Figure 18-1).

The lack of specific medications for children under age 4 is a serious concern for doctors and parents. This age group has experienced the highest increases in asthma rates in recent years, yet is the last group to receive attention in the development of new asthma medications.

Fortunately, the U.S. Congress has established a program of incentives to encourage pharmaceutical manufacturers to conduct clinical trials of medications, including those for asthma, in the pediatric age group. In fact, FDA regulations require pharmaceutical companies to submit detailed plans for studying formulations specifically for children (for example, syrups and chewable tablets) when seeking approval for development of new drugs. With hope, this program can lead to improved medical treatments for young children with asthma and other allergic diseases.

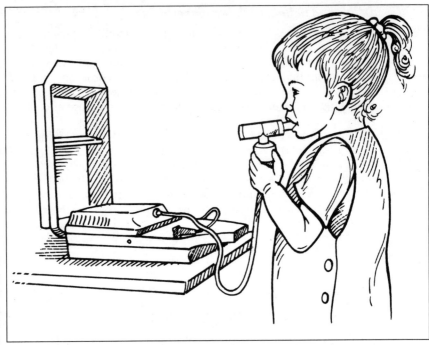

Figure 18-1:
Young child
using a
nebulizer.

Because very few effective asthma medications have gone through the drug development process for FDA approval for use with children under 4 years of age, many doctors prescribe drugs that haven't been studied extensively for use in that age group. Therefore, determining the appropriate dosages of asthma medications for toddlers can prove challenging. Children react differently to medications than do adults, and determining the correct dosage for children isn't as simple as assuming that the toddler receives half of an adult dose.

Peak-flow meters and school-age children (ages 5 to 12)

By the time children reach age 5, they can generally use a peak-flow meter at home. This device allows you and your doctor to assess the state of your child's lungs. Using a peak-flow meter each morning and night can help you and your child manage his or her asthma in the following ways:

✔ Educate both you and your child about what works in terms of treatment and what triggers may cause problems

✔ Enable you to discuss your child's condition in terms of specific criteria, thus enhancing communication between you and your child's doctor

Getting kids into clinical trials

Conducting clinical trials with young children — especially those under 4 years — is very costly and time-consuming compared to clinical trials involving children older than 12 years and adults. Because of the great need for pediatric patient participation, make a commitment to enroll your asthmatic infant and toddler for clinical trials. Doing so can help develop new and better medications that benefit all children. In addition, you and your child can probably discover a great deal about asthma and its management, and you may love all the extra attention while participating in these studies. In addition, the medicines being tested are free, and patients are reimbursed for their time and travel while participating in a clinical trial.

Pharmaceutical companies also need to make a commitment to conduct trials for younger children. These trials may cost more and prove difficult, but the lives and health of young children depend on such studies.

> ✔ Provide an objective way of tracking your child's response to his or her asthma medications
>
> ✔ Warn you and your child that an asthma episode is looming

Establishing your child's personal best peak-flow rate enables you and your child to tell when problems occur, because you can note when the rate goes down according to the green, yellow, and red zones of the peak-flow zone system. For more information on using peak-flow meters, turn to Chapter 4.

Using inhalers: Teens and asthma

Many teens with asthma feel different and insecure because of their disease. Unfortunately, adolescent anxieties about fitting in and being cool can result in teen asthmatics ignoring or not properly managing their disease. In some cases, adolescents may even allow their symptoms to worsen rather than simply taking a whiff or two from their inhalers.

To avoid these types of potentially dangerous asthmatic situations, allow your teenager a voice in the management of his or her asthma. Depending on the severity of your adolescent's asthma, your doctor and teenager can work together to develop a plan for adjusting medication therapy in order to control symptoms, thus avoiding serious episodes that may seem especially embarrassing for a teen. Some asthma medications last 12 hours (see Chapter 15), and therefore your adolescent can use them at home in the morning and the evening, minimizing the need for your teen to be seen using medication while at school.

Your child may also benefit from participating in a support group with other teenage asthmatics. Encourage open and honest discussions with your children about their conditions to ensure that they feel better informed and more respected. Participation in setting goals for therapy, developing a treatment plan, and reviewing its effectiveness can also help teenagers build a positive self-image, increase personal responsibility, and gain problem-solving skills, thus making them more likely to make better decisions about managing their condition.

Handling Asthma at School and Daycare

If your child has asthma, inform the teachers, administrators, and school nurse about your child's condition. Some schools and daycare centers institute asthma management programs that provide the following:

✔ Policies and procedures for administering students' medications.

✔ Specific actions for staff members to perform within the program.

These actions may include establishing clear policies on taking medications during school hours, designating one person on the school staff to maintain each student's asthma plan, and generally working with parents, teachers, and the school nurse (if one is available) to provide the most support possible for students with asthma, especially so they can have access to medications they may need while at school.

✔ An action plan for treating students' asthma episodes.

Whether or not the school or daycare center administers such a program, take the following steps to ensure that your child's school days are as healthy, safe, and fulfilling as possible:

• Meet with school staff to inform them about any medications your child may need to take while on campus, as well as any physical activity restrictions that your doctor may advise. (Properly managing their condition allows most children with asthma to participate in sports and PE classes.)

• File treatment authorization forms with the school office and discuss what school personnel must do if your child suffers an asthma emergency. Also, provide instructions on how to reach you and your child's physician during an emergency.

• Inform school personnel of allergens and irritants that can trigger your child's asthma symptoms, such as pets in the classroom, and request that the school remove the sources of those triggers, if possible.

Make sure your child understands that everyone's asthma is different and that asthma medications shouldn't be shared. Exchanging asthma medications among kids can cause dangerous problems because individual prescriptions vary according to the severity of each child's asthma and other factors. Don't let children use each other's inhalers, because doing so can also spread potential infections, such as colds and flu. Chapters 15 and 16 contain specific information about controller (long-term) and rescue (short-term) asthma medications.

Indoor air quality (IAQ) at school and daycare

From about the age of 2, most children spend the majority of their waking hours at school or daycare. Therefore, ensuring that these environments are as free of potential asthma triggers as possible is essential to your child's health.

According to the Environmental Protection Agency (EPA), recent studies indicate that indoor pollutant levels can often be two to five times higher than outdoor levels, occasionally as much as 100 times higher. Irritants and allergens that can affect your child at school often include the following:

✔ Outdoor smoke, soot, chemicals, pollens, and mold spores

✔ Animal dander from a furry classroom pet

✔ Indoor mold from ventilation ducts as well as indoor irritants such as tobacco smoke, scents from printers and copiers, and fumes from heating, ventilation, and air conditioning (HVAC) systems

Asthmatic symptoms related to poor *indoor air quality* (IAQ) may resemble those that you typically associate with colds, allergic rhinitis, fatigue, or flu. For this reason, you may not as easily realize that your child's asthma suffers as a consequence of poor IAQ at school and daycare. However, the following tips may provide clues that can help you decide whether IAQ is a factor:

✔ Many students, teachers, administrators, and other personnel experience similar symptoms.

✔ Your child's symptoms (and those of other affected people) improve or disappear after school or daycare.

✔ Symptoms begin to appear rapidly following physical changes, such as construction work, painting, or pesticide use at the school or daycare.

✔ Your child and other people with allergies or asthma only experience symptoms inside the building.

If you think that your child may experience symptoms related to poor IAQ at school or daycare, contact an appropriate staff member. Your child's school (or school system) may staff an IAQ coordinator or health and safety coordinator to respond to your concerns.

Participating in PE — exercise and asthma

Living with asthma doesn't mean that your child needs to sit on the sidelines. Participating in PE and other opportunities for exercise are vital for a child's development, regardless of whether or not the youngster has asthma. Nonetheless, make sure that the school's PE instructors are aware of your child's condition and that they know what to do in case an asthma episode develops.

PE instructors and coaches should encourage your asthmatic child to participate actively in sports, but they must also realize and respect your child's limitations. In addition, extended running and any exercise that takes place in cold, dry air appears to trigger asthma flare-ups, known as exercise-induced bronchospasms (EIB) or exercise-induced asthma (EIA). Exercise is one of the most common precipitants of asthma symptoms that most doctors see in clinical practice. More than 90 percent of patients identify physical exertion as a major cause of their asthma symptoms. Although EIA can develop at any age and occurs equally among adults and children, it is a much greater problem in kids because of their characteristically greater degree of physical activity. (See Chapter 9 for more information on EIA.)

Your child's doctor may prescribe medications to control and prevent EIA, as well as advise appropriate warm-up and cool-down activities that can also reduce the risk of EIA. Having an action plan in place prior to an emergency can ensure that your child receives the proper treatment when he or she needs it most. Part of that plan should include providing immediate access to your child's rescue drug in case it's needed to treat the onset of any acute respiratory symptoms.

As long as your child sticks to his or her asthma management plan, the disease shouldn't preclude your child from enjoying or even excelling at a wide range of physical activities. Consider the example of Olympic Gold medalist Jackie Joyner-Kersee and many other top athletes with asthma.

Chapter 19

Pregnancy and Asthma

· ·

In This Chapter

▶ Controlling asthma while pregnant

▶ Maintaining healthy lung functions for you and your baby

· ·

*I*f you have asthma and you're pregnant or considering pregnancy, I have some good news for you: With appropriate care, the vast majority of women with asthma have uncomplicated pregnancies.

Although treatment issues related to asthma affect approximately 4 percent of all pregnancies in the United States, very few of these cases involve situations that imperil either the mother or the child she carries. However, the potential for serious asthma-related complications exists if you don't control your asthma during pregnancy.

Therefore, continuing treatment for your disease — under your doctor's supervision — with an appropriate and effective asthma management plan is vital to

✔ Avert sudden aggravations of your asthma symptoms, thus minimizing the need for emergency care and hospitalizations

✔ Maintain as close to normal lung functions as possible

✔ Prevent chronic and troublesome symptoms of asthma, such as coughing, shortness of breath, wheezing — especially upon awakening in the morning, and episodes that disturb your sleep at night

✔ Provide the most effective medication therapy that results in minimal or no adverse side effects

✔ Sustain near-to-normal levels of exercise and other physical activities

✔ Give birth to a healthy, beautiful baby

In spite of what some people may think, most asthmatics go through pregnancy and labor well. Although I'm sure it has happened somewhere, in my more than 25 years practicing as an allergist, I've never seen labor or delivery set off a severe asthma attack.

Identifying Special Issues with Asthma during Pregnancy

Although one-third of pregnant women don't experience any change in asthma severity levels during pregnancy, another third of expectant mothers suffer from more severe asthma. For the remaining third, their condition may actually improve. In most cases, asthma severity returns to pre-pregnancy levels by the third month after delivery. Your asthma's severity can vary from one pregnancy to another, and neither you nor your doctor can predict how pregnancy may affect your condition.

Your hormones and your asthma

For some women, pregnancy seems to trigger asthma symptoms. In fact, you may not realize that you have asthma until it shows up during your pregnancy, because the significant hormonal changes your body experiences during pregnancy may cause increased airway congestion. Your body's hormonal changes can also induce or aggravate allergic and nonallergic rhinitis and sinusitis during pregnancy. These conditions can, in turn, increase your asthma's severity.

Therefore, you also need to address allergies and related conditions when you're expecting a child. If you have *allergic rhinitis* (hay fever) or *allergic conjunctivitis* (red, itchy eyes), both of which affect many people with allergic asthma, work with your doctor to control those symptoms while you're pregnant.

The basics of managing asthma while pregnant

The first step in avoiding asthma-related complications during your pregnancy is to make sure that your doctor properly diagnoses your respiratory symptoms. (See Chapter 2 for more information.)

If the diagnosis reveals that you have asthma, your doctor should help you develop an effective asthma management plan. This plan should consist of specific avoidance strategies, medications, monitoring, and assessment measures. Your management plan should also provide you with steps to take in case your asthma symptoms suddenly worsen.

Make sure that you (and your doctors) integrate your asthma management plan and any treatment that you may receive from an asthma specialist (such as an allergist or pulmonologist) with obstetric care from your obstetrician, family doctor, and/or primary care physician. A team approach by your physicians helps eliminate the risk of different doctors prescribing different treatments that can, in combination, produce adverse side effects for you and your baby. Integrated treatment can also ensure more effective control of any other condition or complications, besides asthma and related disorders that you may experience during pregnancy.

Breathing for Two

During your pregnancy, you're not only eating for two but also breathing for two — yourself and your baby. Contrary to what some people believe, the greatest danger to your unborn child isn't the preventive (or controller) medication your doctor prescribes to help manage your asthma, but rather the adverse effects that oxygen deprivation can have on your baby if you suffer severe or repeated asthma episodes during pregnancy.

In order to avoid adverse effects during your pregnancy, your asthma management plan needs to

- ✔ **Assess your condition with appropriate pulmonary function tests.** With these tests, you can establish benchmark results against which your doctor can compare later tests to determine your condition's severity.

- ✔ **Avoid or at least minimize exposure to allergens or irritants that may cause asthma flare-ups.** In many cases, effective avoidance measures can reduce the possibility of asthma episodes that require you to take additional medications, especially the frequent need for rescue (or *quick-relief*) drugs.

- ✔ **Treat your condition with appropriate preventive medications to ensure that you adequately maintain your lung functions and that your baby receives a sufficient supply of oxygen.** Preventive medications can also minimize the possibility of asthma episodes that may require emergency treatment or drugs.

Mother Nature's milk

Breastfeeding provides nutritional, immuno-logic, and psychological benefits for your new-born child. Breast milk, in contrast to cow's milk in infant formulas, may decrease the potential for allergic sensitization by reducing your baby's exposure to ingested food allergens. In addition, breast milk may reduce the incidence of bronchiolitis (see Chapter 18) and infection-induced asthma during infancy, because the baby receives antibodies against viral infections through the mother's breast milk.

Avoiding asthma triggers, allergens, and irritants during pregnancy

During your pregnancy, avoid precipitating factors that may trigger asthma episodes. See Chapter 5 for extensive details on asthma triggers and precipi-tating factors.

If you suffer from allergic asthma, implement (under your doctor's supervi-sion) an avoidance and allergy-proofing plan that limits your exposure to inhalant allergens as well as airborne irritants, especially tobacco smoke. Furthermore, a comprehensive avoidance strategy can help to alleviate symptoms of allergic rhinitis and/or allergic conjunctivitis. Effective allergy-proofing focuses on your home in general and your bedroom in particular. I provide extensive information and tips on allergy-proofing in Chapter 10.

Undergoing allergy testing and immunotherapy during pregnancy

If you're already receiving *immunotherapy* (allergy shots) when you become pregnant, your doctor may advise you to continue with the treatment because, in many cases, it can help prevent allergy attacks that may make your asthma worse. Stopping immunotherapy may result in your symptoms worsening, thus requiring additional medication therapy. Frequently, your doctor may advise reduced doses of immunotherapy to minimize potential risks of allergy-shot reactions.

If you're already pregnant and are considering having allergy testing to determine which allergens trigger your symptoms, or if you're thinking about starting immunotherapy, your doctor will probably advise you to wait until after your baby is born.

Managing nasal conditions associated with pregnancy

Expectant women often experience worsening of their pre-existing rhinitis or develop certain nasal and upper respiratory symptoms for the first time. As with the changes in asthma severity levels that I explain in "Your hormones and your asthma," earlier in this chapter, in many cases these increased or newly acquired nasal symptoms result from hormonal changes that occur only during pregnancy.

Poorly managing these nasal conditions can complicate your asthma and, in severe cases, interfere with sleeping, eating, your emotional well-being, and your overall quality of life. Contending with the unpleasantness of impaired sleep, sneezing, runny nose, itchy eyes, inflamed sinuses, ear infections, and sinus headaches while pregnant is a challenge that you (and your family) want to avoid.

The following sections provide information and tips for managing the most common nasal conditions associated with pregnancy.

Allergic rhinitis (Hay fever)

If avoidance and allergy-proofing don't provide sufficient control of your hay fever symptoms, your doctor may advise using nasal cromolyn spray. However, avoid using oral decongestants during the first trimester of your pregnancy. Sometime after the first trimester, your doctor may consider prescribing antihistamines, such as chlorpheniramine (Chlor-Trimeton) and tripelennamine, as well as decongestants such as pseudoephedrine (Sudafed), depending on your condition, the development of your baby, and the severity of your allergy symptoms.

Many people treat hay fever symptoms with over-the-counter (OTC) decongestants and antihistamines. But during your pregnancy, check with your doctor before taking any medications, including OTC products. In many cases, particularly with antihistamines, second-generation products, such as Claritin (now available OTC) and Zyrtec (available by prescription), are actually safer and cause less drowsiness than many of the first-generation antihistamines. In addition, OTC Nasalcrom is considered the safest nasal spray for treating allergic rhinitis during pregnancy.

Vasomotor rhinitis of pregnancy

Vasomotor rhinitis of pregnancy is a nonallergic upper respiratory syndrome that usually only develops during pregnancy, mostly from the second month to term. The associated symptoms of nasal congestion, nasal dryness, and nosebleeds usually disappear after delivery.

Buffered saline nose sprays can provide effective relief for vasomotor rhinitis of pregnancy. Exercise can sometimes help relieve this condition. If nasal congestion persists, however, your doctor may advise using pseudoephedrine (Sudafed) as a decongestant.

Sinusitis

The incidence of sinusitis in pregnant women is six times higher than in the rest of the population. These often-painful sinus infections can develop as complications of rhinitis and viral upper respiratory infections, such as the common cold. Sinusitis can trigger asthma symptoms and, in some cases, may complicate your asthma to the point that it doesn't respond to treatment. Poorly managed sinusitis can also worsen to the point where sinus surgery becomes necessary.

To reduce the risk of sinus infections, your doctor may advise using a nasal douche cup, nasal bulb syringe, or other type of nasal wash device at home to irrigate your nostrils with warm saline solution, thus relieving pressure and congestion in your nasal passages. Ask your doctor for specific instructions on using these devices.

If your doctor prescribes medication to clear a sinus infection, amoxicillin is probably her first choice, unless you're allergic to penicillin. If you're allergic to penicillin, your doctor may prescribe some type of erythromycin-based medication.

Exercising with asthma during pregnancy

Most asthmatics experience some degree of exercise-induced asthma (EIA), particularly as a result of activities that involve breathing cold, dry air (such as running outdoors). Consult with your doctor to evaluate what level and type of exercise benefits you most during your pregnancy.

Activities that allow you to breathe warmer, humidified air (such as swimming in a heated pool) may be less likely to trigger EIA symptoms. In order to lessen the occurrence of EIA episodes, ask your doctor about medications that can help control airway inflammation when you exercise and prevent symptoms of this condition. (See Chapters 15 and 16 for information on these products.)

With proper treatment and management, asthma doesn't have to keep you from your regular physical activities during pregnancy.

Assessing your asthma during pregnancy

In addition to closely monitoring your lung functions through office spirometry (see Chapter 2 for an explanation of this process), your doctor may also advise measuring your airflow at home using a portable peak-flow meter to assess your peak expiratory flow rate (PEFR).

Although PEFR measurements generally don't provide complete information by themselves to fully evaluate your asthma's severity, they certainly can provide a valuable insight into the daily course of your asthma. (I provide detailed instructions on using peak-flow meters in Chapter 4.)

Monitoring your baby's condition

During the beginning of your second trimester, your doctor may use an ultrasound to establish a benchmark for assessing your baby's growth. If your asthma is moderate or severe, your doctor may advise further ultrasound scans during your third trimester.

During the third trimester, your doctor should assess your baby weekly. However, if your doctor suspects problems, she may need to check the baby's well-being more often. Your doctor should encourage you to record the baby's activity, or kick counts, on a daily basis.

During labor, your doctor needs to closely monitor the baby. In most cases, doctors follow the baby's progress through close electronic monitoring. Also, make sure that the staff measures your PEFR when you're first admitted to the hospital for labor and again every 12 hours thereafter until you deliver.

In rare cases, mothers who enter labor with severe or uncontrolled asthma may require more intensive monitoring, either by continuous, electronic monitoring of the baby's heart rate or relatively frequent *auscultation* (listening through a stethoscope to the baby's heart rate).

Taking asthma medications while pregnant

In general, continue your course of asthma medications through your pregnancy, labor, and delivery. The specific medication plan that your doctor prescribes depends on your asthma's severity.

The primary goal of pharmacological asthma management during pregnancy is to use the minimum level of medication necessary — with minimal risk of adverse side effects — to control the underlying airway inflammation.

The preferred medications for treatment of asthma while pregnant are

- ✔ Inhaled products that deliver the drug directly to your airway in higher, and thus more effective, concentrations than oral medications. Inhaled drugs also reduce the risk of systemic side effects. To find out more about asthma medications, their use, and their side effects, turn to Chapters 15 and 16.

- ✔ Drugs, such as cromolyn (Intal), that have a long history of safe use in pregnant women and have been studied extensively in published clinical trials. Budesonide (Pulmicort) is also considered a safe inhaled medication for treatment of asthma during pregnancy.

The drugs your doctor prescribes in order to safely control your asthma during pregnancy may include the following:

- ✔ An inhaled beta$_2$-adrenergic (beta$_2$-agonist) bronchodilator to use in case your asthma symptoms suddenly worsen, or preventively as needed prior to exercise.

  For mild asthma, occasionally using inhaled beta$_2$-adrenergics usually suffices for asthma control. In some cases, your doctor may also recommend regularly using inhaled cromolyn sodium (Intal).

- ✔ Sustained-release theophylline or a long-acting oral or inhaled beta$_2$-adrenergic if your asthma symptoms primarily show up at night.

- ✔ A regimen of constant preventive doses of inhaled corticosteroids, sometimes in combination with a long-acting bronchodilator.

  In milder cases, your doctor may prescribe theophylline, as well as cromolyn sodium, as alternate choices. However, in more severe cases, you may require short bursts of oral prednisone if a combination of bronchodilators, inhaled corticosteroids, and cromolyn sodium fails to keep your asthma symptoms under control.

  Managing severe persistent asthma may require higher doses of inhaled corticosteroids, often in combination with long-acting bronchodilators. Maintaining this aggressive regimen usually allows your doctor to minimize your use of oral corticosteroids.

  In rare cases of uncontrolled asthma during pregnancy, you may require an alternate-day or single-daily morning dose of oral corticosteroids to re-establish control of your symptoms. Make sure that an asthma specialist, in consultation with an obstetrician who specializes in high-risk pregnancies, monitors this course of medication. As soon as your symptoms are under control, your doctors should taper off the dosage of oral corticosteroids and gradually replace them with the regular use of inhaled corticosteroids to reduce the risk of adverse side effects to you or your baby.

Handling asthma emergencies while pregnant

Your doctor should instruct you how to recognize the signs of worsening asthma and how to treat these episodes early with appropriate medications. Also, make sure that you can tell when a deteriorating situation may require emergency medical attention, and know what you need to do if that happens. (Chapter 4 provides details on the emergency management of asthma.)

The most important points to keep in mind when dealing with an asthma emergency during pregnancy are

✔ If you're exposed to any allergens or irritants (especially tobacco smoke), get away from those allergy triggers as quickly as possible. Otherwise, your condition may deteriorate.

✔ Even if you have days when you're feeling better, don't stop taking your preventive medications during your pregnancy, unless your doctor instructs otherwise.

✔ If your symptoms worsen, don't resort to frequently overusing your beta$_2$-adrenergic (beta$_2$-agonist) inhaler. Doing so probably won't improve your condition and may even make matters worse.

✔ If your condition doesn't improve rapidly after one or two doses of your beta$_2$-adrenergic inhaler or if your condition continues to deteriorate, seek appropriate medical care, as detailed in your asthma management plan.

Chapter 20

Asthma and the Elderly

· ·

In This Chapter

▶ Seeking an accurate diagnosis of your condition

▶ Avoiding adverse drug interactions and side effects

· ·

*P*eople are living longer than ever before, especially in developed countries, such as the United States, Canada, and most European Union members. However, people's increased life spans have also been paralleled by an unfortunate rise in the incidence of asthma worldwide among people older than 65.

For seniors, dealing with asthma can present unique challenges due to the following reasons:

✔ Many elderly patients are first diagnosed with asthma only in their later years, after their respiratory symptoms have become increasingly severe and their health, as a result, has deteriorated.

✔ The process of adjusting to life with asthma can be more complex for an older person than for a younger patient, because in many cases, older patients have multiple medical problems.

✔ In many cases, seniors' asthma management plans are more intricate than those of younger asthmatics, and may require more frequent medication adjustments due to potential adverse interactions with drugs that many older patients take for their other medical conditions, such as heart disease, high blood pressure, or diabetes (see "Watching out for adverse side effects," later in this chapter).

Recognizing Asthma Later in Life

Asthma once had a reputation as a disease that primarily affected children and young adults. A common misconception about asthma was that it was a "kid's disease." However, as I explain throughout the book, your respiratory symptoms may vary widely and may first appear at any age over your lifetime.

In fact, the incidence of asthma among the elderly in the United States is second only to that found in children under 18 (called *extrinsic* or *allergic* asthma). Recent studies show that the condition can actually develop later in life, which explains why some doctors use the term *late-onset adult asthma* (*intrinsic* or *nonallergic* asthma) to describe the ailment.

Keep these important facts in mind when dealing with asthma among older asthmatics:

✔ Many elderly patients with late-adult onset asthma aren't diagnosed until their condition has deteriorated, because they initially assume their respiratory symptoms are due to a greater susceptibility to colds and bronchial infections later in life. Wheezing can also be a symptom of other underlying conditions, such as heart failure or vocal chord dysfunction (VCD).

✔ Allergic conditions that frequently coexist with asthma in younger patients, such as *allergic rhinitis* (hay fever; see Chapter 7) and *atopic dermatitis* (eczema; see Chapter 1), aren't present as often in elderly asthmatics, which can further increase the challenge of correctly diagnosing asthma in seniors.

✔ Late-adult onset asthma affects older women to a greater degree than older men. Studies indicate that hormonal changes during menopause may account for this disparity.

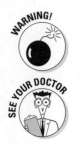

✔ Some seniors are at increased risk for severe, even fatal asthma attacks because they don't perceive a worsening of their respiratory symptoms, such as shortness of breath or chest constriction, and thus fail to use prescribed short-relief medications or seek medical help in time.

✔ For this reason, making sure elderly asthmatics properly monitor their lung functions with peak-flow meters (see Chapter 4) is vital, in order to accurately and objectively assess their condition. Lung-function tests should be part of any checkups and medical exams that seniors receive.

Taking Asthma Medications When Older

Just in case the previous section seemed to raise some serious concerns, the good news is that many elderly asthmatics show remarkable improvement in their respiratory condition when treated with appropriate asthma medications. The challenge in some cases may be to find the best combination of therapies to achieve the desired result.

Because asthma often coexists with chronic bronchitis in elderly patients, your doctor may prescribe a one-to-two-week trial therapy with oral corticosteroids to determine the extent of improvement from spirometry (see Chapter 4) before prescribing appropriate and effective long-term asthma medications.

Your asthma management plan may include a mix of short-term and long-term medications. Your doctor may periodically adjust and refine this multiple drug therapy based on how well you respond to the treatment and also on what other medications you're taking for other medical conditions. And, because many elderly patients take a variety of prescribed medications, make sure you keep an accurate medication record (see Chapter 3) to reduce the risk of potential adverse interactions between certain drugs.

Using more effective delivery devices

As part of your asthma *pharmacotherapy* (treatment with medications), your physician may prescribe a recently developed breath-activated metered-dose inhaler (MDI) such as Maxair Autohaler as a short-term rescue medication, and possibly a dry-powder inhaler (DPI) such as Advair Diskus as a long-term controller medication (see Chapter 14).

These types of newer inhalation devices are usually easier to operate properly and also deliver medication to the airways more effectively than older, generic MDIs, which some seniors find challenging to use. Incorrectly using an older, generic MDI can lead to ineffective administration of the medication, eventually resulting in poor control and worsening of respiratory symptoms.

Watching out for adverse side effects

Although pharmacotherapy is a vital aspect of effective asthma treatment in nearly all cases, elderly patients need to understand that they can be at an increased risk for potential adverse side effects from asthma medications for the following reasons:

- ✔ As you age, your response to the use of bronchodilators may change. For this reason, elderly asthma patients may experience increased sensitivities to adverse side effects of beta$_2$-adrenergic medications, including tremors and an increased heart rate. If you have cardiovascular disease, your doctor may consider prescribing a combination inhaler containing a beta$_2$-adrenergic medication (a short-acting bronchodilator) with an anticholinergic (for example, Combivent; see Chapter 16) as an alternative to additional doses of only beta$_2$-adrenergics.

- ✔ High-dose inhaled corticosteroid use may predispose patients to cataract formation in the eyes and can potentially reduce the bone mineral content in some asthma patients (particularly the elderly) who may have pre-existing osteoporosis and/or a sedentary lifestyle. If this concern pertains to you, your doctor may recommend calcium supplements, vitamin D, and (for women) estrogen-replacement therapy.

  And (for men), inform your doctor of any type of past or current prostate condition before taking any anticholinergic medications, such as ipratropium bromide (Atrovent), because these drugs may potentially aggravate a pre-existing prostate problem.

- ✔ Because they're more likely to use beta-blockers, elderly patients are potentially at risk for worsening of asthma due to the blocking activity of these drugs, which prevents beta$_2$-adrenergic medications from relieving bronchospasms. In addition, many seniors take aspirin daily to prevent heart problems, and can have idiosyncratic adverse drug interactions to aspirin and also to nonsteroidal anti-inflammatory drugs (NSAIDs) taken to relieve arthritis. For more information on drug sensitivities and adverse drug reactions that can affect your asthma, see Chapter 5.

- ✔ Some older patients who may have impaired liver functions may require a reduced dose of theophylline in order to prevent accumulation of this drug in the bloodstream, which can lead to potential side effects. In addition, drug interactions that can cause problems with asthma medications in this age group include some commonly prescribed antibiotics (erythromycin) and cimetidine (Tagamet). Always make sure your doctor is aware of any possible liver conditions that may be affecting you, especially if you take theophylline.

Part VI
The Part of Tens

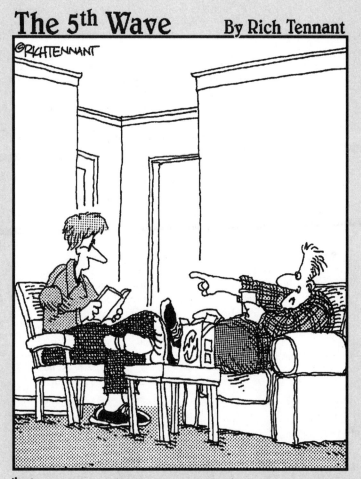

The 5th Wave   By Rich Tennant

"C'mon, Darrel! Someone with asthma shouldn't be lying around all day. Whereas someone with no life, like myself, has a very good reason."

In this part . . .

The Part of Tens is a tradition in *For Dummies* books. In these two chapters, I provide material about asthma that lends itself to an informal "top ten" list presentation.

Thinking of getting your asthma together and taking it on the road? Before you pack up your old kit bag, make sure you read Chapter 21. In this chapter, I discuss what you should take with you — and what you should take into account — when traveling with asthma.

In Chapter 22, I offer examples of significant people from ancient times to today who have excelled in many impressive ways in spite of their asthma. I hope this chapter inspires you to further seek out the care that you deserve, which can give you the freedom to pursue your own personal goals and aspirations.

Chapter 21

Ten Tips for Traveling with Asthma

*I*f only airlines could lose your asthma the way they sometimes lose your baggage. Imagine if you could leave your wheezing instead of your heart in San Francisco. And wouldn't waking up in the city that never sleeps because the Big Apple stirs you to the very core — instead of an asthma episode interrupting a good night's rest — be nice?

Of course, getting away from asthma isn't that easy. Extensive studies over the past 15 years show that this respiratory ailment is an ongoing condition that you usually don't outgrow, although its symptoms can certainly vary in character and severity throughout your lifetime.

Think of asthma, and often-related conditions, such as *allergic rhinitis* (hay fever), as constant companions. Wherever you may roam, these conditions will be along for the ride. Knowing how to control the symptoms of these ailments is vital to ensuring that no matter what else may go wrong during your travel, your respiratory condition won't complicate or ruin your plans.

Planning a Safe, Healthy Trip

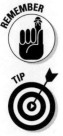

A key element in proper travel planning is avoiding places where you know pollens, dander, tobacco smoke, or other allergens and irritants may be prevalent and could, depending on your specific sensitivities, trigger your respiratory and/or allergy symptoms.

The following points are general guidelines for preventing problems frequently associated with these triggers:

- **Dander:** Beware of visiting or staying in homes with cats, dogs, and other animals, including rabbits, birds, and gerbils and other domesticated rodents. Even if the animal lover removes the pet from the area, you can still suffer an adverse reaction because of the residual dander and/or hair in the room. Horseback riding also may not be advisable. Before you saddle up for a dude ranch out West, make sure you can control any symptoms that Trigger's horsehair may just trigger. Consult your doctor about preventive medications (and see Chapters 5 and 10).

- **Food allergens:** The foods that trigger allergic reactions most frequently in adults with food hypersensitivities include fish, shellfish, peanuts, and tree nuts. For children, the most common triggers are milk, eggs, peanuts, tree nuts, fish, soy, and wheat (see Chapter 8). Because of the swiftness and severity with which a food allergy reaction can strike (especially with peanuts), be especially vigilant in avoiding these triggers when traveling. In particular, if you or your child is sensitive to peanuts and you're planning to travel where these seemingly harmless legumes are a regular part of local cuisine (many parts of East Asia, for example), ask your doctor about additional precautions you can take. Although you can clearly identify peanuts in many dishes, they may be a hidden part of the cooking process itself in many cases (for example, foods cooked alongside dishes prepared with peanut products). When in doubt, avoid local fare in these parts of the world, rather than risk reactions such as an asthma attack, hives, or worse yet, a potentially life-threatening case of anaphylaxis (see Chapter 8).

- **Ragweed:** Avoiding travel to the eastern half of the United States and Canada from mid-August through October is probably advisable (assuming you don't already live there) if you're sensitized to ragweed pollen. If you must travel to those areas during ragweed season, ask your physician about preventive medications that you can take to keep your symptoms under control (see Chapter 10). Also, the National Allergy Bureau (NAB) of the American Academy of Allergy, Asthma, and Immunology (AAAAI) has seasonal allergen maps that chart the prevalence of allergenic pollens, as well as several other allergens around the country throughout the year. Check out the NAB Web site at www.aaaai.org/nab or call 414-272-6071. (See Chapter 10 for more information on pollens.)

Adjusting Treatment for Travel

Prevention is the key to a safe and trouble-free trip, which usually means consulting your physician ahead of time to evaluate your asthma management and to make any advisable adjustments, based on where and when you're going and what you'll be doing while traveling. You may need to adjust your medication because of increased exposures to triggers. In addition, remember that changes in time zones may affect the dosage schedule of some medications you're taking (for any ailment, not just asthma or allergies).

You'll also need to make sure that you'll be able to stick with the program that your physician advises. If possible, get a letter from your doctor summarizing your medical history, as well as the treatments and medications you're currently taking. If you're at risk of acute asthma or allergy attacks, ask your physician about wearing a MedicAlert pendant on your wrist or around your neck. (See the appendix for information on this and other valuable asthma and allergy products.)

Taking Medications and Other Essentials

Make sure you have all your necessary medical supplies, devices, and prescriptions with you when traveling. If flying (or riding on a train or bus), keep these items in your carry-on bag. After you arrive at your destination, keep your essentials with you instead of leaving them in your hotel room (or other accommodation) when you're out and about. If you need to leave your medications in the room (for example, while using hotel recreational facilities), make sure you store these products in a safe and secure location, such as the room safe or in a locked suitcase, instead of leaving them out on the bathroom countertop.

Keep medications in their original containers and never mix pills of different types into one receptacle. By keeping them in their original containers, you'll have the proper dosage information readily available, which is especially important if someone else needs to administer your medication to you. Also, if you're traveling internationally, customs officials are generally less suspicious of pills and capsules in their original containers.

If you or your child uses a nebulizer at home, ask your doctor about taking one with you on your trip. If you're traveling overseas, don't forget to bring whatever adapters and converters (available in most luggage, electronics, and travel stores) you may need in order to use your domestic devices in different countries. The electric current in many other parts of the world is 220 volts rather than the 110 volts that is standard in the United States and Canada. If you have a portable nebulizer, don't forget extra batteries.

Getting Medications and Medical Help Abroad

Ask your doctor about special medical considerations for specific countries and areas. Some countries require that you take certain vaccine shots before your visit. As for medications, don't assume that every place you visit has pharmacies stocked with the supplies you need. Write down both the brand names of your medications and their generic names. In a pinch, having both names available may allow a local pharmacist to find what you need.

When planning your trip, you may want to obtain a booklet that lists qualified, English-speaking physicians in just about every country of the world. The International Association for Medical Assistance to Travelers (IAMAT), a voluntary organization based in Canada, offers this booklet. You can contact them in the United States at 716-754-4883 or via their Web site at www.iamat.org for further information.

Also, if you're a U.S. citizen, the U.S. State Department's American Citizens Services can provide help in case of an emergency. Call the State Department's Hotline for American Travelers, 202-647-5225, or check the State Department's Web site, www.state.gov, before your departure to receive information on contacting U.S. embassies and consulates for assistance with medical matters.

Flying with Allergens and Irritants

Sad to say, but your fellow airplane passengers may make you sick. Studies show that airplane passenger cabins are some of the worst indoor dust mite and animal dander sites. Because airliners are tightly sealed environments that often lack adequate air filtering or cleaning, they often concentrate sky-high quantities of allergens and irritants that hundreds, even thousands, of passengers constantly track in with them. So be advised: Your seat may already be occupied by frequent-flier allergens.

Many airplane seats house thriving colonies of dust mites and their allergenic waste products. In addition, although all U.S., Canadian, and many European flights ban smoking anywhere on the aircraft (and in most parts of airport terminals), some international flights still allow smoking.

If exposure to tobacco smoke triggers your asthma symptoms, find out as much as possible about an air carrier's smoking policies. If your travel includes flying an airline that permits smoking, try to get seating as far away from the smoking section as possible.

Take my advice when you're planning air travel:

✓ **Pack your medications in a carry-on bag so they're immediately available in the event of a serious asthma episode and/or allergic reaction and in case the airline loses your luggage.** (You want to avoid finding yourself in strange territory without your medications.)

✓ **Stay hydrated during your flight.** Avoid alcohol and drink plenty of water. Not only does drinking water help minimize potential asthma and allergy problems, but it also can put a dent in whatever jet lag you may otherwise develop.

✓ **If you have the opportunity/financial ability, consider upgrading to first or business class.** If available, the leather seats may be less likely to harbor allergy triggers, and at the very least, you'll give yourself more breathing (and leg) room.

Considering Allergy Shots and Travel

When you're traveling, I usually recommend transferring your immunotherapy (allergy shots) program to another location only if you'll be gone at least a month or more (if you're a snowbird from the North wintering in southern California or southern Florida, for example). If you'll be gone for a month or more, ask your physician for a referral to a doctor in the area where you'll be staying and have that physician administer your shots in a medical facility.

Although practices vary in different areas of the United States and the world, don't give yourself allergy shots. The risk, although low, of a bad reaction or even anaphylactic shock means you need qualified medical personnel around you, just in case (see Chapter 11).

When visiting the physician in the new location, bring your allergy serum (vaccine) vials in a refrigerated or ice-insulated pack, and make sure you have clear written instructions from your doctor regarding your dose.

Reducing Trigger Exposures in Hotels and Motels

Tobacco smoke and its lingering traces can cause problems, especially outside the United States or Canada, where hotels and other accommodations are less likely to restrict smoking. Wherever you stay, reserve a room on a smoke-free floor. Likewise, if feathers pose a potential allergy problem for you, bring your own pillow and pillowcase (see Chapter 10).

Inspect the room before you occupy it, looking for signs of animal hair, dirty air vents, dust, or mold. If you find evidence suggesting that staying in the room will lead to breathing problems, ask for another room that appears safer and more comfortable. In some cases, your doctor may advise bringing along a portable HEPA air filter system (see Chapter 5). Check to see if your hotel offers allergy-free rooms, which may even come with HEPA filters and allergy covers on the mattresses.

Avoiding Food Allergies during Your Trip

In your travels, you may come into contact with foods to which you have an allergy (not just an intolerance — see Chapter 8 for the difference between the two conditions). In some cases, the menu in a given restaurant, hotel, or cafe reveals all you need to know about potentially problematic ingredients. But more often than not, you need to ask a lot of questions about the cuisine and how it's prepared. Don't be rude, but definitely don't be shy.

As I explain in Chapter 8, you may need to do more than simply determine that a particular dish doesn't contain foods to which you're allergic. For example, in many restaurants, various dishes are all prepared on the same grill. In this case, if you're allergic to shellfish, for example, make sure that the cooking surface and utensils used to prepare your food haven't also been previously used to prepare shellfish. If they have, allergens from the shellfish may end up in your meal, potentially causing a distressful dining experience.

If your food hypersensitivities put you at risk for anaphylaxis, wear a MedicAlert pendant or bracelet. Also ask your doctor about prescribing an epinephrine kit such as an EpiPen (see Chapter 8), and be sure to carry the kit with you.

Finding Help in Case of Emergencies

Although the local hospital probably isn't at the top of your sightseeing list, find out the location of the nearest medical facility equipped to treat you in case of a serious adverse allergic reaction or severe asthma episode. Knowing where the closest help is available can help ensure that you get effective treatment if you experience a life-threatening reaction.

Depending on your destination, you can easily obtain local hospital locations from the organizations that I list earlier in this chapter (see the section "Getting Medications and Medical Help Abroad") and in the appendix, your doctor, or your travel agent. In some cases, you may need to do more homework; however, your health and safety are worth the effort.

Traveling with Your Asthmatic Child

When traveling with a child who has asthma, many of the same considerations that adults must contend with also apply. These points include the following:

✔ **Pack two containers of all medications, and make sure that you've labeled them properly.** Keep one container as a carry-on with you, and keep the other in a purse, backpack, or briefcase.

✔ **Obtain a MedicAlert bracelet or necklace for your child to wear.** If you're not around, emergency medical personnel will immediately know what to do about your child's condition.

✔ **Show your child how to pack his or her asthma and/or allergy medications properly.** In addition to preparing your child for trips that he or she may take without you, this lesson can also help your youngster find out more about managing his or her condition appropriately.

✔ **Take at least two epinephrine kits (such as an EpiPen or EpiPen Jr. for children under 66 pounds) if your child is at risk for anaphylaxis to ensure that you'll always have one at hand.** Make sure that you and/or your child (depending on the youngster's age) know how to use the kit. Knowing how to use the kit means you should receive instructions on the proper use of the injector in your doctor's office, rather than waiting for a potential emergency to figure it out.

✔ **Ask questions about meals.** If your child has peanut allergies, be especially vigilant on airplanes (particularly with the contents of those appealingly packaged snack bags), where peanuts can be as common as delayed flights (see Chapter 18).

Asthma camps

Children with asthma can benefit from a special type of vacation experience. A number of organizations, including the American Lung Association (ALA), sponsor children's asthma camps throughout the United States and Canada. If your child has asthma, consider sending him or her to one of these camps for a healthy, safe, educational, and fun nature-oriented vacation. Asthma camps generally offer one- to two-week programs that teach children how to recognize the signs of asthma and allergy triggers, use medications and inhaler devices properly, and understand the basics of asthma management. Call the Consortium of Asthma Camps at 651-227-8014, or visit the organization's Web site, www.asthmacamps.org, for a list of asthma camps.

Chapter 22

Ten Famous Folks with Asthma

*R*arely do you think of famous figures such as Augustus Caesar, Ludwig van Beethoven, and Charles Dickens in the same breath — unless you're considering the many great achievers throughout human history who had asthma.

The modern world also abounds with asthmatics who have had a significant impact on human events, including John F. Kennedy, Jackie Joyner-Kersee, Kenny G, and Liza Minnelli, to name only a few. Living with asthma doesn't mean you're sentenced to life's sidelines.

Renowned leaders, writers, musicians, doctors, and athletes have overcome their asthma to achieve greatness — in some cases, long before the development of the medications and therapies that help today's asthmatics.

Imagine Dickens, coughing deeply and incessantly while trying to finish *David Copperfield,* or Beethoven suffering from attacks of *dyspnea* (shortness of breath) and wondering whether he was fated to die from a respiratory disease like his mother did. These brilliant creative spirits persevered, fighting past the asthma's restrictions, and created transcendent literature and music that still speaks to people today.

Perhaps you're a budding Beethoven, a youthful Jackie Joyner-Kersee, or an up-and-coming Teddy Roosevelt. You can accomplish your dreams and hopes for the future, despite having asthma — especially if you and your doctor ensure that you receive the necessary treatment to appropriately and effectively manage your condition. As I explain throughout this book, you can control your asthma; don't let your asthma control you.

Augustus Caesar

The great-nephew of Julius Caesar, Gaius Octavius (63 B.C.–A.D. 14), began his life with a slight advantage over his future rivals. However, when his powerful great-uncle was assassinated on the Ides of March (March 15) in 44 B.C., 18-year-old Octavius could hardly have known that he would someday become the first, and ultimately most famous, ruler of the ancient Roman Empire. Octavius fought battles, both political and military, for 17 years before consolidating his power, eliminating his foes (most notably Mark Antony, who was distracted by Cleopatra, the exotic Egyptian queen), and creating the position of Roman Emperor for himself. When he became emperor, Octavius also took on a new name: Augustus, which means "the Exalted."

Augustus acquired his empire while also fighting asthma, according to ancient writings on his life. However, he didn't use respiratory difficulties as an excuse; no accounts of Augustus saying, "I came, I saw, I coughed," have come to light. He forged an empire that encompassed everything from England to Egypt.

Peter the Great

The youngest son of Czar Alexis, Peter (1672–1725) wasn't expected to become head of state, but when his older half-siblings died early, he became co-ruler at the age of 10 and sole czar at age 24. While his lungs fought asthma, Peter battled the Turks and later the Swedes, eventually winning access to the Baltic Sea and founding Russia's "window on the West," Saint Petersburg.

Peter the Great's early experiences of learning from foreigners, especially Dutch traders and merchants, helped fuel his desire to open Russia to Western trade, inventions, and ideas, setting in motion a process that continues (with considerable challenges) to the present day.

Ludwig van Beethoven

Most people know that Beethoven (1770–1827) contended with the worst affliction any musician could face: deafness. And yet, even as his hearing began to deteriorate at age 29 and continued until he became completely deaf at age 46, Beethoven managed to compose some of the most dramatic and beautiful works ever written in the Western classical music tradition.

Beethoven's hearing wasn't his only challenge: The first recorded account of illness in Beethoven's life was an asthma attack he experienced at age 16. He subsequently suffered "numerous colds and bronchitis" for most of his adult life. However, Beethoven pushed the *Pathetique* side of his existence away and aimed for the *Eroica,* becoming one of the world's greatest composers. (No one knows whether a coughing fit inspired the famous opening motif of Beethoven's Fifth Symphony.)

The great German master may have taken some solace from the fact that the Italian composer Antonio Vivaldi (1678–1741) was also asthmatic. Short of breath or not, Vivaldi composed many wonderful works that music lovers continue to enjoy — most notably, *The Four Seasons.*

Charles Dickens

"Please, sir, I want some more." Although Oliver Twist, hero of one of Dickens's best-loved novels, speaks that famous line, imagining the author himself pleading for a bit more oxygen to reach his lungs without a coughing fit to go with it isn't difficult. Although Dickens (1812–1870) grew up in London, where the air was dank with the Industrial Revolution's smoke and fog (hence, smog), the great writer apparently didn't experience real respiratory trouble until he was 37. A vacation retreat to the seaside town of Bonchurch left him allergy-ridden, coughing, and sick to his stomach. Dickens felt relief only after he departed for the inland country surroundings of Broadstairs in Kent.

Over the next few years, asthmatic characters filled Dickens's novels, from Mr. Omer in *David Copperfield* to Mr. Sleary in *Hard Times.* In his correspondence with friends and relations, the author cited nights in which he couldn't sleep because of constant coughing. Dickens also reported that only opiates, which were popular asthma remedies of the time, helped his symptoms. As I explain in Chapters 15 and 16, more effective medications (with far fewer side effects) now exist for treating asthma. Despite his condition, Dickens wrote dozens of terrific books and stories, becoming (along with Shakespeare) one of the two most popular writers of all time in the English language.

Dickens wasn't the only writer and social commentator who rose above asthma. Other significant literary figures with asthma include French author Marcel Proust (1871–1922), Welsh poet Dylan Thomas (1914– 1953), and American author John Updike (born 1932).

Teddy Roosevelt

Theodore (Teddy) Roosevelt (1858–1919) lived with asthma from infancy but overcame the disease in a big way, becoming a prolific author, military hero, and, at age 42, the 26th president of the United States. Perhaps more important for children, he also provided the namesake for the teddy bear.

Roosevelt did everything in a big way: Throughout his childhood, he dealt with numerous diseases, bad eyesight, and unsuccessful asthma remedies. But a course of vigorous exercise, which "TR," as he was also known, began at age 12, eventually helped lessen his attacks. (See Chapter 18 for more information on how exercise can help youngsters with asthma.)

Roosevelt's positive outlook on life, in spite of the many challenges facing him, also kept him from turning his asthma into an excuse for self-pity or losing his wry sense of humor. Referring to one asthma episode, the 15-year-old Teddy wrote, "Except for the fact that I cannot speak, without blowing like an abridged edition of a hippopotamus, it does not inconvenience me much."

In 1884, a terrible pair of tragedies struck Roosevelt: His first wife and his mother died on the same day. Beset by grief, which may have contributed to the serious asthma episodes that plagued him in the wake of his loss, Roosevelt's doctor advised leaving the cooler, humid weather of upstate New York for the drier climate of the West. Horseback riding and a change in surroundings seemed to help his recovery.

As I explain in Chapter 10, however, relocating to a drier climate rarely works these days because of the abundance of non-native plants that so many settlers and developers introduced to the western parts of North America during the last century.

Roosevelt, who was quite the fun-loving, roughhousing parent, sometimes suffered asthma episodes after pillow fights with his children. Therefore, some medical scholars suggest that Teddy was allergic to feathers. However, old "Rough and Ready" fought his asthma well enough to lead his volunteer troops up San Juan Hill during the Spanish-American War and subsequently become a successful two-term president, with his face carved into Mount Rushmore.

Years after he left office, TR ran for president again, this time as an independent candidate. Although he survived an assassination attempt during that campaign, he eventually lost the election to Woodrow Wilson (1856–1924), also an asthmatic.

John F. Kennedy

So much has been written about John F. Kennedy's tragic and untimely death at the age of 46 that overlooking the many health problems he faced through-out his life is easy. From his early childhood, Kennedy (1917–1963) was prone to disease, including asthma. His medical history also included childhood scarlet fever and diphtheria; adolescent afflictions such as bronchitis, sinusi-tis (see Chapter 13), and an irritable colon; hepatitis in college; malaria during World War II; and struggles with hypothyroidism, ulcers, and urinary tract infections later in life.

In 1954, complications from back surgery led to a staph infection that nearly killed the future president. In addition to these ailments, *atopy* (a genetic predisposition to developing allergic conditions), which ran in the Kennedy family, showed up throughout John's life in the form of food allergies and (most significantly) allergic reactions to animal dander, particularly dog hair and horsehair. These reactions often triggered asthma episodes, which plagued Kennedy throughout his life.

As a result, during Kennedy's teenage years, his family kept their beloved dogs outdoors — a less than adequate attempt at avoidance and allergy-proofing (see Chapter 10). The Kennedys loved dogs: Think of all those images of the clan roughhousing with furry friends in Hyannisport. Therefore, JFK was often exposed to these potent asthma triggers (see Chapter 5), either through direct contact with canines or from dander that invariably collected on the clothes of friends and family members and which then permeated indoor environments.

But JFK was remarkably resilient, fighting through his many obstacles to become a U.S. senator from Massachusetts and, in 1960, the youngest elected president in U.S. history. Kennedy contended with his allergies, the related asthma attacks, and the laryngitis that occasionally followed during his years in public office. Not until his years in the White House was Kennedy able to appreciably reduce his sensitivities to animal dander — thanks to a long course of allergy shots (see Chapter 11) that his allergist, Paul F. de Gara (1903–1991), administered.

Because he also suffered from Addison's disease, a condition marked by insuffi-cient adrenal function, Kennedy required cortisone to boost his adrenal levels. This cortisone therapy may have helped control his asthma, reducing the underlying airway inflammation (see Chapter 2).

Ultimately, Kennedy led an extraordinarily productive and successful life despite his physical ailments, heroically fighting in the Pacific during World War II, championing antidiscrimination policies, supporting the arts and culture, and facing down Soviet missiles in Cuba, all in inspiring fashion. Although a standoff with Khrushchev or Castro may have flustered others, JFK didn't flinch. (And neither did Castro's fellow Latin American revolutionary Ché Guevara [1928–1967], also a longtime asthma sufferer.)

Leonard Bernstein

Arguably the most famous American-born conductor of classical music, and certainly one of the most influential figures in American culture, Leonard Bernstein (1918–1990) made his mark on the world despite living with asthma from infancy. In fact, Bernstein had numerous childhood asthma episodes, sometimes turning blue from lack of oxygen.

Bernstein had an incredible will to learn and succeed, insisting on taking piano lessons even though his father was willing to pay only the tiniest of fees in an ultimately unsuccessful attempt at dissuading his son from a career in music. In his early 20s, Bernstein graduated from Harvard with honors and became the assistant conductor of the New York Philharmonic. His first big break came in 1943, when he replaced ailing music director Bruno Walter on the podium at the last minute, leading a performance that wowed the Big Apple's classical music establishment.

Bernstein impacted the arts in the United States and around the world. He showcased his talent as the composer of dynamic, innovative Broadway musicals, such as *West Side Story* and *Kaddish,* a dramatic, semi-liturgical piece. Likewise, Bernstein flamboyantly conducted symphony orchestras and incisively taught TV audiences about great music.

Bernstein's asthma was a constant presence throughout his success, largely because he aggravated the condition by chain-smoking from early adulthood until the end of his life. His wheezing was often so severe that audiences heard it over the sound of the orchestra during performances.

Because of his incessant smoking, Bernstein developed emphysema, which, unlike asthma, often leads to irreversible, destructive lung damage. (See Chapter 5 for more reasons why smoking is a bad idea, especially if you have a respiratory condition like asthma.) When he finally succumbed to a heart attack in 1990, Bernstein was suffering from asthma complicated by emphysema, a lung tumor, and progressive heart failure.

Liza Minnelli

"What good is sitting alone in your room? Come hear the music play," sang Liza Minnelli (born 1946) in her Academy Award–winning performance from the 1972 film *Cabaret*. Throughout her life, Minnelli has followed that advice and then some, as one of the few performers in history to win the triple-stakes of an Oscar, an Emmy, and a Tony, in addition to building a worldwide following of devoted fans.

Beginning in early childhood, Minnelli performed in films and on stage, first as a guest of her legendary mother, Judy Garland, and on her own in her late teens. Considering the extraordinary vocal power that Minnelli displays night after night in concert, you may not suspect that she has asthma or other lung problems.

Although she has dealt with bouts of bronchitis in recent years and several physical mishaps have sidelined her at times, Minnelli continues to make the music "play," as a committed singer, actress, and humanitarian who inspires others rather than "sitting alone in her room."

Kenny G

Despite his asthma, inhaling enough oxygen to make his instrument sing doesn't seem to be a problem for the soprano saxophonist Kenny Gorelick (born 1956), better known as Kenny G. Likewise, asthma hasn't stopped this tuneful reed player from becoming the most commercially successful instrumental artist in recorded music history.

In fact, one of the biggest-selling albums of all time by an instrumentalist is Kenny G's ironically titled *Breathless*. More than 18 years into his solo career, Kenny G continues his string of chart-topping releases and has recently dedicated efforts to raise money for school music programs, helping students discover the power of music.

On the other side of the musical coin, veteran shock-rocker Vincent Furrier, better known as Alice Cooper (born 1947), has also carved out a long career despite having asthma.

Jackie Joyner-Kersee

Growing up in a rough East St. Louis neighborhood, Jackie Joyner (born 1962) had plenty to overcome as a child. She avoided drugs and violence, and she struggled to find money to support her athletic training. Joyner persevered and concentrated her considerable abilities on several sporting pursuits at once, becoming a high school basketball star, excelling in various track and field events, and playing volleyball. She graduated in the top 10 percent of her class and won a basketball scholarship to UCLA, where she met her track-and-field coach and future husband, Bob Kersee.

In 1983, a year before she competed in her first Olympics, Joyner-Kersee was diagnosed with asthma. Although she began taking medication for her condition soon afterward, she often used her prescribed products only when she thought she needed them rather than following her doctor's instructions for regular use. A serious asthma episode during Olympic training in 1988 — triggered by breathing cold air — made her realize the vital importance of using her medication as prescribed, on a consistent basis, to keep her condition under control. (See Chapter 9 for more information on exercise-induced asthma, or EIA.)

Neither her respiratory condition nor her related allergies have kept Joyner-Kersee from reaching the pinnacle of her sport. She won three gold medals in track and field and still holds the world record for the heptathlon, a demanding seven-part grouping of events. She is the only woman to have received the *Sporting News Man of the Year* award. Many sports analysts consider Joyner-Kersee the world's greatest woman athlete, perhaps of all time.

Likewise, other famous athletes have also overcome asthma to reach the top of their fields. Some of these stellar achievers include

- Jerome Bettis, a top NFL running back who has rushed for more than 1,000 yards per season for several years

- Nancy Hogshead, Olympic swimming gold medalist

- Al Joyner, Olympic triple jump gold medalist (and Jackie Joyner-Kersee's brother; remember that asthma runs in families but doesn't have to keep you on the sidelines)

- Greg Louganis, Olympic diving gold medalist

- Art Monk, one of the most successful wide receivers in NFL history

- Dennis Rodman, a leading rebounder in the NBA and a key member of several championship teams (also part-time actor and fashion trendsetter)

- Amy Van Dyken, Olympic swimming gold medalist

Appendix

Asthma Resources

● ●

*T*his appendix lists organizations and publications (books and periodicals) related to the subjects that I discuss throughout this book, and suppliers and manufacturers of asthma and allergy products.

Organizations

The organizations in this section, listed in alphabetical order, can provide you with valuable information about many aspects of dealing with asthma.

Allergy and Asthma Network
Mothers of Asthmatics
2751 Prosperity Ave., Suite 150
Fairfax, VA 22031
800-878-4403; 703-641-9595
www.breatherville.org

American Academy of Allergy,
Asthma, and Immunology
611 East Wells St.
Milwaukee, WI 53202
800-822-2762; 414-272-6071
www.aaaai.org

American College of Allergy,
Asthma, and Immunology
85 W. Algonquin Road, Suite 550
Arlington Heights, IL 60005
847-427-1200
www.acaai.org

American College of
Chest Physicians
3300 Dundee Road
Northbrook, IL 60062
800-842-7777; 847-498-1400
www.chestnet.org

American Dietetic Association
120 South Riverside Plaza, Suite 2000
Chicago, IL 60606
800-877-1600
www.eatright.org

American Lung Association
61 Broadway, 6th floor
New York, NY 10006
212-315-8700
www.lungusa.org

American Thoracic Society
1740 Broadway
New York, NY 10019
212-315-8700
www.thoracic.org

Asthma and Allergy Foundation of
America
1233 20th St. NW, #402
Washington, DC 20036
800-727-8462; 202-466-7643
www.aafa.org

Environmental Protection Agency
Indoor Air Quality Information
Clearinghouse
401 M St. SW
Washington, DC 20460
800-438-4318; 703-356-4020
www.epa.gov
E-mail: iaqinfo@aol.com
Contact this EPA office for information
on indoor air quality.

The Food Allergy & Anaphylaxis
Network
10400 Eaton Place, Suite 107
Fairfax, VA 22030
800-929-4040; fax: 703-691-3179
www.foodallergy.org
E-mail: faan@foodallergy.org

Food and Drug Administration FDA,
HFI-40
Rockville, MD 20857
310-827-6250; 888-463-6332
(INFOFDA)
www.fda.gov

Immune Deficiency Foundation
401 W. Chesapeake Ave., Suite 308
Towson, MD 21204
800-296-4433
www.primaryimmune.org
E-mail: idf@ primaryimmune.org

International Food Information Council
1100 Connecticut Ave. NW, Suite 430
Washington, DC 20036
202-296-6540
www.ific.org
E-mail: foodinfo@ific.org

Joint Council of Allergy, Asthma, and
Immunology
50 N. Brockway, Suite 33
Palatine, IL 60067
847-934-1918
www.jcaai.org
E-mail: info@jcaai.org
Guidelines for allergy and asthma
treatment are located at this Web site.

Journal of the American Medical
Association
JAMA Asthma Information Center
515 N. State St.
Chicago, IL 60610
800-262-2350
www.ama-assn.org

National Allergy Bureau
611 E. Wells St.
Milwaukee, WI 53202
414-272-6071
www.aaaai.org/nab/index.cfm
E-mail: nab@aaaai.org
Contact the NAB for information on its
bureaus throughout the United States
and Canada and in many other coun-
tries that report on local pollen and
mold conditions.

National Asthma Education and
Prevention
NHLBI Information Center
P.O. Box 30105
Bethesda, MD 20824
301-592-8573
www.nhlbi.nih.gov

National Jewish Medical and
Research Center
1400 Jackson St.
Denver, CO 80206
303-388-4461; 800-222-LUNG (5864)
www.njc.org

Asthma and Allergy Environmental-Control Products

This section provides contact information for manufacturers and suppliers of the items that I mention throughout the book, especially for devices to control exposure to allergens (see Chapters 5 and 10), to inhale asthma medications (Chapter 14), and to test your lung function at home (Chapter 4).

Suppliers

The following companies distribute allergy and asthma control products, including allergen barrier encasings for mattresses, box springs, comforters, and pillows; allergenic blankets and linens; HEPA and ULPA air filters, filters, and vacuum cleaners; humidifiers and inhaled medication delivery systems; nebulizers and spacers; and numerous mold, dust mite, and dander-control products.

Allerguard, Inc.
40 Cindy Lane
Ocean, NJ 07712
732-988-6868
www.allerguard-us.com
E-mail: info@allerguard-us.com

Allergy Asthma Technology, Ltd.
8224 Lehigh Ave.
Morton Grove, IL 60053
800-621-5545; 847-966-2952
www.allergyasthmatech.com

Allergy Clean Environments
P.O. Box 9067
San Rafael, CA 94912
800-882-4110; 415-459-4003
www.allergyclean.com

Allergy Control Products, Inc.
96 Danbury Rd.
Ridgefield, CT 06877
800-422-3878; 203-438-9580
www.allergycontrol.com

American Allergy Supply
P.O. Box 722022
Houston, TX 77272
800-321-1096; 713-995-6110
www.americanallergy.com

Enviro Remedies Allergy Relief Products
693 West Reading Ave.
West Reading, PA 19611
800-315-3461
www.enviro-remedies.com

National Allergy Supply, Inc.
1620-D Satellite Blvd.
Duluth, GA 30097
800-522-1448
www.natlallergy.com

Manufacturers of asthma and allergy products

The following list provides contact information for manufacturers that sell specific allergy and asthma products, which I describe throughout this book, directly to consumers.

Ferraris Medical, Inc. (Manufacturers of Pocket Peak-Flow Meters and distributors of Mini-Wright Peak-Flow Meters)
908 Main Street
Louisville, CO 80027
800-205-7187
www.ferrarismedicalusa.com

Honeywell (Manufacturers of HEPA and ULPA air filtration systems)
101 Columbia Road
Morristown, NJ 07962
973-455-2000
www.honeywell.com

MedicAlert Foundation (Manufacturers of emergency medical information necklaces and bracelets. Ask your doctor about wearing a medical tag if you're at risk of anaphylaxis from a life-threatening allergic reaction.)
2323 Colorado Ave.
Turlock, CA 95382
800-432-5378; 209-668-3333
www.medicalert.org

Respironics Health Scan Asthma Allergy Products (Manufacturers of Assess Peak-Flow Meters)
908 Pompton Ave.
Cedar Grove, NJ 07009
800-962-1266; 973-857-3414
www.respironics.com

Vitaire Corporation (Manufacturers of Vitaire HEPA air purifiers and allergen barrier encasings for mattresses, box springs, and pillows)
141 Lanza Ave.
Garfield, NJ 07026
800-552-5533
www.vitaire.com

Other Writings and Media about Asthma and Allergies

The books and periodicals in this section cover a wide range of topics related to asthma and allergies. All these titles are great sources of valuable information.

Books

A Parent's Guide to Asthma:
How You Can Help Your Child
Control Asthma at Home,
School, and Play
Nancy Sander
Plume/Penguin, 1994

Asthma & Exercise
Nancy Hogshead and
Gerald Couzens
Henry Holt and Company, 1990

Asthma — An Emerging Epidemic
Paul J. Hannaway, MD
Lighthouse Press, 2002
P.O. Box 602
Marblehead, MA 01945
800-225-9886
E-mail: Lhtpress@aol.com

Dr. Tom Plaut's Asthma Guide for
People of All Ages
Thomas F. Plaut, MD, with
Teresa B. Jones
Pedipress, Inc., 1999
125 Red Gate Lane
Amherst, MA 01002
800-611-6081
www.pedipress.com

One Minute Asthma: What You Need
to Know (also available in Spanish as
El asma en un minuto: Lo que usted
necesita saber)
Thomas F. Plaut, MD
Pedipress, Inc., 1998

Taking Charge of Asthma
Betty B. Wray, MD
John Wiley & Sons, 1997

Periodicals

Allergy and Asthma Today
The MA Report
Allergy and Asthma Network
Mothers of Asthmatics
2751 Prosperity Ave., Suite 150
Fairfax, VA 22031
800-878-4403
www.breatherville.org
Allergy and Asthma Today is a quarterly, full-color magazine that provides in-depth coverage of allergy and asthma issues from leading medical and consumer experts. Free to members of AANMA.
The MA Report is AANMA's newsletter, published eight times a year.

Asthma Magazine
Periodicals Order Fulfillment Dept.
Mosby Elseveir Science
6277 Sea Harbor Dr.
Orlando, FL 32821
800-654-2452
Six issues per year: $23.00

The Reporter and Breathing Matters
Asthma and Allergy Foundation of
America (AAFA) newsletters
1233 20th St. NW, Suite 402
Washington, DC 20036
800-7-ASTHMA (727-8462)
www.aafa.org

Index

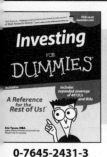
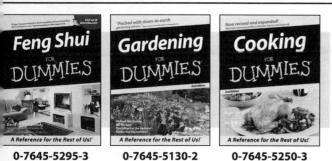
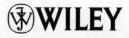

FOR DUMMIES®

A world of resources to help you grow

TRAVEL

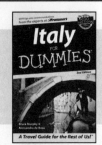

0-7645-5453-0

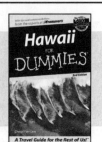

0-7645-5438-7

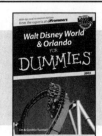

0-7645-5444-1

Also available:

America's National Parks For Dummies
(0-7645-6204-5)

Caribbean For Dummies
(0-7645-5445-X)

Cruise Vacations For Dummies 2003
(0-7645-5459-X)

Europe For Dummies
(0-7645-5456-5)

Ireland For Dummies
(0-7645-6199-5)

France For Dummies
(0-7645-6292-4)

Las Vegas For Dummies
(0-7645-5448-4)

London For Dummies
(0-7645-5416-6)

Mexico's Beach Resorts For Dummies
(0-7645-6262-2)

Paris For Dummies
(0-7645-5494-8)

RV Vacations For Dummies
(0-7645-5443-3)

EDUCATION & TEST PREPARATION

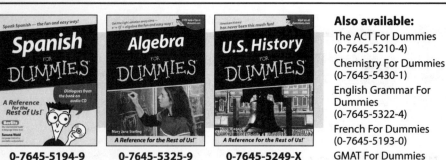

0-7645-5194-9   **0-7645-5325-9**   **0-7645-5249-X**

Also available:

The ACT For Dummies
(0-7645-5210-4)

Chemistry For Dummies
(0-7645-5430-1)

English Grammar For Dummies
(0-7645-5322-4)

French For Dummies
(0-7645-5193-0)

GMAT For Dummies
(0-7645-5251-1)

Inglés Para Dummies
(0-7645-5427-1)

Italian For Dummies
(0-7645-5196-5)

Research Papers For Dummies
(0-7645-5426-3)

SAT I For Dummies
(0-7645-5472-7)

U.S. History For Dummies
(0-7645-5249-X)

World History For Dummies
(0-7645-5242-2)

HEALTH, SELF-HELP & SPIRITUALITY

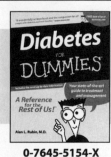

0-7645-5154-X

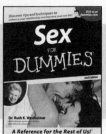

0-7645-5302-X

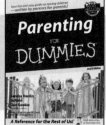

0-7645-5418-2

Also available:

The Bible For Dummies
(0-7645-5296-1)

Controlling Cholesterol For Dummies
(0-7645-5440-9)

Dating For Dummies
(0-7645-5072-1)

Dieting For Dummies
(0-7645-5126-4)

High Blood Pressure For Dummies
(0-7645-5424-7)

Judaism For Dummies
(0-7645-5299-6)

Menopause For Dummies
(0-7645-5458-1)

Nutrition For Dummies
(0-7645-5180-9)

Potty Training For Dummies
(0-7645-5417-4)

Pregnancy For Dummies
(0-7645-5074-8)

Rekindling Romance For Dummies
(0-7645-5303-8)

Religion For Dummies
(0-7645-5264-3)

FOR DUMMIES®

Plain-English solutions for everyday challenges

HOME & BUSINESS COMPUTER BASICS

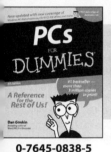 **0-7645-0838-5**

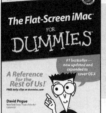 **0-7645-1663-9**

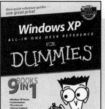 **0-7645-1548-9**

Also available:

Excel 2002 All-in-One Desk Reference For Dummies (0-7645-1794-5)

Office XP 9-in-1 Desk Reference For Dummies (0-7645-0819-9)

PCs All-in-One Desk Reference For Dummies (0-7645-0791-5)

Troubleshooting Your PC For Dummies (0-7645-1669-8)

Upgrading & Fixing PCs For Dummies (0-7645-1665-5)

Windows XP For Dummies (0-7645-0893-8)

Windows XP For Dummies Quick Reference (0-7645-0897-0)

Word 2002 For Dummies (0-7645-0839-3)

INTERNET & DIGITAL MEDIA

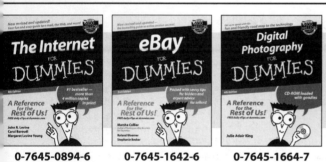

0-7645-0894-6 **0-7645-1642-6** **0-7645-1664-7**

Also available:

CD and DVD Recording For Dummies (0-7645-1627-2)

Digital Photography All-in-One Desk Reference For Dummies (0-7645-1800-3)

eBay For Dummies (0-7645-1642-6)

Genealogy Online For Dummies (0-7645-0807-5)

Internet All-in-One Desk Reference For Dummies (0-7645-1659-0)

Internet For Dummies Quick Reference (0-7645-1645-0)

Internet Privacy For Dummies (0-7645-0846-6)

Paint Shop Pro For Dummies (0-7645-2440-2)

Photo Retouching & Restoration For Dummies (0-7645-1662-0)

Photoshop Elements For Dummies (0-7645-1675-2)

Scanners For Dummies (0-7645-0783-4)

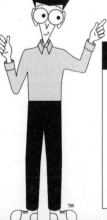

Get smart! Visit www.dummies.com

- **Find listings of even more Dummies titles**
- **Browse online articles, excerpts, and how-to's**
- **Sign up for daily or weekly e-mail tips**
- **Check out Dummies fitness videos and other products**
- **Order from our online bookstore**

Available wherever books are sold. Go to www.dummies.com or call 1-877-762-2974 to order direct

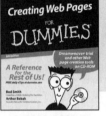
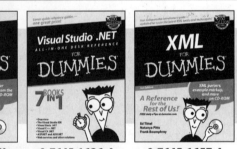
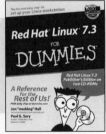
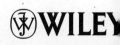